CAMBRIDGE STUDIES
IN MATHEMATICAL BIOLOGY: 15
Editors
C. CANNINGS
University of Sheffield, UK
F. C. HOPPENSTEADT
Arizona State University, Tempe, USA
L. A. SEGEL
Weizmann Institute of Science, Rehovot, Israel

EPIDEMIC MODELLING: AN INTRODUCTION

This is a general introduction to the ideas and techniques required to understand
the mathematical modelling of diseases. It begins with an historical outline of some
disease statistics dating from Daniel Bernoulli's smallpox data of 1760. The authors
then describe simple deterministic and stochastic models in continuous and discrete
time for epidemics taking place in either homogeneous or stratified
(non-homogeneous) populations. A range of techniques for constructing and
analysing models is provided, mostly in the context of viral and bacterial diseases of
human populations. These models are contrasted with models for rumours and
vector-borne diseases like malaria. Questions of fitting data to models, and the use
of models to understand methods for controlling the spread of infection are
discussed. Exercises and complementary results at the end of each chapter extend
the scope of the text, which will be useful for students taking courses in
mathematical biology who have some basic knowledge of probability and statistics.

CAMBRIDGE STUDIES
IN MATHEMATICAL BIOLOGY

D. J. DALEY and J. GANI
Australian National University

Epidemic Modelling:
An Introduction

PUBLISHED BY THE PRESS SYNDICATE OF THE UNIVERSITY OF CAMBRIDGE
The Pitt Building, Trumpington Street, Cambridge, United Kingdom

CAMBRIDGE UNIVERSITY PRESS
The Edinburgh Building, Cambridge CB2 2RU, UK
40 West 20th Street, New York, NY 10011–4211, USA
10 Stamford Road, Oakleigh, VIC 3166, Australia
Ruiz de Alarcón 13, 28014 Madrid, Spain
Dock House, The Waterfront, Cape Town 8001, South Africa

http://www.cambridge.org

First published 1999
Reprinted 2001
First paperback edition 2001

Printed in the United Kingdom at the University Press, Cambridge

Typeset in Computer Modern 10/13pt by the authors using Plain TEX

A catalogue record of this book is available from the British Library

Library of Congress Cataloguing in Publication data
Daley, Daryl J.
    Epidemic modelling : an introduction / D.J. Daley and J.M. Gani.
        p.   cm. – (Cambridge studies in mathematical biology ; 14)
    Includes bibliographical references and index.
    ISBN 0 521 64079 2
    1. Epidemiology–Mathematical models. 2. Epidemiology–
Statistical methods. I. Gani, J. M. (Joseph Mark) II. Title.
III. Series.
RA652.2.M3D34   1999
614.4′01′5–dc21   98-44051   CIP

ISBN 0 521 64079 2 hardback
ISBN 0 521 01467 0 paperback

To Nola, for constant support and understanding [DJD]

To my late wife Ruth, who first directed my interest
to biological problems [JMG]

... The history of malaria contains a great lesson for humanity—that we should be more scientific in our habits of thought, and more practical in our habits of government. The neglect of this lesson has already cost many countries an immense loss in life and in prosperity.

Ronald Ross,
The Prevention of Malaria (1911)

... It follows that epidemic theory should certainly continue to search for new insights into the mechanisms of the population dynamics of infectious diseases, especially those of high priority in the world today, but that increased attention should be paid to formulating applied models that are sufficiently realistic to contribute directly to broad programs of intervention and control.

Norman T. J. Bailey,
The Mathematical Theory of Infectious Diseases (1975, p. 27)

... The level of economic development of communities generally determines the level of health services. The higher the level of economic development, the more effectively did surveillance and containment principles apply and the earlier was *variole major* [smallpox], in particular, eliminated from the country.

F. J. Fenner,
Smallpox and its Eradication (1988)

... Statistical science has made important contributions to our understanding of AIDS. Statistical methods were used in the earliest studies of the etiology of AIDS, and evidence for sexual transmission came from case-control studies among gay men, in which AIDS cases were compared to matched controls. It was found that high numbers of sexual contacts were a risk factor for AIDS.

R. Brookmeyer and M. H. Gail,
in *Chance* **3**(4), 9–14, 1990

Contents

Preface

This monograph is designed to introduce probabilists and statisticians to the diverse models describing the spread of epidemics and rumours in a population. Not all epidemic type processes have been included. With minor exceptions, we have restricted ourselves to the spread of viral and bacterial infections, or to the propagation of rumours, by direct contact between infective and susceptible individuals. Host–vector and parasitic infections have been mentioned only very briefly.

Throughout the book, the emphasis is on the mathematical modelling of epidemics and rumours, and the evolution of this modelling over the past three centuries.

Chapter 1 is a historical introduction to the subject, with illustrations of the most common approaches to modelling. This is followed in Chapter 2 by an account of deterministic models, in both discrete and continuous time. Chapter 3 analyses stochastic models in continuous time, and includes detailed studies of the simple, general and carrier-borne epidemics. In Chapter 4, the main stochastic models in discrete time, namely the chain binomial models are studied, and a pairs-at-parties and related models outlined. Chapter 5 considers models for the propagation and cessation of rumours, and exploits some of the techniques introduced earlier to analyse them; the results highlight differences between these and the classical epidemic models. Chapter 6, which is essentially statistical, is concerned with the fit of various models to observed epidemic data. The book ends with Chapter 7, which describes three main methods of controlling epidemics. A list of references that also incorporates an author index, and a subject index are provided at the end.

While the monograph cannot claim to be comprehensive, our hope is that readers who master its contents should have little difficulty in reading the current literature on epidemic modelling. The two main treatises on the subject are Bailey (1975) and Anderson and May (1991); both are often referred to in the text. The former considers most of the classical epidemic models, both deterministic and stochastic, while the latter concentrates essentially on deterministic results. We believe that both types of models have a role to play in describing the spread of infections in large and small populations, and have attempted to give due weight to each.

Current epidemic modelling relies on a great variety of mathematical methods; we have endeavoured to emphasize the intrinsic interest of such methods, as well as demonstrate their practical usefulness. Exercises and complements have been provided at the end of each Chapter, with the dual intentions of extending the text and of providing opportunities for readers to practise their skills in modelling and the analysis of models. The exercises are not of uniform difficulty.

For those who wish to reach the forefront of current research, the volumes of papers edited by Mollison (1995) and Isham and Medley (1996), both arising from a six-month research programme on Epidemic Models at the Newton Institute in Cambridge in 1993, provide further illustrations of epidemic modelling and many challenging problems in the field.

Finally we thank all of our colleagues who have collaborated with us over many years in both this area of applied probability and others; their contributions are too many to mention individually, save that DJD pays tribute to David Kendall who first introduced him to the topic of this book, and JMG expresses his gratitude to Norman Bailey and Maurice Bartlett, pioneers of stochastic epidemic modelling.

We also thank David Tranah, and the Copy Editor and others at Cambridge University Press for their cooperation in producing this book without invoking LaTeX.

Daryl Daley,   Joe Gani
Canberra,   October 1998

1

Some History

The mathematical study of diseases and their dissemination is at most just over three centuries old. To give a full account of the history of the subject would require a book in itself. The interested reader may refer to Burnet and White (1972) for a natural history of diseases, to Fenner *et al.* (1988) for an account of smallpox and its eradication, and to Bailey (1975) and Anderson and May (1991) for an outline of the development of mathematical theories for the spread of epidemics. We shall be concerned with the more modest task of placing some of the recent epidemic models in perspective. We therefore present a selective account of historical highlights to illustrate the developments of the subject between the seventeenth and early twentieth centuries. Creighton (1894) gives a descriptive account of epidemics in Britain to the end of the nineteenth century, and Razzell (1977) for smallpox.

1.1 An empirical approach

The quantitative study of human diseases and deaths ensuing from them can be traced back to the book by John Graunt (b. 1620, d. 1674) *Natural and Political Observations made upon the Bills of Mortality* (1662). These *Bills* were weekly records of London parishes, listing the numbers and causes of deaths in the parishes. In his book, Graunt discussed various demographic problems of seventeenth century Britain. Four of his twelve chapters deal with the causes of death of individuals whose diseases were recorded in the *Bills*. These death records, kept irregularly from about 1592 onwards and continuously from 1603, provided the data on which Graunt based his observations.

Table 1.1. *Numbers of deaths due to eight causes, and related risks*

Causes	Deaths	Risk
1. Thrush, Convulsion, Rickets, Teeth and Worms; Abortives, Chrysomes, Infants, Liver-grown and overlaid	71,124	0.310
2. Chronical Diseases: Consumptions, Ague and Fever	68,271	0.298
3. Acute Diseases, and Miscellaneous	49,505	0.216
4. Plague	16,384	0.071
5. Small-pox, Swine-pox, Measles and Worms without Convulsions	12,210	0.053
6. Notorious Diseases: Apoplex, Gowt, Leprosy, Palsy, Stone and Strangury, Sodainly, etc.	5,547	0.024
7. Cancers, Fistulae, Sores, Ulcers, Impostume, Itch, King's Evil, Scal'd-head, Wens	3,320	0.014
8. Casualties: Drowned, Killed by Accidents, Murthured	2,889	0.013

Source: Graunt (1662). The figures for Groups 1, 2, 3, 6 and 8 are quoted directly in Graunt's text, while those for Groups 4, 5 and 7 are obtained from his complete table of casualties appended after his comments in 'The Conclusion'.

In the 20 years 1629–36 and 1647–58, there were 229 250 deaths recorded from 81 different causes. Table 1.1 consolidates these data into eight main groups. The relative risks of death from each of the eight causes are indicated in the column furthest to the right in Table 1.1.

The main killers were Groups 1, 2 and 3; Graunt was led to observe that

whereas many persons live in great fear, and apprehension of some of the more formidable, and notorious diseases following [Group 6]; I shall onely [*sic*] set down how many died of each: that the respective numbers, being compared with the Total of 229,250, those persons may the better understand the hazards they are in.

The notorious diseases were further broken up by Graunt into the subcategories of Table 1.2. Among these, apoplexy appears to have been the largest killer. Graunt's analysis of the various causes of death provided the first systematic method for estimating the comparative risks of dying from the plague, as against the chronical or other diseases, for example.

These observations may well be considered to be the first approach to the theory of competing risks, a theory that is now well established among modern epidemiologists.

1.2 A deterministic model

A more theoretical approach to the effects of a disease, namely smallpox, was taken by Daniel Bernoulli (b. 1700, d. 1782) almost a century later. Smallpox was then widespread in many parts of Europe where it affected

Table 1.2. *Deaths due to notorious diseases*

Causes	Deaths	Risk $\times 10^{-3}$
1. Apoplex	1306	5.697
2. Cut of the stone	38	0.166
3. Falling sickness	74	0.323
4. Dead in the streets	243	1.060
5. Gowt	134	0.585
6. Head-ach	51	0.222
7. Jaundice	998	4.353
8. Lethargy	67	0.292
9. Leprosy	6	0.026
10. Lunatique	155	0.676
11. Overlaid, and starved	529	2.308
12. Palsy	423	1.845
13. Rupture	201	0.877
14. Stone and strangury	863	3.764
15. Sciatica	5	0.022
16. Sodainly	454	1.980
Total	5547	24.196

Source: Graunt (1662).

a large proportion of the population, being responsible for around 10% of the mortality of minors (cf. Bernoulli's model-based estimate in the last column of Table 1.3) while those who survived were immune to further attack but left scarred for life. In 1760 Bernoulli read his paper 'Essai d'une nouvelle analyse de la mortalité causée par la petite vérole et des avantages de l'inoculation pour la prévenir' to the French Royal Academy of Sciences in Paris. His intention was to demonstrate that variolation, i.e. inoculation with live virus obtained directly from a patient with a mild case of smallpox, a procedure that usually conferred immunity, would reduce the death rate and increase the population of France. Bernoulli's argument is readily recognized as the following problem in competing risks.

Suppose first that a cohort of individuals born in a particular year has an age-specific *per capita* death rate $\mu(t)$ at age t. Then given an initial population size $\xi(0) \equiv \xi_0$, its size $\xi(t)$ at age t satisfies the equation

$$\dot{\xi}(t) = -\mu(t)\xi(t), \qquad (1.2.1)$$

so

$$\xi(t) = \xi(0) \exp\left(-\int_0^t \mu(u)\, du\right) \equiv \xi(0)e^{-M(t)} \equiv \zeta(t), \qquad (1.2.2)$$

where $M(t)$ is the cumulative hazard. We shall use $\zeta(\cdot)$ below.

Consider another cohort subject to both the general *per capita* death rate $\mu(t)$ as above and a further hazard (infection) like smallpox with a constant infection rate β per individual per unit time. Individuals succumb

Table 1.3. *Age profile of population afflicted with smallpox (Bernoulli)*

Age (yrs) t	Total $\xi_\beta(t)$	Age cohort Immune $z(t)$	Suscept. $x(t)$	Smallpox Incidence	Cumulative Deaths	Annual Mortality Total	Smallpox
0	1,300	0	1,300				
1	1,000	104	896	137	17.1	300	17.1
2	855	170	685	99	29.5	145	12.4
3	798	227	571	78	39.2	57	9.7
4	760	275	485	66	47.5	38	8.3
5	732	316	416	56	54.5	28	7.0
6	710	351	359	48	60.5	22	6.0
7	692	381	311	42	65.7	18	5.2
8	680	408	272	36	70.2	12	4.5
9	670	433	237	32	74.2	10	4.0
10	661	453	208	28	77.7	9	3.5
11	653	471	182	24.4	80.7	8	3.0
12	646	486	160	21.4	83.4	7	2.7
13	640	500	140	18.7	85.7	6	2.3
14	634	511	123	16.6	87.8	6	2.1
15	628	520	108	14.4	89.6	6	1.8
16	622	528	94	12.6	91.2	6	1.6
17	616	533	83	11.0	92.6	6	1.4
18	610	538	72	9.7	93.8	6	1.2
19	604	541	63	8.4	94.8	6	1.0
20	598	542	56	7.4	95.7	6	0.9
21	592	543	48.5	6.5	96.5	6	0.8
22	586	543	42.5	5.6	97.2	6	0.7
23	579	542	37	5.0	97.8	7	0.6
24	572	540	32.4	4.4	98.3	7	0.5

Source: Bernoulli (1760). Note that Halley's table (column 1) starts at $t = 1$; Bernoulli gives reasons for choosing cohort size 1,300 for $t = 0$. Bernoulli used $\alpha = \beta = 1/8$, and obtained his figures by smoothing to the mid-point of the previous year, so his figure 17.1 for $t = 1$, coming from 1017.1, differs from $1014.9 = 8 \times 1000/[7 + \exp(-1/8)]$ as follows from (1.2.6) (cf. Gani, 1978).

only once, the result of such infection being either death in a fraction α of cases or immunity for the remainder of life in the complementary fraction $1 - \alpha$. Denote the number of individuals still susceptible to the disease at age t by $x(t)$, and the total number of the surviving cohort of age t, whether immune or not, by $\xi_\beta(t)$ as shown in Figure 1.1. To simplify the mathematical model, the infectious state is assumed to be instantaneous, so that as soon as an infection occurs, the infective individual either dies or recovers immediately. Then for the $x(t)$ susceptibles and $z(t) \equiv \xi_\beta(t) - x(t)$ immunes in this cohort,

$$\dot{x}(t) = -\big(\mu(t) + \beta\big)x(t) \tag{1.2.3a}$$

and

$$\dot{z}(t) = -\mu(t)z(t) + (1 - \alpha)\beta x(t). \tag{1.2.3b}$$

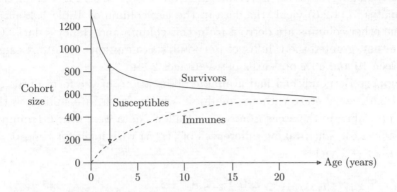

Figure 1.1. Survivors ξ_β (——) and immunes z (- - - -) in cohort of initial size 1300 (data from Table 1.3). The susceptibles of age t in the cohort are $x(t) = \xi_\beta(t) - z(t)$.

These equations are solved via integrating factors. Using $M(t)$ and $x(0) = \xi_\beta(0) = \xi(0) = \xi_0$ as before, we have

$$\frac{d}{dt}\left(e^{M(t)+\beta t}x(t)\right) = 0,$$

whence

$$x(t) = \xi_0 e^{-M(t)}e^{-\beta t}, \tag{1.2.4}$$

and

$$\frac{d}{dt}\left(e^{M(t)}z(t)\right) = (1-\alpha)\beta e^{M(t)}x(t) = (1-\alpha)\beta\xi_0 e^{-\beta t}.$$

Integrating on $(0, t)$ and simplifying,

$$\xi_\beta(t) = e^{-M(t)}\xi_0[e^{-\beta t} + (1-\alpha)(1-e^{-\beta t})]$$
$$= \zeta(t)(1 - \alpha + \alpha e^{-\beta t}), \tag{1.2.5}$$

using (1.2.2); observe that $\zeta(t) = \xi_0(t)$ when the infection rate $\beta = 0$.

Equation (1.2.5) relates the sizes of the surviving cohorts of age t in populations with ($\beta > 0$) and without ($\beta = 0$) smallpox, respectively. Bernoulli used it in the form

$$\zeta(t) = \frac{\xi_\beta(t)}{1 - \alpha + \alpha e^{-\beta t}} \tag{1.2.6}$$

to estimate the size of a surviving cohort $\zeta(t)$ in a 'state without smallpox' on the basis of Halley's (1693) data from Breslau, now Wrocław. This estimation required parameters α and β; on reviewing what evidence he could from a number of areas, Bernoulli fixed on $\alpha = \beta = 0.125$. Use of these estimates in (1.2.6) yields the data in the last column of Table 1.3; entries in the other columns are derived from this column and Halley's data. Observe that, granted the validity of Bernoulli's assumptions, smallpox caused between 10 and 40% of deaths between ages 2 and 23.

Suppose Bernoulli had had available observations of the form of his $\zeta(\cdot)$ at (1.2.6), for a 'state without smallpox' with a death rate similar to that $\mu(\cdot)$ prevailing in the areas from which Halley's data were drawn (column 2 of Table 1.3). Then taking differences of (1.2.5) with itself for times $t = t'$ and $t = t' + 1$ yields

$$\Delta\big(\xi_\beta(t')/\zeta(t')\big) \equiv \frac{\xi_\beta(t')}{\zeta(t')} - \frac{\xi_\beta(t'+1)}{\zeta(t'+1)} = \alpha(1 - e^{-\beta})e^{-\beta t'},$$

so that

$$\ln\Delta\big(\xi_\beta(t')/\zeta(t')\big) = -(a + \beta t'), \tag{1.2.7}$$

where $a = -\ln[\alpha(1 - e^{-\beta})]$. This is the simplest way of expressing the result (1.2.5) for the purpose of estimating β and α *conditional* on such extended data being available. All that Bernoulli could do was to present the advantage of variolation (i.e. absence of deaths due to smallpox) on the basis of his model-based calculations. Note too that the population risk of death from smallpox (cf. Tables 1.1–2) as implied by Table 1.1 is about $100/1300 \approx 7.7\%$, higher than in Table 1.1 because the London population from which Graunt drew his data, included more immigrants than Breslau. In Halley's day Breslau had rather few immigrants, and hence, proportionately more infant and childhood deaths, smallpox being more prevalent amongst children than adults.

1.2.1   The Law of Mass Action

The *Law of Mass Action* has found wide applicability in many areas of science. In chemistry, the idea that a reaction is influenced by the quantities of the reactant materials goes back at least to Boyle (*c*. 1674). Around 1800, C. L. Berthollet emphasized the importance of mass or concentration of a substance on a chemical reaction, but this was not generally accepted for half a century. Ultimately, Guldberg and Waage (1864–1867) postulated that *for a homogeneous system, the rate of a chemical reaction is proportional to the active masses of the reacting substances* (Glasstone (1948, p. 816)).

Applied to population processes, *if the individuals in a population mix homogeneously, the rate of interaction between two different subsets of the population is proportional to the product of the numbers in each of the subsets concerned.* In any population it is possible for several processes to occur concurrently, in which case the effects on the numbers in any given subset of the population from these various processes are assumed to be additive. Thus, in the case of epidemic modelling, the Law is applied to rates of transition of individuals between two interacting categories of the population, such as susceptibles who, as a result of contact with infectives, themselves become infectives; a second simultaneous process is that of the infectives who become removals. These two processes underlie equations (1.3.2a) and (1.3.2c) respectively: when more than one process is involved, as for the numbers of infectives in equation (1.3.2b), the effects are additive.

Application of the Law to transitions that occur in discrete time is not so straightforward, but, subject to certain constraints on the size of the change involved (see e.g. Section 2.8 below), it remains valid.

The Law also has a stochastic version when the process concerned is assumed to be Markovian, and the rate is then interpreted as the infinitesimal transition probability.

Implicit in the 'proportionality' aspect of the Law, is an assumption that the quantities concerned in inducing the transition are subject to *homogeneous mixing* with each other. The Law can then be seen as the result of superposing all possible contributions of the individual components to the interaction, these individuals being regarded as equally likely to interact with each other in a given (small) interval of time.

1.3 From curve-fitting to homogeneous mixing models

First issued in 1837, each *Annual Report of the Registrar-General of Births, Deaths and Marriages in England* included tables of causes of death and commentaries. The *Report* for 1840 includes a contribution from William Farr[1] entitled 'Progress of epidemics', in which Farr attempted to characterize mathematically the smoothed quarterly data for smallpox deaths. Some 26 years later, in a letter to the London *Daily News* of 17 February

---

[1]Farr was appointed compiler of abstracts to the General Register Office in 1839 and remained there until retirement in 1879. Early volumes of the *Annual Reports* contain papers of Farr prefaced by a 'Letter to the Registrar-General'; they cover a variety of issues pertaining to the data in the *Reports*. Thus, in the *Sixth Annual Report* (1842) Farr noted that the annual small-pox death-rates per 10^6 live individuals for the years 1838–42 were 1 101, 604, 679, 408 and 172 respectively, and remarked that 'The reduction in the mortality from small-pox since 1840 was probably the result, at least in part, of the Vaccination Act' [of 1840]. Later he gave the 1850 death-rate as 263.

Table 1.4. *Deaths from smallpox in consecutive quarters 1837–39*

	Sum. 1837	Aut. 1837	Win. 1838	Spr. 1838	Sum. 1838	Aut. 1838	Win. 1839	Spr. 1839	Sum. 1839	Aut. 1839
Observed deaths	2513	3289	4242	4484	3685	3851	2982	2505	1533	1730
Deaths averaged over two consecutive quarters		2901	3766	4365	4087	3767	3416	2743	2019	1637
Percentage change		+30	+16	−6	−8	−9	−20	−26	−19	

Source: Farr (1840).

1866 (quoted by Brownlee, 1915), he attempted to predict the spread of rinderpest among cattle by a similar method.

Table 1.4 gives the observed deaths in the smallpox epidemic of 1837–39 drawn from Farr (1840), together with the average values of consecutive quarters, for 10 quarters in all. Farr concluded that as the epidemic declined, he could detect an approximately steady rate of deceleration in the number of deaths per quarter. Brownlee (1906) later carried out work of a similar type: he fitted Pearson curves to epidemic data for several diseases, and for several different locations.

But these pragmatic approaches were essentially limited, so long as there was not an appropriate theory to explain the mechanism by which epidemics spread. By the beginning of the twentieth century, the idea of passing on a bacterial disease through contact between susceptibles and infectives had become familiar, and Hamer (1906) first foreshadowed the simple 'mass action' principle for a deterministic epidemic model in discrete time. This principle, which incorporates the principle of homogeneous mixing, has been the basis of most subsequent developments in epidemic theory (see Section 1.2.1 above and Anderson and May (1991, p. 7) for discussion).

Hamer, noticing the rise and fall of infectives in the course of a large range of epidemics, argued against variable infectivity. Specifically, he wrote that to explain the eventual decline of an epidemic, 'the assumption of loss of virulence or infecting power on the part of the organism is quite unnecessary'. He also put forward a numerical argument about the initial increase and eventual decline of the number of infectives in a population; this indicates that he was aware that both susceptibles and infectives affected the number of new infectives listed in the weekly reports of measles in London:

Now the outbreak will take much longer to decline to extinction than it took to rise, for those especially exposed have in large part been already attacked and the disease must spread, in the main, among persons whose manner of life brings them comparatively little into contact with their fellows.

Let x_t, y_t be the numbers of susceptibles and infectives respectively at times $t = 0, 1, 2, \ldots$. Hamer's idea was equivalent to expressing the new number of infectives at time $t + 1$ by Δy_t such that

$$\Delta y_t = \beta x_t y_t \qquad (t = 0, 1, 2, \ldots) \qquad (1.3.1)$$

where the constant β is such that $\beta x_t y_t \leq x_t$ for all t, i.e. $\beta \leq 1/(\max_{i \geq 1} y_i)$. These new infectives are a proportion β of the number $x_t y_t$ of contacts between susceptibles and infectives, where β is known as the infection parameter. Because of the constraint on β, it follows that in a closed population in which $y_t = N - x_t$, we have $\beta x_t (N - x_t) \leq x_t$ or $\beta(N - x_t) \leq 1$; this is certainly satisfied if $\beta \leq 1/N$.

Continuous time versions of epidemic equations were used by Ross (1916) and Ross and Hudson (1917) in their studies of populations subject to infection. But the form of equations most commonly used to characterize the typical *general epidemic* with susceptibles $x(t)$, infectives $y(t)$ and immunes $z(t)$ (such as a measles epidemic) is due to Kermack and McKendrick (1927). They assumed a fixed population size $N = x(t) + y(t) + z(t)$, and using the homogeneous mixing principle for continuous time $t \geq 0$ derived the (now) classical equations

$$\frac{\mathrm{d}x}{\mathrm{d}t} = -\beta xy, \qquad (1.3.2a)$$

$$\frac{\mathrm{d}y}{\mathrm{d}t} = \beta xy - \gamma y, \qquad (1.3.2b)$$

$$\frac{\mathrm{d}z}{\mathrm{d}t} = \gamma y, \qquad (1.3.2c)$$

subject to the initial conditions $\big(x(0), y(0), z(0)\big) = (x_0, y_0, 0)$. Here β is[2] the infection parameter, similar to that in (1.3.1), and γ is the removal parameter giving the rate at which infectives become immune. In cases where death or isolation may occur, $z(t)$ represents all removals from the population, including immunes, deaths and isolates.

Dividing equation (1.3.2a) by (1.3.2c) gives

$$\frac{\mathrm{d}x}{\mathrm{d}z} = -\frac{\beta}{\gamma} x = -\frac{x}{\rho} \qquad \text{with} \qquad \rho \equiv \frac{\gamma}{\beta},$$

the parameter ρ being the *relative removal rate*. The solution of this equation is

$$x = x_0 \mathrm{e}^{-z/\rho},$$

---

[2] Some authors write $\beta = \beta'/x(0)$ so (1.3.2a) becomes $\dot{x} = -\beta'(x/x_0)y$.

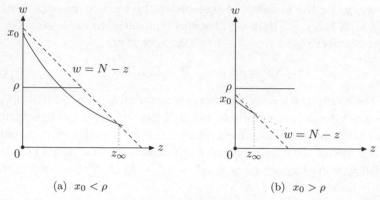

(a) $x_0 < \rho$ (b) $x_0 > \rho$

Figure 1.2. z_∞ as the point of intersection of $w = N - z$ and $w = x_0\,e^{-z/\rho}$.

so that

$$y = N - z - x_0 e^{-z/\rho}.$$

Hence

$$\frac{\mathrm{d}z}{\mathrm{d}t} = \gamma(N - z - x_0 e^{-z/\rho}),$$

with the parametric solution

$$\gamma t = \int_0^z \frac{\mathrm{d}v}{N - v - x_0 e^{-v/\rho}} \qquad (0 \le t < \infty). \tag{1.3.3}$$

Kermack and McKendrick obtained two basic results, referred to as their Threshold Theorem. The first is a criticality statement, and comes from equation (1.3.2b). Writing this equation as

$$\frac{\mathrm{d}y}{\mathrm{d}t} = \beta y(x - \rho)$$

shows that if the epidemic is ever to grow, then we must have $\mathrm{d}y/\mathrm{d}t|_{t=0} > 0$, or $x_0 > \rho$, i.e. *the initial number of susceptibles must exceed a threshold value* ρ. The second, deduced from (1.3.3), states that as $t \to \infty$, $z(t) \to z_\infty < N$. Now in the limit $t \to \infty$, $N - z_\infty - x_0 e^{-z_\infty/\rho} = 0$ (see the graphs in Figure 1.2).

Suppose now that x_0 is close to N; then z_∞ will be the approximate solution of

$$0 = N - z_\infty - N e^{-z_\infty/\rho} \approx N - z_\infty - N\left(1 - \frac{z_\infty}{\rho} + \frac{z_\infty^2}{2\rho^2}\right), \tag{1.3.4}$$

so that if $N = \rho + \nu$ with $\nu \ll \rho$, then

$$z_\infty \approx \frac{2\nu}{1 + \nu/\rho} \approx 2\nu. \tag{1.3.5}$$

Thus, if $x_0 \approx N = \rho + \nu$ with $\nu > 0$, then since $y_\infty = 0$, $x_\infty + z_\infty = N$ gives

$$x_\infty \approx \rho - \nu$$

(see Exercise 1.1 for the next term in the approximation).

Kermack and McKendrick's paper also includes the observation that, according to the model, some susceptibles survive the epidemic free from infection. At the time this was a significant result. We may view these three results, stated formally later at Theorem 2.1, as typical of the qualitative insights which mathematical models of epidemics attempt to achieve.

1.4 Stochastic modelling

The spread of an infectious disease is a random process; in a small group of individuals, one of whom has a cold, some will catch the infection while others will not. When the number of individuals is very large, it is customary to represent the infection process deterministically as, for example, Anderson and May (1991) mostly do. However, deterministic models are unsuitable for small populations, while in larger populations, the mean number of infectives in a stochastic model may not always be approximated satisfactorily by the equivalent deterministic model.

One of the earliest of stochastic models is due to McKendrick (1926), but the most used may well be the chain binomial model of Reed and Frost, put forward in their class lectures[3] at Johns Hopkins University in 1928, and based on one originally suggested by Soper (1929). Reed and Frost never published their work; Helen Abbey (1952) later gave a detailed account of it (see also Wilson and Burke (1942, 1943)). It should however be pointed out that En'ko (1889) anticipated some aspects of Reed and Frost's model by nearly 40 years, fitting data on measles epidemics recorded in St. Petersburg to a discrete time model similar to theirs (see En'ko (1889) and Dietz (1988)).

---

[3] E. B. Wilson records these dates as February 2–3, 1928, and refers to correspondence with Dr Frost shortly thereafter: 'I strongly urged Dr Frost to publish his theory of the epidemic curve, but he thought it too slight a contribution' (Wilson and Burke, 1942, note 3).

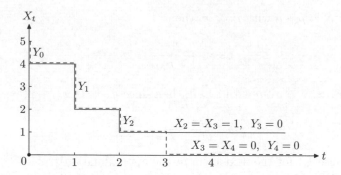

Figure 1.3. Two sample paths of a Reed–Frost epidemic, ending at $t = 3$ (——) and $t = 4$ (- - - -) respectively.

The model is based on the assumption that, in a group of X_t susceptibles and Y_t infectives at times $t = 0, 1, 2, \ldots$, where the time unit is the average length of the serial interval (see Figure 1.3), infection is passed on by 'adequate' contact of an infective with a susceptible in a relatively short time interval $(t, t + \epsilon)$ at the beginning of the period (indeed, instantaneously at $t + 0$). The newly infected individuals Y_{t+1} will themselves become infectious in $(t+1, t+1+\epsilon)$, while the current infectives Y_t will then be removed. Each susceptible is assumed to have the same probability $0 \le q \le 1$ of not making adequate contact with any given infective, or q^{Y_t} of not making contact with any of the Y_t independent infectives during $(t, t + \epsilon)$. Thus, for each susceptible, the probability of infection will be $1 - q^{Y_t}$; assuming the independence of each susceptible, the probability that there will be Y_{t+1} infectives at $t + 1$ can therefore be taken to be the binomial probability

$$P\{X_{t+1}, Y_{t+1} \mid X_t, Y_t\} = \binom{X_t}{X_{t+1}}(1 - q^{Y_t})^{Y_{t+1}}(q^{Y_t})^{X_{t+1}} \tag{1.4.1}$$

where $X_t = X_{t+1} + Y_{t+1}$. Figure 1.3 depicts two possible paths of an epidemic starting from $(X_0, Y_0) = (4, 1)$; for one path, $X_1 > X_2 = X_3 = 1$ and $Y_3 = 0$, so that the epidemic terminates at $t = 3$, while for the other, $X_2 > X_3 = X_4 = 0$ and $Y_4 = 0$ and it terminates at $t = 4$.

Because of the structure of (1.4.1), it is easily seen that the probability of an epidemic such as that in Figure 1.3 would be

$$L = P\{X_1, Y_1 \mid X_0, Y_0\} P\{X_2, Y_2 \mid X_1, Y_1\} P\{X_2, 0 \mid X_2, Y_2\}$$

$$= \binom{X_0}{X_1}(1 - q^{Y_0})^{Y_1} q^{Y_0 X_1} \binom{X_1}{X_2}(1 - q^{Y_1})^{Y_2} q^{Y_1 X_2} \binom{X_2}{X_2}(1 - q^{Y_2})^0 q^{Y_2 X_2}$$

$$= \binom{X_0}{X_1}\binom{X_1}{X_2}(1 - q^{Y_0})^{Y_1}(1 - q^{Y_1})^{Y_2} q^{Y_0 X_1 + Y_1 X_2 + Y_2 X_2}, \tag{1.4.2}$$

i.e. the product of a chain of binomials. Hence the model is referred to as a *chain binomial model*; such models will be discussed in much greater detail in Chapters 4 and 6 below.

Since the later 1940s, when Bartlett (1949) formulated the model for the general stochastic epidemic by analogy with the Kermack–McKendrick deterministic model, stochastic models for epidemic processes have proliferated. Most have relied on discrete or continuous time Markov chain structures, and we shall consider some of these in subsequent chapters. At this stage all that needs to be said is that reviews of the literature of epidemic models (see e.g. Dietz and Schenzle (1985), Hethcote (1994)) indicate that their number has grown very rapidly in the past 50 years.

1.5 Model fitting and prediction

Epidemic modelling has three main aims. The first is to understand better the mechanisms by which diseases spread; for this, a mathematical structure is important. For example, the simple insight provided by Kermack and McKendrick's model that the initial number of susceptibles x_0 must exceed the relative removal rate ρ for an epidemic to grow, could not have been reached without their mathematical equations (1.3.2).

The second aim is to predict the future course of the epidemic. Again using Kermack and McKendrick's general epidemic model as an example, we learn that if $x_0 = \rho + \nu$ is the number of susceptibles at the start of the epidemic and ν is somewhat smaller than ρ, then we can expect their number to be about $x_\infty = \rho - \nu$ at the end. Thus, we could predict that the total number of individuals affected by the epidemic would be about 2ν if we wished to estimate the medical costs of the epidemic, or to assess the possible impact of any outbreak of the disease.

The third aim is to understand how we may control the spread of the epidemic. Of the several methods for achieving this, education, immunization and isolation are those most often used. If one were able, for example, to reduce the number of susceptibles x_0 in the Kermack–McKendrick model by immunization to a level below ρ, the epidemic would be much reduced in size.

In order to make reasonable predictions and develop methods of control, we must be confident that our model captures the essential features of the course of an epidemic. Thus, it becomes important to validate models, whether deterministic or stochastic, by checking whether they fit the observed data. We now outline an example of such model fitting in the case of

Table 1.5. *The Aycock measles epidemic*

t	0	1	2	3	4	5
X_t	117	108	86	25	12	12
Y_t	1	9	22	61	13	0

Source: Abbey (1952).

a measles epidemic. If the model is validated, it can then be used to predict the course of the epidemic in time.

Following the pioneering study of measles and scarlet fever by Wilson *et al.* (1939), Abbey (1952) was among the first to use a stochastic epidemic model for the estimation of a 'contact' parameter, and for testing the validity of the model. Among her many sets of data was one for a particular measles epidemic in 1934 studied by Aycock (1942); to this data set she decided to fit a Reed–Frost model for $t = 0, 1, \ldots, 5$, the unit of time being a 12-day period. Using the same notation as in the previous section, Table 1.5 records the progress of the Aycock epidemic.

From the Reed–Frost model, the probabilities of these results in each individual time interval can be worked out respectively as

$$L_1(q_1) = \binom{117}{108}(1 - q_1)^9 q_1^{108}, \qquad L_2(q_2) = \binom{108}{86}(1 - q_2^9)^{22}(q_2^9)^{86},$$

$$L_3(q_3) = \binom{86}{25}(1 - q_3^{22})^{61}(q_3^{22})^{25}, \quad L_4(q_4) = \binom{25}{12}(1 - q_4^{61})^{13}(q_4^{61})^{12}.$$

$$(1.5.1)$$

Abbey obtained estimates of the probabilities q_i of no contact in each separate interval $i = 1, 2, 3, 4$ by the Maximum Likelihood method as

$$\hat{q}_1 = \frac{108}{117} = 0.9231, \qquad\qquad \hat{q}_2 = \left(\frac{86}{108}\right)^{1/9} = 0.975,$$

$$\hat{q}_3 = \left(\frac{25}{86}\right)^{1/22} = 0.9454, \qquad \hat{q}_4 = \left(\frac{12}{25}\right)^{1/61} = 0.988.$$

$$(1.5.2)$$

If one assumes that the probability of no contact has the same value q throughout all intervals, then the probability of the epidemic is given by

$$L(q) \equiv L_1(q)L_2(q)L_3(q)L_4(q), \tag{1.5.3}$$

with functions L_i as in (1.5.1). The Maximum Likelihood estimator $\hat{q}$ of q satisfies the relation

$$\left.\frac{\partial \ln L}{\partial q}\right|_{q=\hat{q}} \equiv -\frac{9}{1-\hat{q}} - \frac{198\hat{q}^8}{1-\hat{q}^9} - \frac{1342\hat{q}^{21}}{1-\hat{q}^{22}} - \frac{793\hat{q}^{60}}{1-\hat{q}^{61}} + \frac{2320}{\hat{q}} = 0, \quad (1.5.4)$$

which can be solved numerically to yield $\hat{q} = 0.9685$.

The fit of this model to the data turns out to be far from perfect: on a goodness-of-fit test Abbey reported $\chi^2 = 53.1$ on 4 degrees of freedom, and noted a significantly improved fit from estimating (rather than counting) the number of susceptibles. Abbey (1952) found the same true of other measles, chickenpox and German measles data, and investigated variation of the contact rate either with time or between individuals, or both, as other possible reasons for the inadequate fit of the model to the data (see Chapter 4).

1.6 Some general observations and summary

Mathematical techniques and models used in the study of epidemics form a major part of this book. They usually encompass, for any given model, a set of assumptions which can roughly be described as belonging one to each of the categories listed below.

The 'epidemic process' can be characterized as the evolution of some infectious disease phenomenon within a given population of individuals. The properties of the process fall naturally into three categories:

(1) assumptions about the population of individuals within which the disease first manifests itself, and then spreads;

(2) assumptions about the disease mechanism: how it is spread, and the mechanism of recovery or removal, if such occurs; and

(3) mathematical modelling assumptions that allow the specification of the two preceding properties.

So far as the population is concerned, we make assumptions about

(a) its *general structure*: it may be a single homogeneous group of individuals (apart from (c) below), or a collection of several homogeneous strata or subgroups, or else generally heterogeneous so that each individual is different;

(b) the population *dynamics* which specify whether the population is *closed* so that it is a constant collection of the same set of individuals for all time, or *open*, allowing individuals to give birth and die, and to emigrate or immigrate or both; and

(c) a mutually exclusive and exhaustive classification of individuals according to their *disease status*; thus, at any given time, an individual is either susceptible to the disease, or incubating it, or infectious with it, or possibly an infectious carrier without any symptoms of the disease, or a 'removed case.' A removal has been infectious or an infectious carrier but is so no longer, whether by acquired immunity or isolation or death.

Given the population, we next turn to a mathematical description of the mechanism(s) which specify how the disease is spread and how, if at all, individuals may ultimately recover temporarily or permanently from the disease. We mostly restrict ourselves to the assumption that the disease is spread by a *contagious mechanism*, viral or bacterial, so that contact between an infectious individual and a susceptible is necessary. After an infectious contact, the infectious individual or carrier succeeds in changing the susceptible's disease status: there follows an incubation period during part of which the disease is latent within the newly infected susceptible. After this the susceptible itself becomes an infective (see Figure 1.4 and Section 1.6.2).

1.6.1   Methods and models

This monograph is as much about mathematical methods as about the epidemic models themselves. So, unlike Bailey's (1975) classical treatise, it is primarily organized around the various mathematical techniques used to study epidemic models. Consequently some models recur in several places.

Chapter 2 outlines a few deterministic models, after which Chapter 3 describes some stochastic models in continuous time, Chapter 4 others in discrete time, and Chapter 5 models for rumours. Chapter 6 discusses the fitting of models to data. In Chapter 7, three examples are given of how epidemic modelling may help us to control the spread of epidemics.

Our hope is that the reader who masters the methods outlined here will be well prepared to tackle the more comprehensive treatises of Bailey (1975) and Anderson and May (1991), and papers in the recently published volumes edited by Mollison (1995) and Isham and Medley (1996).

1.6.2   Some terminology

It may be useful to clarify some terms commonly employed in epidemic theory: these are illustrated in Figure 1.4 (cf. also Anderson and May, 1991, §§3.1.1 and 3.2.4). We assume that there is an instant at which infection occurs for an individual; this is the start of a latent period during which this individual is not infectious. There then follows an infectious period within which symptoms will appear; the incubation period is the time from first infection to the appearance of symptoms, and this is necessarily greater than or equal to the latent period. The serial interval is the time between first infection and the infection of a second individual; this is again larger than or equal to the latent period, but can be either smaller or larger than

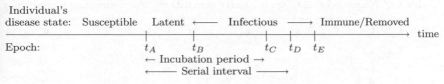

Individual's
disease state: Susceptible   Latent ⟵—   Infectious —⟶   Immune/Removed

Epoch: t_A t_B t_C t_D t_E
                        ← Incubation period →
                    ⟵——— Serial interval ———⟶

t_A: Infection occurs t_B: Latency to infectious transition
t_C: Symptoms appear t_D: First transmission to another susceptible
t_E: Individual no longer infectious to susceptibles (recovery or removal)
Note: t_D is constrained to lie in the interval (t_B, t_E), so $t_D > t_C$ (as shown) and $t_D < t_C$ are both possible.

Figure 1.4. Diagrammatic representation of progress of a disease in an individual.

the incubation period. Often the serial interval and latent period are used interchangeably although their meanings are different. The fundamental quantity in the process of infection is the *serial interval*, but the *latent period* is often used in the literature because it is assumed that a second infection will occur as soon as the first infective becomes infectious. Anderson and May (1991, §3.2.4) use the term *generation time of the disease agent*; in terms of the notation in Figure 1.4 it is the expectation of $(t_B - t_A) + \frac{1}{2}(t_E - t_B)$, i.e. the mean latent period plus half the mean infectious period.

1.7   Exercises and Complements to Chapter 1

1.1   Show that for positive n, ϵ and ρ there exists a unique root of the equation
$$n + \epsilon = z + ne^{-z/\rho}$$
satisfying $0 < z - \epsilon < n$, $z = \zeta$ say. Expand the exponential term to third order and deduce that in the limit $\epsilon \downarrow 0$, $\zeta \approx 2\nu - \frac{2}{3}\nu^2/\rho$ where $0 < \nu = n - \rho = O(\rho^{\frac{1}{2}})$ (cf. Daley and Gani, 1994, §4.1). (The notation here and of equation (1.3.4) is related by $z = z_\infty$, $n = x_0$ and $n + \epsilon = N$.)

1.2   In the general epidemic model sketched in Section 1.3, the quantity $R_0 \equiv n/\rho = \beta n/\gamma = $ (initial no. of susceptibles)/(relative removal rate) coincides with the *Basic Reproduction Ratio* in Section 3.5 below. Show that for $R_0 = 2$ in this model starting from $y_0 \ll x_0$, about 20% of the population survive the epidemic. Bartholomew (1973, p. 346) gives 2% for $R_0 = 4$.

1.3   The data in Table 1.6 come from bar charts labelled a, ..., j in En'ko (transl. 1989). En'ko extracted the daily numbers of measles cases for several years from records at the St Petersburg Alexander Institute, where the date of a measles case was determined by the appearance of a rash on the face, and at the Educational College for the Daughters of the Nobility, where the date was determined by the date of transfer into the infirmary. En'ko allocated cases recorded 0–7, 8–17, 18–29, 30–41, 42–53, 54–65, ... days following the

Table 1.6. *Numbers of cases in successive generations of several measles epidemics*

1st day	0	1	2	3	4	5	6	7	8	9
1865, b										
0	1									
9	1	2	2	4	4					
20	6	5	3	4	3	0	3	0	1	
32	1	4	2	2	0	3				
44	2	0	0	1	0	1				
1875, i										
0	1									
8	5	0	2	3	2					
21	3	0	2	0	1					
1879, c										
0	2									
9	3	5	6	5	0	5	2	1	1	
19	1	1	3	0	2	2	2	2	0	1
37	1									
1882, e										
0	1									
11	2	0	0	0	1					
25	1	0	3	3	3	1	1			
35	1	6	1	1	1	0	1			
1884, f										
0	1									
12	1	1	1	0	1					
24	1	0	0	0	3	1	1	0	1	
37	1	0	0	0	0	0	1	0	1	

1st day	0	1	2	3	4	5	6	7	8	9	10	11
1870, h												
0	1	1	0	0	0	2						
10	2	4	0	0	0	2	1					
22	2	0	2	1	2	1	0	1				
34	2	3	1	4	3	4	4	0	2	0	1	
46	4	2	3	4	2	1	0	1	1			
1874, g												
0	1											
9	1	22	18	7	12	7	17	1	1			
19	1	5	11	4	3	5	5	6	1	2	1	1
35	1	0	1									
1875, a												
0	2	1										
8	2	5	1	4	20	7	5	5	2	1	1	
18	2	3	4	7	6	2	0	1	0	2	0	
32	1											
1888, d												
0	1											
11	1	0	1	0	1	1						
20	2	1	1	1	2	1	2	1				
29	3	1	0	1	0	1	0	1	2	2	1	1
51	1											
Combined counts of 10 epidemics, j												
0	13	2	0	0	0	2	0	1				
8	7	10	34	43	39	25	18	13	6	2	1	
19	5	18	21	18	18	17	12	18	10	13	3	2
31	2	3	7	4	8	6	13	6	7	5	2	2
44	4	0	5	3	4	4	3	1	0	1	1	
60	1											
69	1											
85	1											

Source: From bar charts in En'ko (transl. 1989). See Exercise 1.3 for more explanation.

initial case on day 0, to generation 0, 1, ... respectively. The table gives for each epidemic the first day of observing a case for each generation, and the number of cases reported on the various days within the generation, for as long as there were any such cases.

(a) Investigate whether the spread of the dates of recording cases within an epidemic shows any systematic trend from one generation to another (if not, then periodicity is strong, and identifying a case is variable).

(b) Repeat the analysis of (a) on the combined data: what sort of additional variability does such pooling of data introduce?

(c) The construction of analogues of $\hat{q}_i$ and $\hat{q}$ as in section 1.5 entails the estimation of the population size as well.

(d) If a model is fitted as in (c), then a χ^2 goodness of fit test can be performed.

1.4 Wilson and Burke (1943) list the monthly numbers of measles cases in Providence RI for the years 1917–1940 as in Table 1.7. Plot out the course of the nine epidemics for which the epidemic curves peak around May 1918, Mar. 1921, Mar. 1923, Jan. 1926, Apr. 1928, Jan. 1932, May 1935, Mar. 1937, Mar. 1940. Observe that there is a marked seasonality effect if the dataset is treated as a whole.

(a) Assuming a mean serial interval of 0.5 months and a closed population for the course of the epidemic, investigate how estimates of any or all of N, ρ, β, γ might be constructed.

(b) Repeat this analysis for the record as a whole assuming instead an immigration of 2130 new susceptibles each September (thus, N_{year} varies as each year changes).

(c) Repeat the analysis of (b) but assuming now a steady immigration of 178 new susceptibles per month.

Table 1.7. *Measles cases by months in Providence RI 1917–1940*

Year	Jan.	Feb.	Mar.	Apr.	May	June	July	Aug.	Sep.	Oct.	Nov.	Dec.	Total
1917	33	47	62	109	119	36	13	7	2	1	8	55	492
1918	55	98	373	1232	1299	780	261	23	8	6	5	3	4143
1919	1	4	4	4	5	4	3	3	1	2	1	3	35
1920	125	127	136	279	404	288	146	38	45	53	190	191	2022
1921	329	585	665	390	266	99	28	10	1	2	7	26	2408
1922	89	4	3	26	25	22	23	19	7	16	131	652	1017
1923	680	1228	1470	687	383	117	29	6	3	10	7	7	4627
1924	5	6	3	11	16	30	15	2	2	1	5	2	98
1925	13	11	6	15	18	30	58	50	13	81	417	1224	1936
1926	2057	1360	648	348	196	105	48	8	1	0	0	4	4775
1927	5	2	1	1	2	2	6	2	0	9	7	23	60
1928	45	112	422	1081	883	800	508	77	18	36	36	61	4079
1929	84	189	261	399	276	111	38	4	3	2	0	0	1367
1930	2	0	1	4	23	46	22	8	1	0	2	0	109
1931	1	2	49	158	456	358	179	99	22	191	337	1548	3400
1932	2799	2037	574	199	81	11	2	0	0	0	0	0	5703
1933	0	0	0	3	3	6	5	2	4	0	1	1	25
1934	4	11	21	18	29	106	44	25	8	5	1	7	279
1935	13	57	343	1351	1953	1279	241	17	4	1	0	48	5307
1936	119	74	92	76	83	17	11	4	0	0	9	77	562
1937	422	811	1184	711	472	129	31	4	0	2	3	3	3772
1938	2	5	4	2	0	0	0	3	1	0	0	3	20
1939	33	35	40	118	317	286	157	64	20	89	267	446	1872
1940	569	495	530	462	543	372	121	20	1	0	1	1	3113
Total	7485	7300	6890	7684	7852	4934	1989	495	165	507	1435	4385	51221

Source: Wilson and Burke (1943).

2

Deterministic Models

In deterministic models, population sizes of susceptibles, infectives and removals are assumed to be functions of discrete time $t = 0, 1, 2, \ldots$ or differentiable functions of continuous time $t \geq 0$. Such approximations to the true, integer-valued numbers of individuals involved in an epidemic, allow us to derive sets of difference or differential equations governing the process. The evolution of this epidemic process is deterministic in the sense that no randomness is allowed for; the system develops according to laws similar to those for dynamical systems. It is usual to regard the results of a deterministic process as giving an approximation to the mean of a random process: there are examples related to this in the next chapter (see equations (3.2.4) and (3.3.6), and Exercises 3.1, 3.2, 3.5 and 3.11).

2.1 The simple epidemic in continuous time

A *simple epidemic* is one where the population consists only of susceptibles and infectives; once a susceptible is infected, it becomes an infective and remains in that state indefinitely. A simple epidemic may be thought of as one where

(a) the disease is highly infectious but not serious, so that infectives remain in contact with the susceptibles for all time $t \geq 0$;

(b) the infectives continue to spread their infection until the end of the epidemic (see equation (2.1.2) and below for interpretations of the 'end' of the epidemic).

An infection which may approximate these conditions is the common cold over a period of a few days. This simple epidemic model is the same as the logistic model of population growth, attributed[1] to Verhulst (1838).

---

[1]Miner (1933) remarks that 'Verhulst's work was generally forgotten until after the

We suppose that the total population is closed, i.e.

$$x(t) + y(t) = N \quad \text{(all } t \geq 0)$$

where, as throughout this chapter, $x(t)$ and $y(t)$ denote the numbers of susceptibles and infectives at time t, with initial conditions $\big(x(0), y(0)\big) = (x_0, y_0)$ with $y_0 \geq 1$. Then assuming that the individuals of the population mix homogeneously, we can write

$$\frac{dy}{dt} = \beta xy = \beta y(N - y), \tag{2.1.1}$$

where β is the pairwise rate of infection (i.e. *infection parameter*) and, in contrast to the discrete time case (cf. (1.3.1)), the condition $\beta \leq 1/N$ is no longer needed. This differential equation, the so-called logistic growth equation, is readily solved, since

$$\frac{dy}{y(N - y)} = \Big(\frac{1}{y} + \frac{1}{N - y}\Big)\frac{dy}{N} = \beta \, dt,$$

so integrating on $(0, t)$,

$$\ln \frac{y(t)}{N - y(t)} - \ln \frac{y_0}{N - y_0} = \beta N t.$$

Hence

$$y(t) = \frac{y_0 N}{y_0 + (N - y_0)e^{-\beta N t}}. \tag{2.1.2}$$

As $t \to \infty$, equation (2.1.2) shows that $y(t) \to N$, so that according to the model all individuals in the population eventually become infected, thus causing the end of the epidemic (in the mathematical sense).

In this *model* we have both $x(t) > 0$ and $y(t) > 0$ for *all* finite positive t, so the question arises as to when we may consider the epidemic to have terminated in practical terms. Realistically, we could define the 'end' of the epidemic to occur at $T_1 \equiv \inf\{t : y(t) > N - 1\}$, i.e. when the number of infectives is within 1 of its final value. Since the function $y(\cdot)$ has a positive

---

independent rediscovery of the logistic curve by Pearl and Reed in 1920', and that to his knowledge 'the only reference to the work of Verhulst in modern times prior to [1920] is [a paper in 1918 by Du Pasquier]'. Bailey (1975) gives no account of its emergence in epidemic theory; Bailey (1955) attributes the stochastic version of the model to Bartlett's 1946 lecture notes (see Bartlett, 1947).

derivative for finite t, T_1 is determined by $y(T_1) = N - 1$. It follows from (2.1.2) that

$$\frac{y_0 N}{y_0 + (N - y_0)e^{-\beta N T_1}} = N - 1,$$

so

$$T_1 = \frac{1}{\beta N} \ln \left(\frac{(N - 1)(N - y_0)}{y_0} \right). \tag{2.1.3}$$

Table 2.1 illustrates the values of T_1 for various values of y_0 when $N = 24, 50, 100, 1000$ for the simple case where $\beta = 1/N$.

Table 2.1. T_1 *determined from* $y(T_1) = N - 1$ *when* $\beta = 1/N$

y_0	$N =$	24	50	100	1000
1		6.2710	7.7836	9.1902	13.8135
10		3.3979	5.2781	6.7923	11.5019
$\frac{1}{2}N$		3.1355	3.8918	4.5951	6.9068

Observe that as y_0 increases from 1 to $\frac{1}{2}N$, the time T_1 taken to reach $N - 1$ is halved, as follows from the symmetry about $y = \frac{1}{2}N$ of the derivative at (2.1.1). Also, as N increases from 24 to 1000, T_1 increases rather slowly for, as (2.1.3) shows, $T_1 = O\big((\ln N)/\beta N\big)$.

Thus, if the unit of time is the day, in a classroom of 50 schoolchildren of whom one has a cold initially, the infection spreads among the whole class in fewer than eight days if $\beta N = O(1)$.

Sometimes epidemiologists are more interested in the *epidemic curve*, which is the rate of occurrence of new infectives, here dy/dt. We see from (2.1.1) that

$$\frac{dy}{dt} = \frac{\beta N^2 y_0(N - y_0)e^{\beta Nt}}{[y_0 e^{\beta Nt} + (N - y_0)]^2} = \frac{\beta y_0(N - y_0)}{[\cosh \beta Nt + (1 - 2y_0/N) \sinh \beta Nt]^2}. \tag{2.1.4}$$

It has a maximum when

$$t = \frac{1}{\beta N} \ln \frac{N - y_0}{y_0}.$$

At this time we have $x(t) = y(t) = \frac{1}{2}N$, and $(dy/dt) = \beta(\frac{1}{2}N)^2$. The dashed curve in Figure 2.1 illustrates equation (2.1.4), i.e. the epidemic curve for the deterministic model of a simple epidemic (cf. also Figure 2.12 below).

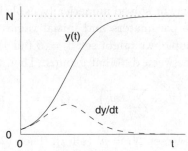

Figure 2.1. $y(t)$ (———) and dy/dt (– – –) for the simple epidemic.

2.2 The simple epidemic in interacting groups

We suppose in this section that a closed population now consists of m groups of sizes $N_1, \ldots, N_m$, in each of which a simple epidemic may break out. Assume that these groups interact with each other as follows. In place of the single pairwise infection rate β as in (2.1.1), suppose that susceptibles in the jth group are subject to infection from infectives in the ith group at rate β_{ij} per interacting pair; for $i = j$ we set $\beta_j = \beta_{jj}$ ($j = 1, \ldots, m$). Figure 2.2 illustrates the model, which is due to Rushton and Mautner (1955).

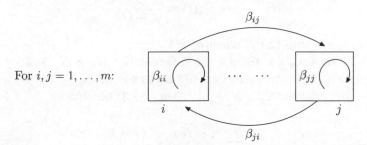

Figure 2.2. Infection rates in interacting communities $i, j = 1, \ldots, m$.

Let $x_j(t)$, $y_j(t)$ denote the numbers of susceptibles and infectives in each of the groups $j = 1, \ldots, m$ respectively. Then we readily see that when infection is transmitted both within and between groups, equation (2.1.1) can be generalized to the set of equations

$$\frac{dy_j}{dt} = \beta_j y_j x_j + \sum_{i \neq j} \beta_{ij} y_i x_j \qquad (j = 1, \ldots, m), \qquad (2.2.1)$$

subject to the initial conditions $y_j(0) = y_{j0}$ and $x_j(0) = N_j - y_{j0}$, as follows from $x_j = N_j - y_j$.

While these equations may be solved numerically, explicit algebraic results are obtainable only if the parameters and initial values have a relatively simple structure. For example, we might set $\beta_j = \beta$ (all j) and $\beta_{ij} = \beta\kappa$ for some $\kappa \neq 1$ for infection between different groups. Then (2.2.1) becomes

$$\frac{dy_j}{dt} = \beta(N_j - y_j)\left(y_j + \sum_{i \neq j} \kappa y_i\right) \qquad (j = 1, \ldots, m). \qquad (2.2.2)$$

A further simplification is to set $N_j = N$ (all j). Then (2.2.2) becomes

$$\frac{dy_j}{dt} = \beta(N - y_j)\left(y_j + \sum_{i \neq j} \kappa y_i\right) \qquad (j = 1, \ldots, m). \qquad (2.2.3)$$

If all the initial values $y_{j0} = y_0$ are the same, this set of equations basically reduces to the single equation

$$\frac{dy}{dt} = \beta(N - y)y[1 + (m - 1)\kappa] = \beta'(N - y)y,$$

where $\beta' \equiv \beta[1 + (m - 1)\kappa]$ and

$$y(t) = y_1(t) = \cdots = y_m(t) = \frac{y_0 N}{y_0 + (N - y_0)e^{-\beta' Nt}},$$

as is consistent with (2.1.2) when $m = 1$.

We now show that if the y_{j0} are different but $N_j = N$ for all j, there exist explicit parametric solutions of (2.2.3) for the $y_j(t)$. Write $\tau = \beta t$, $a = 1 + (m - 1)\kappa$ and $x_j = N - y_j$. Then (2.2.3) becomes

$$\frac{d}{d\tau} \ln x_j = x_j + \kappa \sum_{i \neq j} x_i - Na \qquad (j = 1, \ldots, m). \qquad (2.2.4)$$

The further transformations $U_j = e^{aN\tau}(x_j/N)$ and $v = (1 - e^{-aN\tau})/a$ lead to

$$\frac{d}{dv} \ln U_j = U_j + \kappa \sum_{i \neq j} U_i \qquad (j = 1, \ldots, m), \qquad (2.2.5)$$

or in terms of m-vectors $\mathbf{U}$ and $\ln \mathbf{U}$ and the $m \times m$ matrix $\mathbf{B} = (b_{ij})$ defined by

$$\mathbf{U} = \begin{pmatrix} U_1 \\ U_2 \\ \vdots \\ U_m \end{pmatrix}, \qquad \ln \mathbf{U} = \begin{pmatrix} \ln U_1 \\ \ln U_2 \\ \vdots \\ \ln U_m \end{pmatrix}, \qquad \mathbf{B} = \begin{pmatrix} 1 & \kappa & \cdots & \kappa \\ \kappa & 1 & \cdots & \kappa \\ \vdots & \vdots & \ddots & \vdots \\ \kappa & \kappa & \cdots & 1 \end{pmatrix},$$

where $\ln \mathbf{U}$ involves an abuse of notation,

$$\frac{d}{dv} \ln \mathbf{U} = \mathbf{B}\mathbf{U}. \tag{2.2.6}$$

Note that for $t = 0$, $\tau = 0$, $v = 0$ and $x_{j0} = N - y_{j0} \equiv N U_j(0)$.

This matrix equation can be solved as follows. First use the inverse $\mathbf{B}^{-1} = (b^{ij})$ of $\mathbf{B}$ (assuming $|\mathbf{B}| \neq 0$) to give

$$\frac{d}{dv} \mathbf{B}^{-1} \ln \mathbf{U} = \mathbf{U},$$

i.e.

$$\frac{d}{dv} \sum_{i=1}^{m} b^{ji} \ln U_i = U_j \qquad (j = 1, \dots, m).$$

Define $\mathbf{X}$ by setting $\ln \mathbf{X} = \mathbf{B}^{-1} \ln \mathbf{U}$, so that $\ln \mathbf{U} = \mathbf{B} \ln \mathbf{X}$. These relations are equivalent to

$$X_j = \prod_{i=1}^{m} U_i^{b^{ji}} \quad \text{and} \quad U_j = \prod_{i=1}^{m} X_i^{b_{ji}}, \tag{2.2.7}$$

from which it follows that

$$\frac{d}{dv} \ln X_j = U_j = \prod_{i=1}^{m} X_i^{b_{ji}} = (X_1 \dots X_m)^{\kappa} X_j^{1-\kappa}.$$

Then for all $j = 1, \dots, m$,

$$X_j^{\kappa-2} \frac{dX_j}{dv} = \left(\prod_{i=1}^{m} X_i \right)^{\kappa} \equiv F(v) \quad \text{say.} \tag{2.2.8}$$

Hence on integration,

$$X_j^{\kappa-1}(v) - X_j^{\kappa-1}(0) = (\kappa - 1) \int_0^v F(u) \, du \equiv G(v),$$

or

$$X_j(v) = \left[X_j^{\kappa-1}(0) + (\kappa-1) \int_0^v F(u) \, du \right]^{1/(\kappa-1)} = \left[X_j^{\kappa-1}(0) + G(v) \right]^{1/(\kappa-1)},$$

where $X_j(0) = \prod_{i=1}^{m} U_i^{b^{ji}}(0) = \prod_{i=0}^{m} (x_{j0}/N)^{b^{ji}}$. Now from (2.2.7), for all $j = 1, \dots, m$,

$$U_j(v) = \left(\prod_{i=1}^{m} X_i^{\kappa} \right) X_j^{1-\kappa} = \frac{F'(v)}{X_j^{\kappa-1}(0) + G(v)}. \tag{2.2.9}$$

But from (2.2.8),

$$F(v) = \prod_{j=1}^{m} \left[X_j^{\kappa-1}(0) + G(v) \right]^{\kappa/(\kappa-1)} = \frac{1}{\kappa-1} \frac{dG}{dv},$$

whence

$$v = \frac{1 - e^{-aN\beta t}}{a} = \frac{1}{\kappa-1} \int_0^G \prod_{j=1}^{m} \left[X_j^{\kappa-1}(0) + g \right]^{\kappa/(1-\kappa)} dg, \qquad (2.2.10)$$

so that the time is given parametrically in terms of G. We can now find the solutions for $U_j(v)$ and hence for the original $y_j = N - Ne^{-aN\beta t}U_j$.

These computations simplify as follows in the special case where $y_{10} = 1$ and $y_{j0} = 0$ for $j = 2, \ldots, m$, so the $y_j(t)$ for $j = 2, \ldots, m$ are identical for all $t \geq 0$, and equations (2.2.4) reduce to the two equations

$$\begin{aligned}
\frac{d\ln x_1}{d\tau} &= x_1 + (m-1)\kappa x_2 - Na, \\
\frac{d\ln x_2}{d\tau} &= \kappa x_1 + [1 + (m-2)\kappa]x_2 - Na.
\end{aligned} \qquad (2.2.11)$$

Further transformations as in (2.2.5) lead to

$$\frac{d}{dv} \begin{pmatrix} \ln U_1 \\ \ln U_2 \end{pmatrix} = \begin{pmatrix} 1 & (m-1)\kappa \\ \kappa & 1 + (m-2)\kappa \end{pmatrix} \begin{pmatrix} U_1 \\ U_2 \end{pmatrix} = \mathbf{B} \begin{pmatrix} U_1 \\ U_2 \end{pmatrix}. \qquad (2.2.12)$$

We note that

$$\mathbf{B}^{-1} = \frac{1}{K} \begin{pmatrix} 1 + (m-2)\kappa & -(m-1)\kappa \\ -\kappa & 1 \end{pmatrix}$$

where

$$K \equiv |\mathbf{B}| = 1 + (m-2)\kappa - (m-1)\kappa^2 = (1-\kappa)[1 + (m-1)\kappa],$$

so that

$$X_1 = U_1^{[1+(m-2)\kappa]/K} U_2^{-(m-1)\kappa/K}, \qquad X_2 = U_1^{-\kappa/K} U_2^{1/K}.$$

It follows that when $t = 0$, $v = 0$ and

$$\begin{aligned}
X_1(0) &= U_1^{[1+(m-2)\kappa]/K}(0) U_2^{-(m-1)/K}(0) = (1 - N^{-1})^{[1+(m-2)\kappa]/K}, \\
X_2(0) &= U_1^{-\kappa/K}(0) U_2^{1/K}(0) = (1 - N^{-1})^{-\kappa/K}.
\end{aligned}$$

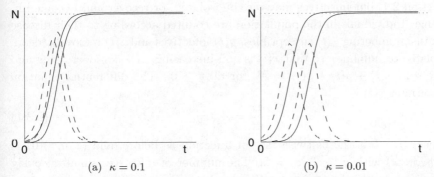

(a) $\kappa = 0.1$ (b) $\kappa = 0.01$

Figure 2.3. Numbers of infectives y_1 and y_2 (———), and infection rates $\dot{y}_1$ and $\dot{y}_2$ ($---$), for a Rushton–Mautner simple epidemic spreading in two communities, with $x_1(0) = x_2(0) = N$, $y_1(0) = 1$ and $y_2(0) = 0$, and κ as shown.

Hence

$$X_1(v) = \left((1 - N^{-1})^{-1+\{\kappa/[1+(m-1)\kappa]\}} + G(v)\right)^{1/(\kappa-1)},$$

$$X_2(v) = \left((1 - N^{-1})^{-1/[1+(m-1)\kappa]} + G(v)\right)^{1/(\kappa-1)},$$

where

$$
\begin{aligned}
v &= \frac{1 - e^{-aN\beta t}}{a} = \frac{1}{\kappa - 1} \int_0^{G(v)} \left((1 - N^{-1})^{-1+\{\kappa/[1+(m-1)\kappa]\}} + g\right)^{\kappa/(1-\kappa)} \\
&\qquad\qquad\qquad\qquad\qquad \times \left((1 - N^{-1})^{-1/[1+(m-1)\kappa]} + g\right)^{\kappa/(1-\kappa)} dg \\
&= \frac{1}{\kappa - 1} \int_0^{G(v)} \left[(\alpha_1 + g)(\alpha_2 + g)\right]^{\kappa/(1-\kappa)} dg. \qquad (2.2.13)
\end{aligned}
$$

Hence, for any time v, $G(v)$ is known by (2.2.13), and thus also $X_1(v)$ and $X_2(v)$. From these $U_1(v)$ and $U_2(v)$ are obtained as $U_1 = X_1 X_2^{(m-1)\kappa}$ and $U_2 = X_1^\kappa X_2^{1+(m-2)\kappa}$, and thus x_j and $y_j = N - x_j$ $(j = 1, 2)$.

Figure 2.3 depicts the spread of infection in a population of two equally sized strata. For larger κ as in (a), the outbreaks largely overlap and reinforce each other, whereas in (b) the epidemics occur more slowly and approximately in sequence.

2.3   The general epidemic in a homogeneous population

In the classical model for a *general epidemic* that we now describe, the size of the population N is assumed to be fixed as for the simple epidemic of

Section 2.1, but infectives may die, be isolated, or recover and become immune. Individuals in the population are counted according to their disease status, numbering $x(t)$ susceptibles, $y(t)$ infectives and $z(t)$ removals (dead, isolated or immune), so that $x(t)$ is non-increasing, $z(t)$ non-decreasing and the sum $x(t) + y(t) + z(t) = N$, for all $t \geq 0$. The differential equation governing $x(t)$ is

$$\frac{dx}{dt} = -\beta xy, \tag{2.3.1}$$

where $\beta > 0$ is the pairwise rate of infection as before, and $(x, y, z)(0) = (x_0, y_0, z_0)$ with $y_0 \geq 1$, $z_0 = 0$. The number of infectives simultaneously increases at the same rate as the number of susceptibles decreases, and decreases through removal (by death, isolation or immunity) at a *per capita* rate $\gamma > 0$, so that

$$\frac{dy}{dt} = \beta xy - \gamma y. \tag{2.3.2}$$

Finally the number of removals increases at exactly the same rate as the loss of infectives, so that

$$\frac{dz}{dt} = \gamma y. \tag{2.3.3}$$

Observe that $(d/dt)\big(x(t) + y(t) + z(t)\big) = 0$, as is consistent with the total population size remaining fixed at N.

In their first paper entitled 'A contribution to the mathematical theory of epidemics', Kermack and McKendrick (1927) proposed these equations as a simple model describing the course of an epidemic. We can write (2.3.1) and (2.3.3) as

$$\frac{1}{x} \cdot \frac{dx}{dt} = -\frac{\beta}{\gamma} \cdot \frac{dz}{dt} = -\frac{1}{\rho} \cdot \frac{dz}{dt}, \tag{2.3.4}$$

where $\rho \equiv \gamma/\beta$ is the *relative removal rate*. Integrating this differential equation directly, and using the initial values x_0 and $z_0 = 0$ as above, we obtain

$$x(t) = x_0 e^{-z(t)/\rho}. \tag{2.3.5}$$

A second integral is also readily obtained: equations (2.3.1–2) imply that $x(t)$ and $y(t)$ satisfy

$$\frac{dy}{dx} = -1 + \frac{\rho}{x},$$

so

$$x(t) + y(t) - \rho \ln x(t) = x_0 + y_0 - \rho \ln x_0. \tag{2.3.6}$$

Within the region where x, y and z are non-negative, equation (2.3.2) yields the inequality $\dot{y} \geq -\gamma y$, which in turn implies that $y(t) \geq y_0 e^{-\gamma t} > 0$

(all $0 < t < \infty$). Similarly, $\dot{x} \geq -\beta x(x_0 + y_0)$ so that $x(t) \geq x_0 e^{-\beta(x_0 + y_0)t} > 0$ (all $0 < t < \infty$). However, from (2.3.1), $x(t)$ is strictly decreasing for all such t. Consequently, $x(t)$ and $z(t)$, and hence $y(t)$ as well, converge to finite limits x_∞, z_∞ and y_∞ as $t \to \infty$, with $y_\infty = 0$ as we would have $\lim_{t \to \infty} \dot{z} > 0$ otherwise. Further, from (2.3.5), $x_\infty = x_0 e^{-z_\infty / \rho}$. Because $z_\infty \leq x_0 + y_0 < \infty$, $x_\infty > 0$, and equation (2.3.2) then implies that $\dot{y}$ is ultimately monotonic decreasing; it is in fact monotonic decreasing for all $t > 0$ if and only if $x_0 \leq \gamma/\beta = \rho$.

Kermack and McKendrick's results constitute a benchmark for a range of epidemic models, so we state them formally for later reference.

Theorem 2.1 (Kermack–McKendrick). *A general epidemic evolves according to the differential equations (2.3.1–3) from initial values $(x_0, y_0, 0)$, where $x_0 + y_0 = N$.*

(i) (Survival and Total Size). *When infection ultimately ceases spreading, a positive number x_∞ of susceptibles remain uninfected, and the total number z_∞ of individuals ultimately infected and removed equals $x_0 + y_0 - x_\infty$ and is the unique root of the equation*

$$N - z_\infty = x_0 + y_0 - z_\infty = x_0 e^{-z_\infty / \rho}, \tag{2.3.7}$$

where $y_0 < z_\infty < x_0 + y_0$, $\rho = \gamma/\beta$ being the relative removal rate.

(ii) (Threshold Theorem). *A major outbreak occurs if and only if $\dot{y}(0) > 0$; this happens only if the initial number of susceptibles $x_0 > \rho$.*

(iii) (Second Threshold Theorem). *If x_0 exceeds ρ by a small quantity ν, and if the initial number of infectives y_0 is small relative to ν, then the final number of susceptibles left in the population is approximately $\rho - \nu$, and $z_\infty \approx 2\nu$.*

The major significance of these statements at the time of their first publication was a mathematical demonstration that even with a major outbreak of a disease satisfying the simple model, *not all susceptibles would necessarily be infected.* Conditions were given for a major outbreak to occur, namely that the number of susceptibles at the start of the epidemic should be sufficiently high; this would happen, for example, in a city with a large population. These conclusions were consistent with observation, such as had been noted by Hamer in his 1906 lectures.

It remains to demonstrate part (iii) of the theorem. Kermack and McKendrick did so by first finding an approximation to $x(t)$ as an explicit function of t. To this end, observe that substituting from (2.3.5) into (2.3.3) together with the constraint on the population size yields

$$\frac{dz}{dt} = \gamma(N - z(t) - x_0 e^{-z(t)/\rho}). \tag{2.3.8}$$

This differential equation does not have an explicit solution for z in terms of t. However, using the expansion $e^{-u} = 1 - u + \frac{1}{2}u^2 + O(u^3)$ and neglecting the last term, yields the approximate relation

$$\frac{dz}{dt} \approx \gamma\left[N - x_0 + z\left(\frac{x_0}{\rho} - 1\right) - \frac{z^2 x_0}{2\rho^2}\right] \tag{2.3.9}$$

which can be solved. First express the right-hand side as in

$$\frac{dz}{dt} \approx \frac{\rho^2 \gamma}{2x_0}\left[(N - x_0)\frac{2x_0}{\rho^2} + \left(\frac{x_0}{\rho} - 1\right)^2 - \left(\frac{x_0}{\rho^2}\left[z - \frac{\rho^2}{x_0}\left(\frac{x_0}{\rho} - 1\right)\right]\right)^2\right].$$

Now setting

$$\alpha = \left[\frac{2x_0}{\rho^2}(N - x_0) + \left(\frac{x_0}{\rho} - 1\right)^2\right]^{\frac{1}{2}} \tag{2.3.10}$$

this reduces to

$$\frac{dz}{dt} \approx \frac{\rho^2 \gamma}{2x_0}\left[\alpha^2 - \left(\frac{x_0}{\rho^2}\left[z - \frac{\rho^2}{x_0}\left(\frac{x_0}{\rho} - 1\right)\right]\right)^2\right]. \tag{2.3.11}$$

Substitute

$$\alpha \tanh v = \frac{x_0}{\rho^2}\left[z - \frac{\rho^2}{x_0}\left(\frac{x_0}{\rho} - 1\right)\right]$$

where at time $t = 0$, $z_0 = 0$, so that $\alpha \tanh v_0 = -[(x_0/\rho) - 1]$. Then we can readily see with this substitution in (2.3.11) that

$$\frac{dz}{dt} \approx \frac{\rho^2 \gamma}{2x_0}(\alpha^2 - \alpha^2 \tanh^2 v) = \frac{\rho^2}{x_0}\alpha \operatorname{sech}^2 v \frac{dv}{dt}.$$

Hence

$$\frac{dv}{dt} \approx \tfrac{1}{2}\gamma\alpha, \qquad \text{so} \quad v \approx \tfrac{1}{2}\gamma\alpha t + v_0$$

and

$$z(t) \approx \frac{\rho^2}{x_0}\left(\frac{x_0}{\rho} - 1\right) + \frac{\alpha\rho^2}{x_0}\tanh\left(\tfrac{1}{2}\gamma\alpha t - \varphi\right) \tag{2.3.12}$$

with $\varphi = \tanh^{-1}\left[(1/\alpha)((x_0/\rho) - 1)\right]$.

Equation (2.3.12) yields an approximation to $z_\infty \equiv \lim_{t\to\infty} z(t)$, namely

$$z_\infty \approx \frac{\rho^2}{x_0}\left(\frac{x_0}{\rho} - 1 + \alpha\right). \tag{2.3.13}$$

Now from equation (2.3.10) for α, when $2x_0(N - x_0) \ll (x_0 - \rho)^2$ and $x_0 > \rho$,

$$z_\infty \approx 2\rho\left(1 - \frac{\rho}{x_0}\right), \tag{2.3.14}$$

or, writing $x_0 = \rho + \nu$ for some positive ν,

$$z_\infty \approx 2\nu.$$

Equivalently, $x_\infty \approx \rho + \nu - 2\nu = \rho - \nu$. Note that this result is obtained from the approximation (2.3.9) to the differential equation (2.3.8).

Another route to part (iii) of Theorem 2.1 is to analyse equation (2.3.5) more directly. Observe that the function $f(z) = x_0 e^{-z/\rho}$ is convex monotonic non-increasing for $z > 0$, so it intersects the line $g(z) = N - z = x_0 + y_0 - z$ at most twice. In fact, since $g(0) > f(0)$, there is exactly one point of intersection z_∞ say, in $z > 0$ unless $y_0 = 0$, in which case $z = 0$ is also a point of intersection. Now if $f'(0) = -x_0/\rho \geq -1$, the point of intersection in $z > 0$ is necessarily close to the origin; conversely, z_∞ is much larger than zero if $f'(0) \leq -1$. This effectively substantiates (ii). For (iii), again use an expansion of the exponential function, this time in (2.3.7), so that for $z_\infty > 0$ and $y_0 \approx 0$,

$$z_\infty \approx x_0\left[\frac{z_\infty}{\rho} - \frac{1}{2}\left(\frac{z_\infty}{\rho}\right)^2\right],$$

which in fact is the same as (2.3.14).

We now analyse this model more carefully using Kendall's (1956) methods. Kendall noted that Kermack and McKendrick's approximate results would in fact be exact if the infection parameter β were not constant but rather a function of z, namely

$$\beta(z) = \frac{2\beta}{\left(1 - \frac{z}{\rho}\right) + \left(1 - \frac{z}{\rho}\right)^{-1}} \qquad \left(0 < z < \rho, \ \rho = \frac{\gamma}{\beta}\right). \tag{2.3.15}$$

Note that z cannot be allowed to be equal to or larger than ρ, otherwise $\beta(z)$ becomes zero or negative. We see that $\beta(0) = \beta$, and that as z increases, $\beta(z)$ decreases monotonically as shown in Figure 2.4, so that the *per capita* infection rate decreases as the number of removals increases. For $\beta(z)$ to remain within 20% of the initial value β, it is enough that $z \leq \frac{1}{2}\rho$.

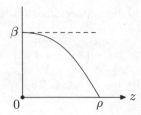

Figure 2.4. Kendall's modified infection parameter $\beta(z)$ (——) and β (- - - -).

The solution of equation (2.3.4) with $\beta(z)$ in place of β is

$$x = x_0 \exp\left(-\frac{1}{\gamma}\int_0^z \beta(w)\,dw\right) = x_0 \exp\left(-\frac{2\beta}{\gamma}\int_0^z \frac{1-w/\rho}{1+(1-w/\rho)^2}\,dw\right)$$

$$= \tfrac{1}{2}x_0\left[\left(1-\frac{z}{\rho}\right)^2 + 1\right] = x_0\left[1 - \frac{z}{\rho} + \tfrac{1}{2}\left(\frac{z}{\rho}\right)^2\right]. \tag{2.3.16}$$

This equation is precisely the case $t \to \infty$ of equation (2.3.12), obtained from (2.3.7) using the expansion of the exponential function to the second order. Thus, the approximate solution (2.3.12) for z underestimates the number of removals, since the infection parameter $\beta(z)$ is always less than its initial value β as in (2.3.1–3).

Returning to equation (2.3.7) for constant β, Kendall (1956) viewed the epidemic rather more generally, first from time $t = 0$ to $t = \infty$, with

$$t = \frac{1}{\gamma}\int_0^z \frac{dw}{N - w - x_0 e^{-w/\rho}} \qquad (0 \le z < z_\infty \equiv z(\infty)), \tag{2.3.17}$$

where $t \to \infty$ as $z \uparrow z_\infty$. We have already noted in (ii) of Theorem 2.1 that z_∞ is a positive root of (2.3.6); this is illustrated in Figure 2.5 (see also Figure 1.2).

Notice that there is a second root $z_{-\infty} < 0$. Now we can imagine the epidemic as starting at time close to $t = -\infty$ with a very small number ϵ of infectives and $N + |z_{-\infty}| - \epsilon$ susceptibles, and evolving to 0 infectives and $N - z_\infty$ susceptibles at time $t = \infty$. The total number of removals would then be $z_\infty + |z_{-\infty}|$ from a total population $N' \equiv N + |z_{-\infty}|$.

In order to consider the evolution of the equations (2.3.1–3) on the whole real line as time interval, it is convenient to take as the time origin the epoch t_1 corresponding to $x(t_1) = \rho$ susceptibles because the peak of the epidemic curve occurs at this instant. Indeed, we can see directly from (2.3.2) that $\dot{y} = 0$ for $x = \rho$, so that $y(t)$ is at a maximum there, as asserted. Note that from (2.3.5) the corresponding value of z is $z(t_1) = \rho\ln(x_0/\rho) = z_\rho$.

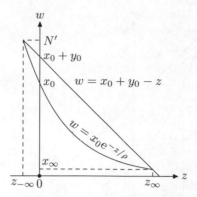

Figure 2.5. z_∞ and $z_{-\infty}$ as points of intersection of
$w = x_0 + y_0 - z$ and $w = x_0 e^{-z/\rho}$.

We remark that in plotting the evolution of several epidemics of a given disease in different time periods, a useful common origin is exactly such a time where the epidemic curve is believed to have peaked. For example, Wilson and Burke's (1943) data given in Exercise 1.4 could be plotted in this way.

In terms of the functions x, y and z satisfying (2.3.1–3), $x(t_1) = \rho$ corresponds from (2.3.17) to the time

$$t_1 \equiv \frac{1}{\gamma} \int_0^{\rho \ln(x_0/\rho)} \frac{dw}{N - w - x_0 e^{-w/\rho}} ;$$

we now define $(x'(u), y'(u), z'(u)) \equiv (x(t_1+u), y(t_1+u), z(t_1+u) - z_\rho)$. Such functions satisfy the equations (2.3.1–3) with (x, y, z) replaced by (x', y', z'), and initial conditions

$$(x_0', y_0', z_0') = (\rho, N - \rho - z_\rho, 0) = (\rho, N - \rho - \rho \ln(x_0/\rho), 0),$$

except that we consider them as being defined for all $-\infty < t < \infty$, and satisfying $(x' + y' + z')(u) = N - z_\rho$ (all u). The limiting values at $u = -\infty$, ∞ are $(N', 0, -|z'_{-\infty}|)$ and $(N' - |z'_{-\infty}| - z'_\infty, 0, z'_\infty)$ respectively, where $z'_{-\infty} = z_{-\infty} - z_\rho$, $z'_\infty = z_\infty - z_\rho$. Note that $|z'_{-\infty}| + z'_\infty = |z_{-\infty}| + z_{-\infty}$. These quantities are illustrated in Figure 2.6.

This information can be interpreted conveniently in terms of the *intensity* of the epidemic, defined by

$$i = \frac{|z_{-\infty}| + z_\infty}{N'}, \tag{2.3.18}$$

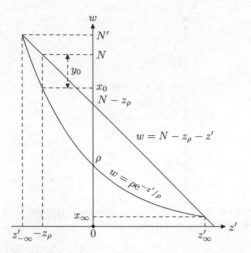

Figure 2.6. Some relations between $(x_0, y_0; N)$, $(x_\infty, z_\infty, z_{-\infty}; N)$ and $(x'_\infty, z'_\infty, z'_{-\infty}; N')$.

using $x' = \rho e^{-z'/\rho}$, $N' = \rho e^{|z'_{-\infty}|/\rho}$, and $N' - |z'_{-\infty}| - z'_\infty = \rho e^{-z'_\infty/\rho}$. Hence

$$\frac{N'(1 - i)}{N'} = \frac{\rho e^{-z'_\infty/\rho}}{\rho e^{|z'_{-\infty}|/\rho}} = e^{-(|z'_{-\infty}| + z'_\infty)/\rho}$$

or

$$1 - i = e^{-N'i/\rho}. \qquad (2.3.19)$$

Further, since $N' = \rho e^{|z'_{-\infty}|/\rho}$, or $|z'_{-\infty}| = \rho \ln(N'/\rho)$, then

$$\frac{|z'_{-\infty}|}{z'_\infty + |z'_{-\infty}|} = \left(\frac{\rho}{N'i}\right)^{\ln(N'/\rho)}. \qquad (2.3.20)$$

Table 2.2 lists various indicators of the characteristics of an epidemic in terms of the intensity. Note that an epidemic of zero intensity represents the limiting case where $i \downarrow 0$.

We can see from Table 2.2 that for all i in $0 < i < 1$, or equivalently, for $0 < \rho < N' < \infty$, there are more removals after $u = 0$ than before. For example, if $N' = 1000$ and $\rho = 896$, so $N'/\rho = 1.116$ and $i = 0.2$, then about 20% of the population become infected and thus about 800 susceptibles remain at the end of the epidemic. On the other hand, with the same N' but now $\rho = 390$ so that $N'/\rho = 2.564$ and $i = 0.9$, about 90% of the population are affected by the disease and only 100 remain susceptible at the end of the epidemic. Broadly speaking, while a small major outbreak occurs when the population size parameter N' is in the

Table 2.2. Characteristics of a general epidemic in terms of the intensity i

Intensity i	Relative size N'/ρ	Peak incidence $y'(0)/N'$	Severity before peak $z'_\infty/(\lvert z'_{-\infty}\rvert + z'_\infty)$
0	1	0	(0.5000)
0.2	1.1157	0.0056	0.5094
0.4	1.2771	0.0254	0.5212
0.6	1.5272	0.0679	0.5379
0.8	2.0118	0.1556	0.5657
0.9	2.5584	0.2418	0.5921
0.99	4.6517	0.4546	0.6662

Notes. For given i, $N'/\rho = \lvert\ln(1-i)\rvert/i$, $y'(0)/N' = 1 - (\rho/N')[1 + \ln(N'/\rho)]$, and $\lvert z'_{-\infty}\rvert/(z'_\infty + \lvert z'_{-\infty}\rvert) = (\rho/N'i)\ln(N'/\rho) = [\ln(N'/\rho)]/\lvert\ln(1-i)\rvert$. See text.

region of the critical threshold size ρ, most of the population is affected (i.e. a large major outbreak occurs) as soon as N' is 3 or more times ρ.

Table 2.2 can also be used to relate the measures (x_0, y_0) in the original time scale t to the 'standardized' measures of the table. For, supposing that (x_0, y_0), ρ and N are given, then we can solve equation (2.3.5) to find the value z_ρ for which $x_0 = \rho$, namely $z_\rho = \rho\ln(x_0/\rho)$, and hence obtain $z' = z - z_\rho$. Then $z_{-\infty}$ and z_∞ are the two roots of

$$N - z - x_0 e^{-z/\rho} = 0,$$

and finally $N' = N + \lvert z_{-\infty}\rvert$. All the quantities of Table 2.2 can now be found.

For example, $(x_0, y_0) = (800, 100)$, $N = 900$ and $\rho = 390$ gives $z_\rho = 280.2$, $z_{-\infty} = -78.6$, $z_\infty = 796.1$, so $N' = 978.6$ and $i = (78.6 + 796.1)/978.6 = 0.8938$, i.e. close to 90% of the population are infected by the epidemic.

Note that the epidemic is skewed about the central value z_ρ: in the example just given, $z'_\infty = z_\infty - z_\rho = 796.1 - 280.2 = 515.9$, while $-z'_{-\infty} = \lvert z_{-\infty} - z_\rho\rvert = 78.6 + 280.2 = 358.8$, which is about two-thirds of 515.9. The corresponding values of the susceptibles x' are $x'_\infty = 103.9$ and $x'_{-\infty} = 978.6$. The value ν discussed after (2.3.14) could be estimated as either $800 - 390 = 410$ or $390 - 103.4 = 286.6$, again differing appreciably. In other words, in terms of $x_0 = \rho + \nu$, the rough approximation $x_\infty \approx \rho - \nu = x_0 - 2\nu$ holds at best for a small range of intensities i.

2.4 The general epidemic in a stratified population

A major aim of this section is to indicate how Kermack and McKendrick's results as stated in Theorem 2.1 extend to the more general setting of Section 2.2 in which an epidemic spreads in a stratified population (hence,

non-homogeneous). We do not need to specify here the basis of the stratification: it may be spatial (i.e. geographical), behavioural, cultural or socio-
economic, for example. In this section, in addition to the pairwise infectious
contact rates β_{ij} for an infective in the ith sub-population or stratum to
infect a susceptible in the jth stratum, for $i, j = 1, \ldots, m$, we also suppose
that there are *per capita* removal rates γ_j for the removal of infectives from
the jth stratum; $z_j(t)$ denotes the cumulative total of such removals by
time t. Then by analogy with the basic equations (2.4.1–3), again by the
Law of Mass Action, we have the differential equations (d.e.s)

$$\dot{x}_j = -x_j(\beta_{1j}y_1 + \cdots + \beta_{mj}y_m), \tag{2.4.1}$$

$$\dot{y}_j = x_j(\beta_{1j}y_1 + \cdots + \beta_{mj}y_m) - \gamma_j y_j, \tag{2.4.2}$$

$$\dot{z}_j = \gamma_j y_j, \tag{2.4.3}$$

for each $j = 1, \ldots, m$, with initial conditions $(x_j, y_j, z_j)(0) = (x_{j0}, y_{j0}, 0)$.
These equations are expressed more compactly using vector notation similar
to that of Section 2.2, extended to include the vectors

$$\mathbf{x} = \begin{pmatrix} x_1 \\ x_2 \\ \vdots \\ x_m \end{pmatrix}, \quad \mathbf{y} = \begin{pmatrix} y_1 \\ y_2 \\ \vdots \\ y_m \end{pmatrix}, \quad \mathbf{z} = \begin{pmatrix} z_1 \\ z_2 \\ \vdots \\ z_m \end{pmatrix}, \quad \boldsymbol{\gamma} = \begin{pmatrix} \gamma_1 \\ \gamma_2 \\ \vdots \\ \gamma_m \end{pmatrix}.$$

We indulge in the same sort of abuse of notation for $\ln \mathbf{x}$ as with $\ln \mathbf{U}$ in
(2.2.6), and extend it to the use of $\operatorname{diag} \boldsymbol{\gamma}^{-1} \equiv \operatorname{diag}(\gamma_1^{-1}, \gamma_2^{-1}, \ldots, \gamma_m^{-1})$ for
the diagonal matrix whose elements are the reciprocals of the elements of
a vector like $\boldsymbol{\gamma}$. In this vector notation, with $\mathbf{B} = (\beta_{ij})$, the differential
equations (d.e.s) (2.4.1–3) are expressible as

$$\dot{\mathbf{x}} = -\operatorname{diag}(\mathbf{x})\mathbf{B}'\mathbf{y}, \quad \dot{\mathbf{y}} = \operatorname{diag}(\mathbf{x})\mathbf{B}'\mathbf{y} - \operatorname{diag}(\boldsymbol{\gamma})\mathbf{y}, \quad \dot{\mathbf{z}} = \operatorname{diag}(\boldsymbol{\gamma})\mathbf{y}. \tag{2.4.4}$$

Writing $\mathbf{B}_\gamma = \mathbf{B}' \operatorname{diag}(\boldsymbol{\gamma}^{-1})$, the first and third of these give (cf. (2.3.4))

$$\frac{\mathrm{d}\ln \mathbf{x}}{\mathrm{d}t} = -\mathbf{B}' \operatorname{diag}(\boldsymbol{\gamma}^{-1})\dot{\mathbf{z}} \equiv -\mathbf{B}_\gamma \dot{\mathbf{z}}.$$

Integration on $(0, t)$ coupled with the initial conditions leads to

$$\ln[x_j(t)/x_{j0}] = -\sum_{i=1}^{m} \beta_{ij}z_i(t)/\gamma_i \equiv -[\mathbf{B}_\gamma \mathbf{z}]_j \qquad (j = 1, \ldots, m), \tag{2.4.5}$$

provided that this solution curve or *trajectory* lies in the region $\mathcal{X}$ defined by

$$x_j, y_j, z_j \geq 0, \qquad x_j + y_j + z_j = x_{j0} + y_{j0} \quad (j = 1, \ldots, m). \qquad (2.4.6)$$

It is not difficult to check that the trajectory does indeed lie in $\mathcal{X}$: it follows from (2.4.1) that trajectories in $\mathcal{X}$ are monotonic in each x_j, and $y_j(t) > 0$ for $0 < t < \infty$ assuming the matrix $\mathbf{B}$ is primitive (i.e. for sufficiently large n, all components of $\mathbf{B}^n$ are strictly positive). Then using the boundedness as well, it follows that the component vectors of $\lim_{t \to \infty}(\mathbf{x}, \mathbf{y}, \mathbf{z}) \equiv (\mathbf{x}^\infty, \mathbf{y}^\infty, \mathbf{z}^\infty)$ exist and satisfy

$$\mathbf{y}^\infty = \mathbf{0}, \qquad \mathbf{x}^\infty = \mathbf{x}_0 + \mathbf{y}_0 - \mathbf{z}^\infty,$$
$$x_j^\infty = x_{j0} \exp\left(-[\mathbf{B}_\gamma \mathbf{z}^\infty]_j\right) \quad (j = 1, \ldots, m). \qquad (2.4.7)$$

Thus, the d.e. system (2.4.1–3) yields a unique limit point $(\mathbf{x}^\infty, \mathbf{y}^\infty, \mathbf{z}^\infty)$. Further analysis completes the proof of part (i) of the following statement, which is an analogue of the Kermack–McKendrick Theorem 2.1.

Theorem 2.2. *A general epidemic evolves in a stratified population according to the differential equations (2.4.1–3) in the region $\mathcal{X}$, starting from initial values $(\mathbf{x}_0, \mathbf{y}_0, \mathbf{0})$, where the transmission matrix $\mathbf{B}$ is primitive and the removal rate vector $\boldsymbol{\gamma}$ has all components positive.*
(i) *(Survival and Total Size). When infection ultimately ceases spreading, positive numbers of susceptibles x_j^∞ remain in each of the strata $j = 1, \ldots, m$. The numbers of removals z_j^∞ constitute the unique solution in $\mathcal{X}$ of the equations (2.4.7). If $\mathbf{x}_0$ is replaced by any $\mathbf{x}_0'$ that is componentwise larger than $\mathbf{x}_0$, i.e. $\mathbf{x}_0' \succeq \mathbf{x}_0$, then $\mathbf{z}^\infty$ is replaced by $\mathbf{z}'^\infty \succeq \mathbf{z}^\infty$.*
(ii) *(Threshold Theorem). A major outbreak occurs if and only if the eigenvalue $\lambda_{\max}$ of the non-negative matrix $\operatorname{diag}(\mathbf{x}_0)\mathbf{B}_\gamma$ with largest modulus, lies strictly outside the unit circle, where $\mathbf{B}_\gamma = \mathbf{B}' \operatorname{diag}(\boldsymbol{\gamma}^{-1})$.*
(iii) *(Second Threshold Theorem). If $\mathbf{x}_0 = \boldsymbol{\xi} + \Delta\mathbf{x}$, where the components of $\Delta\mathbf{x}$ are non-negative and sufficiently small and $\lambda_{\max}(\operatorname{diag}(\boldsymbol{\xi})\mathbf{B}_\gamma) = 1 < \lambda_{\max}(\operatorname{diag}(\mathbf{x}_0)\mathbf{B}_\gamma)$, then*

$$z_j^\infty \approx \sum_{i=1}^{m} 2\Delta x_i v_j / v_i, \qquad (2.4.8)$$

i.e. $\mathbf{z}^\infty \approx 2[\mathbf{1}' \operatorname{diag}(\mathbf{v}^{-1})(\mathbf{x}_0 - \boldsymbol{\xi})]\mathbf{v}$, where $\mathbf{v}$ is the right eigenvector of the eigenvalue 1 of the matrix $\operatorname{diag}(\boldsymbol{\xi})\mathbf{B}_\gamma$.

The detailed proof of this theorem can be found in Daley and Gani (1994); we confine ourselves here to some indicative comments. Watson (1972) treats special cases of the model.

Equations (2.4.7) can be solved iteratively via the transformation T : $\mathbf{z}^{(n)} \mapsto \mathbf{z}^{(n+1)}$ defined componentwise by

$$z_j^{(n+1)} = y_{j0} + x_{j0}\big(1 - \exp[-(\mathbf{B}_\gamma \mathbf{z}^{(n)})_j]\big), \qquad (2.4.9)$$

starting from any convenient $\mathbf{z}^{(0)} \in \mathcal{X}$ such as $\mathbf{z}^{(0)} = \mathbf{y}_0$. Thus, the vector $\mathbf{z}^\infty$ is a fixed point for T, i.e. $T\mathbf{z}^\infty = \mathbf{z}^\infty$, and under the stated conditions it is the only fixed point in $\mathcal{X}$.

The criticality statement (ii) is motivated in part by recalling that for a general epidemic in a homogeneous population, the initial point (x_0, y_0) is close to the singular point $(x_0, 0)$ for the pair of d.e.s (2.3.1–2) describing the evolution of the process. The linear d.e. system approximating (2.3.1–2) at that singular point either diverges when $x_0 > \rho$ or converges when $x_0 < \rho$. A linear approximation to (2.4.1–3) in the neighbourhood of $(\mathbf{x}_0, \mathbf{y}_0) \approx (\mathbf{x}_0, \mathbf{0})$ leads to a similar divergent/convergent dichotomy, determined here by the dominant eigenvalue of the matrix analogous to the product $x_0 \beta \gamma^{-1}$ of the Kermack–McKendrick Threshold Theorem. We shall meet λ_{max} again in Section 3.5 in the context of the Basic Reproduction Ratio.

The approximation in (2.4.8) is derived by a power series expansion in the solution equations (2.4.7), much along the lines of the argument below (2.3.14) based on (2.3.5).

The description we have given for an epidemic in a stratified population is not the only possibility. For example, Ball and Clancy (1993) and Clancy (1994) allow individuals to move between strata, hence offering a more general cross-infection mechanism than our formulation with the matrix $\mathbf{B}$ allows. Exercise 2.4 sketches details of a special case of Theorem 2.2, and Exercise 3.9 evaluates λ_{max} for a special case of $\mathbf{B}$.

Exercise 2.5 discusses briefly the question of stratified population analogues of the 'other' root $z_{-\infty}$ (see Figure 2.5) and the standardized intensity measure i at (2.3.18). Certainly, $\mathbf{B}_\gamma^{-1}$ is well-defined when $\mathbf{B}_\gamma$ is primitive.

2.5   Generation-wise evolution of epidemics

One can envisage an infection in a population as spreading along a sequence of links from any given individual to a number of others. If for example the infection is 'psychological' like a rumour or item of important news (cf. Chapter 5), then there may be a strong interest in knowing how many individuals are infected direct from the initial infective(s): this is the number of first-generation infectives. Individuals infected first-hand from one of these first-generation infectives are then second-generation infectives, and so on through to the jth generation. The accuracy of the 'infection' may be affected by the closeness or otherwise of the source of an individual's infection to the initial infective(s). In the case of the simple and general epidemic models of Sections 2.1 and 2.3 the proportion of jth-generation infectives can be derived algebraically. To the extent that this involves considering sub-divisions of the population, there is some overlap with the analysis in Sections 2.2 and 2.4.

For clarity below and consistency with all of our later exposition, we set $N = x_0$ and $I = y_0$ in notation used up to this point, and $N' = N + I$.

Consider first the simple epidemic model of Section 2.1. Use $y_j(t)$ to denote the number of infectives at time t who have acquired their infection by contact with some $(j-1)$th infective, i.e. with an infective counted amongst the $y_{j-1}(u)$ infectives of the $(j-1)$th generation at some earlier time $u < t$, the instant of contact for the individual concerned. So, in a simple epidemic in a population of size N', there is a constant number $y_0 = I$ of initial infectives, $y_1(t)$ who by time t have been infected first-hand from these y_0, and so on up to $y_j(t)$ jth-generation infectives who by time t have been infected from the $y_{j-1}(t)$.

We assume homogeneous mixing of the population, with the infection spread from one individual to another. Then, when the size N of the closed population is large, the equations describing the spread are

$$\dot{y}_j(t) = \beta x y_{j-1}(t) \qquad (j = 1, 2, \ldots), \tag{2.5.1}$$

with

$$y(t) = y_0 + \sum_{j=1}^{\infty} y_j(t) = N + I - x(t) \equiv N' - x(t); \tag{2.5.2}$$

note that the number of generations j must in fact be finite. In addition to the equations at (2.5.1) we also have the relation $\dot{y} = \beta x y = \beta(N' - y(t))y(t)$ as at (2.1.1), from which we know that $y(t) = IN'/(I + Ne^{-\beta N't})$ (see (2.1.2)).

To solve the d.e.s (2.5.1), rewrite them as

$$\dot{y}_{j+1}(t) = \frac{\dot{y}(t)}{y(t)} y_j(t) \tag{2.5.3}$$

so

$$y_{j+1}(t) = \int_0^t \mathrm{d}y_{j+1}(u) = \int_0^t y_j(u_j) W(u_j) \, \mathrm{d}u_j \qquad (j = 0, 1, \ldots),$$

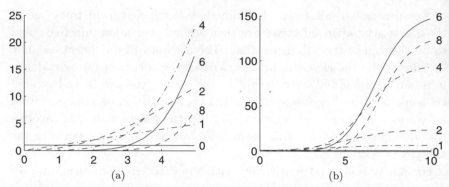

Figure 2.7. Growth of 'generations' 0, 1, 2, 4, 6, 8 of infectives in a simple epidemic with $(N, I) = (1000, 1)$, $\beta = 0.0001$, on $0 < \beta N' t < 10$; part (a) is an enlargement of the start of (b). The number at the right-hand end of the curve shows the generation number; generation 6 is the modal generation for large t.

where $W(u_j) = \dot{y}(u_j)/y(u_j) = (\mathrm{d}/\mathrm{d}t) \ln y(t)\big|_{t=u_j}$. Thus,

$$y_{j+1}(t) = \iint\limits_{0 \le u_{j-1} \le u_j \le t} y_{j-1}(u_{j-1}) W(u_{j-1}) W(u_j)\, \mathrm{d}u_{j-1} \mathrm{d}u_j$$

$$= \int \cdots \int\limits_{0 \le u_0 \le u_1 \le \cdots \le u_j \le t} y_0(u_0) W(u_0) W(u_1) \ldots W(u_j)\, \mathrm{d}u_0\, \mathrm{d}u_1 \ldots \mathrm{d}u_j.$$

Here, $y_0(u) = I$ (all $u > 0$), and the $(j+1)$-fold integral is symmetric in its arguments, so with

$$\ln U(t) = \int_0^t W(u)\, \mathrm{d}u = \int_0^t \frac{\mathrm{d} \ln y(u)}{\mathrm{d}u}\, \mathrm{d}u = \ln\left(\frac{y(t)}{I}\right),$$

we have

$$y_j(t) = y_0 \frac{\left[\int_0^t W(u)\, \mathrm{d}u\right]^j}{j!} = \frac{I\, [\ln U(t)]^j}{j!}$$

$$\to I \frac{[\ln(1 + N/I)]^j}{j!} \qquad (t \to \infty).$$

(2.5.4)

Equation (2.5.4) shows that the sequence $\{y_j(t)\}$ is proportional to the terms of a Poisson distribution with increasing mean $\ln U(t)$ (cf. Daley, 1967a). For small t (meaning, $\beta N' t = o(1)$), $\ln U(t) \approx (1 - I/N')\beta N' t$. Figure 2.7 illustrates the growth of the 'generation sizes' in the case $(N, I) = (1000, 1)$, $\beta = 0.0001$ and $\beta N' t < 10$. Part (a) of the figure shows the behaviour for smaller t.

To study the generation-wise evolution for the general epidemic model of Section 2.3, we continue to use the functions $y_j(t)$ as defined above (2.5.1), and introduce the function $z_j(t)$ to denote the number of jth generation infectives removed by time t. In place of the d.e.s (2.5.1), we define $y_{-1} \equiv 0$ and now have for $j = 0, 1, \ldots$,

$$\dot{x} = -\beta xy,$$
$$\dot{y}_j = \beta xy_{j-1} - \gamma y_j, \qquad (2.5.5)$$
$$\dot{z}_j = \gamma y_j,$$

where $y = \sum_{j=0}^{\infty} y_j$ as before, and $\dot{y} = (\beta x - \gamma)y$. Thus, $\beta x = \gamma + \dot{y}/y$, and the second of the equations at (2.5.5) becomes

$$\dot{y}_j = \left(\gamma + \frac{\mathrm{d}\ln y}{\mathrm{d}t}\right) y_{j-1} - \gamma y_j,$$

or equivalently,

$$\dot{w}_j(t) = \frac{\mathrm{d}\ln w(t)}{\mathrm{d}t}\, w_{j-1}(t) \qquad (j = 1, 2, \ldots).$$

Here we have written $w_j(t) = \mathrm{e}^{\gamma t} y_j(t)$ $(j = 0, 1, \ldots)$ and $w(t) = \mathrm{e}^{\gamma t} y(t)$, for which $w_0(t) = I$ $(0 \leq t \leq \infty)$ and $w_j(0) = 0$ $(j = 1, 2, \ldots)$. Setting $W(t) = \mathrm{d}\ln w(t)/\mathrm{d}t$, we see that the functional form of these equations is exactly the same as in (2.5.1), with solution

$$w_j(t) = \frac{I\left[\int_0^t W(u)\,\mathrm{d}u\right]^j}{j!},$$

similar to (2.5.4). Then, since $\int_0^t W(u)\,\mathrm{d}u = \ln[w(t)/w(0)] = \gamma t + \ln[y(t)/I]$,

$$y_j(t) = I\mathrm{e}^{-\gamma t}\frac{(\gamma t + \ln[y(t)/I])^j}{j!}. \qquad (2.5.6)$$

Thus, as for (2.5.4), the relative frequencies of the generation types among the infectives at time t are proportional to the terms of a Poisson distribution. However, since from (2.5.5),

$$z_j(t) = \gamma \int_0^t y_j(u)\,\mathrm{d}u = \gamma I \int_0^t \mathrm{e}^{-\gamma u}\frac{(\gamma u + \ln[y(u)/I])^j}{j!}\,\mathrm{d}u, \qquad (2.5.7)$$

we see that for the removals at time t, the numbers in the various generations are proportional to the terms of a mixed Poisson distribution. The mixing

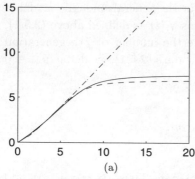
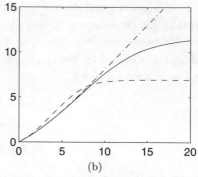

(a)   (b)

Figure 2.8. Average generation number among removals in a general epidemic (——), deaths in a linear birth-and-death process ($-\cdot-\cdot-$) and 'aged' infectives in a simple epidemic ($-\,-\,-$) with $(N, I) = (1000, 1)$, $\beta N' t < 20$ and (a) $\gamma = 0.01$ (hence, $\rho = 100$, $R_0 \equiv N/\rho = 10$), and (b) $\gamma = 0.05$ (hence, $\rho = 500$, $R_0 = 2$). See Section 3.5 for discussion concerning the Basic Reproduction Ratio R_0.

factor $\gamma e^{-\gamma u}\, du$ arises from the distribution of the time an individual, once infected, remains so until it is removed.

As a measure of the average number of generations represented among the removals we use

$$m(t) \equiv \frac{\sum_{j=0}^{\infty} j z_j(t)}{\sum_{j=0}^{\infty} z_j(t)}. \tag{2.5.8}$$

The denominator here is $z(t) = N + I - x(t) - y(t) = \rho \ln[N/x(t)]$, while the summation in the numerator yields, on simplification,

$$m(t) = \frac{\beta}{\ln[N/x(t)]} \int_0^t \left(\gamma u + \ln[y(u)/I]\right) y(u)\, du. \tag{2.5.9}$$

This function is conveniently studied numerically by means of the three d.e.s

$$\dot{x} = -\beta x y, \qquad \dot{y} = \beta x y - \gamma y, \qquad \dot{m} = \frac{\gamma y}{z}\left[-m + \gamma t + \ln\frac{y}{I}\right]. \tag{2.5.10}$$

The function $m(t)$ is plotted in Figure 2.8 together with the corresponding functions from the simple epidemic and linear birth-and-death processes (see Exercises 2.6 and 3.5 respectively).

We see that the ultimate 'average' generation number of those infected in a general epidemic is larger than the corresponding 'average' in a simple epidemic. This occurs because in the former the number of infectives is reduced by removal, thereby slowing down the rate of spread of infection (so, the pool of susceptibles remains larger). Thus the difference in the ultimate averages reflects the later occurrence of infection in the general epidemic as against the simple epidemic. These interpretations are further borne out by the comparison of the two sets of averages for the same initial conditions and pairwise infection rate, but increased removal rate of (b) over (a) in Figure 2.8.

It follows from (2.5.7) that $z_j^\infty \equiv \lim_{t\to\infty} z_j(t)$ equals the limit as $t \to \infty$ of the given integral. Recall from (2.3.6) that $x(t)$ and $y(t)$ are related by

$$y(t) = C + \rho \ln x(t) - x(t) \qquad \text{where} \quad C \equiv N + I - \rho \ln N. \qquad (2.5.11)$$

Also, from Kendall's argument referred to following (2.3.17), the monotonic function $x(t)$ has inverse $\tau(x)$, given by $\tau(N) = 0$ and for $N > x > x_\infty$,

$$\tau(x) = \int_x^N \frac{\mathrm{d}x}{|\dot{x}|} = \int_x^N \frac{\mathrm{d}x}{\beta xy} = \int_x^N \frac{\mathrm{d}u}{\beta u(C + \rho \ln u - u)}. \qquad (2.5.12)$$

Writing $v(x) = \int_0^{\tau(x)} W(u)\,\mathrm{d}u$, the limit of the integral (2.5.7) after a change of variable from t to x gives

$$z_j^\infty = \gamma I \int_{x_\infty}^N \frac{[v(u)]^j}{j!} \cdot \frac{\mathrm{e}^{-\gamma\tau(u)}}{\beta u\,(C + \rho \ln u - u)}\,\mathrm{d}u = \rho \int_{x_\infty}^N \mathrm{e}^{-v(u)} \frac{[v(u)]^j}{j!}\,u^{-1}\,\mathrm{d}u, \qquad (2.5.13)$$

where

$$v(x) = \gamma\tau(x) + \ln\left(\frac{y(\tau(x))}{I}\right) = \int_x^N \frac{\mathrm{d}u}{C + \rho \ln u - u}. \qquad (2.5.14)$$

Dunstan (1982) used Daley's (1967b) result (2.5.7) to show that for fixed I and j and large N, with $N \gg \rho$,

$$z_j^\infty \approx I\frac{[\ln(N/I)]^j}{j!}, \qquad (2.5.15)$$

irrespective of the infection and removal rates β and γ. This right-hand side is the same as $\lim_{t\to\infty} y_j(t)$ in the simple epidemic (see (2.5.4)), and hence is a limit property of $\{z_j^\infty\}$ when $\rho \downarrow 0$. To explain this coincidence, observe from the d.e.s at (2.5.1–2) and (2.5.5) that the simple and general epidemic models with the same initial conditions and pairwise infection rate β, have

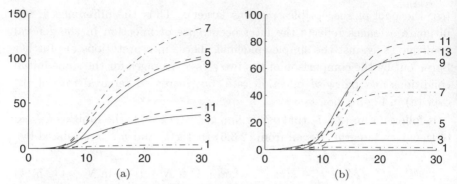

Figure 2.9. Growth of odd-numbered 'generations' in a general epidemic
on $\beta N't < 30$ with $(N, I) = (1000, I)$, $\beta = 0.0001$ and (a) $\gamma = 0.01$
(hence, $\rho = 100$, $R_0 = 10$), (b) $\gamma = 0.05$ (hence, $\rho = 500$, $R_0 = 2$).
Generation number shown at right.

approximately the same behaviour for $0 < t < o(\gamma^{-1}/N) = o(1/(\gamma N))$.
Then for sufficiently small γ, at the end of this 'initial' phase, the population
in the general epidemic will consist almost entirely of infectives for which
the generation-type will be the same as under the simple epidemic. The
simple epidemic by this time has essentially reached its final state, while
in the general epidemic model each j th-generation infective subsequently
becomes a j th-generation removal.

Let us now review both these results and the properties of birth-and-
death processes (see Exercise 3.5), in conjunction with the fact that for a
discrete time Galton–Watson branching process the mean sizes of successive
generations form a geometric rather than Poisson sequence. We see that
the Poisson nature is attributable to the modelling assumption that any
infective, irrespective of 'age', is as likely as any other to infect a susceptible.
The mixed Poisson characteristic in the proportions of removals, comes from
the delay between an individual's being counted first as an infective and
subsequently as a removal in the general epidemic, or a death in the birth-
and-death process. The finiteness of the population reduces the average
generation number from a linear function, as in the linear birth-and-death
process, to either $\ln U(t)$ or $\int_0^t W(u)\,du$, both of which have finite limits as
$t \to \infty$.

Figure 2.9 shows how the odd-numbered $z_j(t)$ evolve in general epidemics
for the same models and initial conditions as in Figure 2.8.

Exercise 2.7 sketches another model for the generation-wise evolution of
an epidemic in which successive generations are non-overlapping.

2.6 Carrier models

A major complication with certain diseases such as typhoid, tuberculosis and poliomyelitis is that the infectives who are the source of infection in the community, may be individuals who do not display any symptoms and are apparently healthy. It may take the detection of a geographical pattern of infection, or a mass screening programme before such infectives are identified and removed from contact with susceptibles. We call such infectives *carriers* to distinguish them from susceptibles who, on being infected, may be quickly recognized by their symptoms and removed from the population.

This type of situation requires a somewhat different model. The infection of a susceptible through contact with a carrier, in the simplest model, now results in the removal of the infected susceptible while the number of carriers remains unaltered. Carriers are distinct, and their numbers are diminished by an independent removal process. Applying the Law of Mass Action, the numbers of carriers $w(t)$ and susceptibles $x(t)$ follow the differential equations

$$\dot{x} = -\beta x w \qquad \text{and} \qquad \dot{w} = -\gamma w. \tag{2.6.1}$$

These are easily solved, given initial conditions $\big(x(0), w(0)\big) = (x_0, w_0)$, as

$$w(t) = w_0 e^{-\gamma t} \qquad \text{and} \qquad x(t) = x_0 \exp\big(-(\beta w_0/\gamma)(1 - e^{-\gamma t})\big). \tag{2.6.2}$$

In practice, when a carrier-borne disease is recognized in a community where it is normally absent, measures are quickly taken to locate the source or sources of infection. Suppose then that the introduction into the community of w_0 carriers occurs at time $t = 0$, and that the identification of the disease through some susceptibles who have developed symptoms occurs at some time t_0 later, at which point the removal rate γ increases to γ' say. The result of such activity is that the d.e. for w is no longer as at (2.6.1) but

$$\dot{w} = \begin{cases} -\gamma w & (0 < t \le t_0), \\ -\gamma' w & (t > t_0), \end{cases} \tag{2.6.3}$$

while the d.e. for x is unchanged. Then the solution is now that in (2.6.2) for $0 < t \le t_0$, while for $t > t_0$ it is

$$w(t) = w_0 e^{-\gamma t_0 - \gamma'(t - t_0)},$$
$$x(t) = x(t_0) \exp\big(-(\beta w(t_0)/\gamma')(1 - e^{-\gamma'(t - t_0)})\big). \tag{2.6.4}$$

Carrier models have a much simpler structure than the general epidemic model, due to the fact that the process $w(t)$ in the model is independent of $x(t)$; $x(t)$, however, depends on the evolution of $w(t)$. See also Exercise 2.8.

2.7 Endemicity of a vector-borne disease

The development of epidemic modelling owes much to the work of malariologists Ronald Ross (1857–1932) and George Macdonald (1903–1967); see e.g. Macdonald (1973). Malaria, unlike viral diseases such as measles, mumps and HIV which spread by contact between infectives and susceptibles, is caused by a parasite whose life-cycle is spent partly in an intermediate host, the *Anopheles* mosquito. The mechanism of infection in this case is different from that which we have so far studied; we must now track the disease-status of both human and mosquito populations. Our aim is to model the progress of an outbreak of malaria, and thereby describe conditions for its endemicity. We outline briefly a simple deterministic model, noting that it is capable of considerable refinement, in both deterministic and stochastic settings (see e.g. Anderson and May (1991, Chapter 14) and, particularly, Bailey (1982)).

The life-span of malarial infection is relatively short compared with the human life-span, and a mosquito population is typically unaffected by the prevalence or absence of malaria. Thus, it suffices to consider two populations of constant sizes N_1 humans and N_2 mosquitoes, in both of which individuals are either infected or not, the numbers of susceptibles and infectives being $X_k(t)$ and $Y_k(t)$ respectively, $X_k(t) + Y_k(t) = N_k$ $(k = 1, 2)$. A human infective with malaria loses infectivity (and is again susceptible) at rate μ_1; similarly a mosquito infective dies at rate μ_2 and is immediately replaced by a new-born susceptible. A mosquito depends on biting a human for a blood-meal during which it can ingest infected blood if the blood-source is malarial; in its turn it will infect a human susceptible when it is infective (see the cited references for more biological detail). Then the human malaria-infected population, neglecting any latent period, changes at rate

$$\frac{dY_1(t)}{dt} = \beta\gamma_{21}Y_2(t)\frac{X_1(t)}{N_1} - \mu_1Y_1(t),$$

and similarly, for the $Y_2(t)$ malaria-carrying mosquitoes,

$$\frac{dY_2(t)}{dt} = \beta\gamma_{12}X_2(t)\frac{Y_1(t)}{N_1} - \mu_2Y_2(t),$$

where β denotes the feeding rate per mosquito and γ_{ij} the infection transmission rate from an infective of type i to a susceptible of type j $(i, j = 1, 2)$.

In terms of proportions $x_k = X_k/N_k = 1 - y_k$ $(k = 1, 2)$,

$$\dot{y}_1 = \beta\gamma_{21}\frac{N_2}{N_1}y_2x_1 - \mu_1y_1 = \mu_1(\alpha_1y_2x_1 - y_1),$$

$$\dot{y}_2 = \beta\gamma_{12}x_2y_1 - \mu_2y_2 = \mu_2(\alpha_2y_1x_2 - y_2),$$

$$(2.7.1)$$

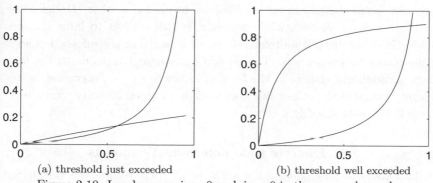

(a) threshold just exceeded   (b) threshold well exceeded

Figure 2.10. Level curves $\dot{y}_1 = 0$ and $\dot{y}_2 = 0$ in the y_1–y_2 phase-plane.

where $\alpha_1 = \beta\gamma_{21}(N_2/N_1)/\mu_1$, $\alpha_2 = \beta\gamma_{12}/\mu_2$. By inspection, $y_1 = y_2 = 0$ is a stationary point, as is any solution of the equations $\dot{y}_1 = 0 = \dot{y}_2$, namely

$$y_1 = \alpha_1 y_2(1 - y_1) \qquad \text{and} \qquad y_2 = \alpha_2 y_1(1 - y_2).$$

Thus

$$y_2 = \frac{\alpha_1\alpha_2 - 1}{\alpha_1(\alpha_2 + 1)} \tag{2.7.2}$$

is a possible equilibrium value; it always lies in $(-\infty, 1)$, and in $(0, 1)$ if and only if $\alpha_1\alpha_2 > 1$, i.e.

$$\frac{\mu_1}{\beta\gamma_{21}}N_1 < \frac{\beta\gamma_{12}}{\mu_2}N_2. \tag{2.7.3}$$

Thus, according to the model, if malaria is to remain endemic a threshold condition must be satisfied, namely that the relative recovery rate of humans from malarial infection must be smaller than the relative infection rate of the new-born mosquito population. Further, as also noted by Ross (1916), to eradicate malaria, it suffices to reduce the mosquito population sufficiently.

Macdonald (1952) distinguished two types of behaviour of infected populations where malaria was endemic: in some populations malarial infection would ebb and flow quite markedly ('unstable' endemic), while in others it would remain at an approximately constant level. Sketching the curves $\dot{y}_1 = 0$ and $\dot{y}_2 = 0$ from (2.7.1) in the y_1–y_2 plane, and supposing that the system lies above the threshold as at (2.7.3), these curves cross at the stationary point at an angle lying between zero and a right angle. The first extreme, where the curves cross at a small angle, corresponds to a situation where the infection and transmission levels are only just sufficient to yield an endemic situation: small changes in the level of one of y_1 and y_2 (in Figure 2.10 it is y_2, i.e. the fraction of the mosquito population that is infected) determine large changes in the equilibrium level of the other. Under these circumstances the disease, while endemic, is still subject to large changes in infectivity resulting from relatively small changes in the infestation level of the mosquito population. The second extreme corresponds to the case where a significant change in the level of either y_1 or y_2, determines a significant change in the other; this corresponds to an endemicity whose level is sustained quite steadily.

2.8 Discrete time deterministic models

All data available for epidemics are gathered at discrete time intervals, as for example the numbers of infectives recorded in a population on consecutive days, or in consecutive serial intervals. It is therefore proper to examine the principles of deterministic modelling in discrete time, whether as skeletons of continuous processes or as discrete processes in their own right.

Gani (1978) studied a discrete time equivalent of the simple epidemic, where observations are made at the times $t = 0, 1, \ldots$. Let a closed population of size N consist of x_t susceptibles and y_t infectives at time t where $x_t + y_t = N$ and y_0 is given, with $0 < y_0 < N$. One way of describing the progress of a simple epidemic, appealing to the Law of Mass Action, is by the difference equation

$$y_{t+1} = \min(y_t + \beta y_t(N - y_t), N) \qquad (t = 0, 1, \ldots), \qquad (2.8.1)$$

where β represents the pairwise infection rate over the discrete time unit concerned; this parameter is usually different from that for the analogous model in continuous time. Omitting the $\min(\cdot)$ operator and expressing the relation in the form $y_{t+1} - y_t = \beta y_t(N - y_t)$ stresses the analogy with the logistic equation (2.1.1) for population growth.

We study the process $\{y_t\}$ through the function

$$f(y) = \beta y(\beta^{-1} + N - y) = y + \beta y(N - y) \qquad (2.8.2)$$

which is concave, $f(\beta^{-1}) = N = f(N)$, and has 0 and N as fixed points. We use this function because, at least for $0 < y_t < \min(N, \beta^{-1})$, $y_{t+1} = f(y_t)$. Define a sequence $\{y_t^*\}$ by $y_0^* = y_0$, $y_{t+1}^* = f(y_t^*)$ so that $y_t = y_t^*$ provided the right-hand side lies in the range $(0, N)$. There are two cases to consider, according as $\beta N \leq 1$ or $\beta N > 1$. In the former case, this discrete time epidemic parallels the behaviour of the simple epidemic in continuous time as presented in Section 2.1 above. To see this, note that $f(y)$ is a parabola as shown in Figure 2.11(a), and that for $y < N$, $y < f(y) < N$. Thus, starting from positive $y_0 < N$, $y_t^* < N < 1/\beta$ for all $t = 1, 2, \ldots$ so $y_t = y_t^*$, and $y_t \uparrow N$ as $t \to \infty$.

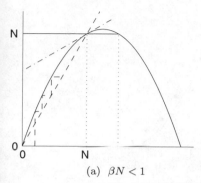

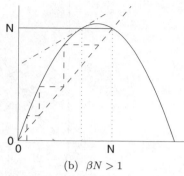

(a) $\beta N < 1$ (b) $\beta N > 1$

Figure 2.11. Discrete time logistic epidemic.

When $\beta N > 1$, it follows from (2.8.2) (cf. Figure 2.11(b)) and the concavity of f that if $\beta^{-1} \le y^* < N$, then $f(y^*) \ge N$, while if $0 < y^* < \beta^{-1}$ then $(\beta N)y^* < f(y^*)$. Consequently, for t such that $\max_{0 \le s \le t}\{y_s^*\} < \beta^{-1}$, $(\beta N)^t y_0^* < y_{t+1}^*$, and therefore for some t sufficiently large, $t = T$ say, we have $y_{T+1}^* > \beta^{-1} > y_T^*$, and thus $y_{T+2}^* > N$. This means that for such y_0^*,

$$y_s = \begin{cases} y_s^* & (s = 0, \ldots, T+1), \\ N & (s = T+2, T+3, \ldots). \end{cases} \qquad (2.8.3)$$

Thus, for $\beta N > 1$, the entire population contracts the disease in a finite time $T + 1$.

This type of behaviour is expressed formally in the theorem below: there is no such analogous behaviour of continuous time deterministic simple epidemics. The result is a consequence of the discretization of time.

Theorem 2.3 (Threshold Theorem for Discrete Time Logistic Equation). *For an epidemic described by the logistic growth process in discrete time as in equation (2.8.1) with an initial number of infectives y_0 in $(0, N)$, either* (a) $\beta \le N^{-1}$, *and at any time $t = 0, 1, \ldots$ after the initial infection, a positive number of susceptibles remains in the population (i.e. $y_t < N$); or* (b) $\beta > N^{-1}$ *and no susceptibles remain after some finite time $T + 1$.*

Spicer (1979) used a discrete time deterministic model for predicting the course of influenza epidemics in England and Wales. It is an analogue of the continuous time general epidemic model of Section 2.3. Let x_t, y_t denote the numbers of susceptibles and *new* infectives on day t, and β the pairwise infection rate as defined at (2.8.1). Removal of infectives occurs daily, with the proportion ψ_j of the new infectives on any given day t remaining in the population j days later. Assume that $0 \le \psi_j \le 1$ (all $j = 0, 1, \ldots$).

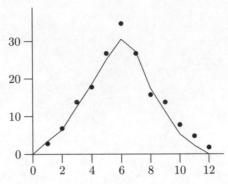

Figure 2.12. Weekly deaths from influenza and influenzal pneumonia in Greater London, 1971–72. (Data from Spicer, 1979.)

Suppose the epidemic starts with x_0 susceptibles and y_0 new infectives on
day 0. Then using the same Mass Action principle as before, the sequence
$\{(x_t, y_t)\}$ evolves according to the law, for $t = 0, 1, \ldots,$

$$y_{t+1} = \beta x_t \sum_{j=0}^{t} \psi_j y_{t-j} \equiv \beta x_t Y_t, \qquad x_{t+1} = x_t - y_{t+1}, \qquad (2.8.4)$$

while the number z_{t+1} of infectives removed on day t is given by

$$z_{t+1} = Y_t - (Y_{t+1} - y_{t+1}) = \sum_{j=0}^{t} (\psi_j - \psi_{j+1}) y_{t-j}.$$

Spicer used the estimated proportions $\psi_0, \ldots, \psi_5 = 1.0, 0.9, 0.55, 0.3, 0.15$
and 0.05, with $\psi_j = 0$ for $j = 6, 7, \ldots,$ to predict the progress of influenza
epidemics in Greater London in 1958–73, and hence to estimate the number
of deaths (as a proportion of the number of infectives) from influenza and
influenzal pneumonia in that period. The important factor was to obtain
an estimate of βx_0; this was found to range between 4.5 and 7.7 in the
period 1958–73. Figure 2.12 illustrates the quality of the fit of the model to
the data (see also Section 6.1 and Exercise 6.1 below). If we assume that
deaths are proportional to the number of new infections in any week, then
the plotted points and fitted curve of Figure 2.12 are proportional to the
epidemic curve defined around (2.1.4).

Saunders (1980) used a slightly different approach to study the spread
of myxomatosis among rabbits in Australia. After infection, a rabbit goes
through a latent period of about 7 days, followed by an infectious period of
about 9 days during which symptoms can be observed. Nearly all infectives

die, so that removals in this case are due to death. The model postulates that a rabbit infected on day t enters and remains in the latent period until day $t + \ell - 1$ ($\ell = 7$). It then becomes infectious on day $t + \ell$ and remains so until day $t + \ell + k - 1$ ($k = 9$), after which it dies.

Let $y_1(t)$ denote the number of rabbits first observed to be infectious on day t; these were infected on day $t - \ell$, and remain infectious and in the population until day $t + k - 1$. Hence on day t, the total number of infectives is

$$y(t) \equiv \sum_{j=0}^{k-1} y_1(t - j), \qquad (2.8.5)$$

since any rabbits becoming infectious before day $t - k + 1$ have died by day t. Starting with x_0 susceptibles at time $t = 0$, the number of remaining susceptibles at time t is

$$x(t) = x_0 - \sum_{j=1}^{t+\ell} y_1(j), \qquad (2.8.6)$$

while the number of those in the latent state is

$$w(t) = \sum_{j=1}^{\ell} y_1(t + j). \qquad (2.8.7)$$

The total number of rabbits alive on day t is

$$p(t) = x(t) + y(t) + w(t).$$

Saunders used the homogeneous mixing model

$$y_1(t + \ell) = \beta y(t) x(t) \qquad (2.8.8)$$

with an estimated $\beta = 0.0031$, $\ell = 7$, $k = 9$, but the fit of the model proved unsatisfactory (see Figure 2.13(a)). An improved fit results from using a population dependent model in which

$$y_1(t + \ell) = \frac{a}{p(x(t))} \, y(t) x(t), \qquad (2.8.9)$$

i.e. β has been replaced by $a/p(x(t))$, on the assumption that each infected rabbit makes contact with a constant number a of rabbits each day. An estimate of a gave $a = 0.34$, and this change with $p(n) = \sqrt{n}$, resulted in better agreement with data, as can be seen from Figure 2.13(b). Saunders also used a goodness-of-fit criterion to discriminate between possible density-dependence functions $p(n) = c$, $\sqrt{n}$ and n, where c is a constant.

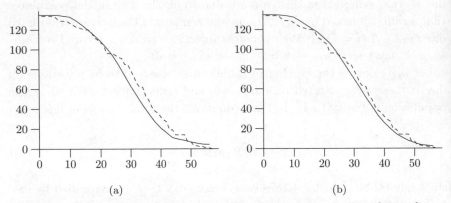

Figure 2.13. Rabbit population affected by myxomatosis: observed
data (----) and fitted models (——): (a) homogeneous mixing, and
(b) population dependent model. (Data from Saunders, 1980.)

It is possible to develop a discrete time model equivalent to the general
epidemic model of Section 2.3 in which for $t = 0, 1, \ldots,$

$$x_{t+1} - x_t = \beta x_t y_t, \quad y_{t+1} - y_t = \beta x_t y_t - \gamma y_t, \quad z_{t+1} - z_t = -\gamma y_t, \quad (2.8.10)$$

with $x_t + y_t + z_t = N$, and β, γ are the infection and removal parameters
which may differ from those in the continuous time model. More correctly,
to avoid negative values of x_t, one should rewrite the first two of these
relations as

$$x_{t+1} = \max(0, x_t - \beta y_t x_t), \quad y_{t+1} = y_t - \gamma y_t + \min(x_t, \beta x_t y_t) \quad (2.8.11)$$

and restrict the value of γ to $(0, 1)$. This model was studied in detail by
de Hoog, Gani and Gates (1979) who derived an analogue of the classical Kermack–McKendrick theorem, but it is somewhat more complex than
Theorem 2.3; we refer the reader to the 1979 paper for details.

Enough has been said to indicate that while it is mathematically more
convenient and elegant to deal with deterministic models in continuous time,
their discrete time analogues are used fairly often when it comes to analysing
data collected daily, or at other serial intervals. The examples sketched
above are intended to indicate both the usefulness and the complexity of
discrete time deterministic models.

2.9   Exercises and Complements to Chapter 2

2.1   Mimic the solution of Section 2.2 in the two special cases:
(a) For the simple epidemic model in a homogeneously mixing population of Section 2.1, put $m = 1$ and $\kappa = 0$ in Section 2.2, and deduce that $F(v) = 1$.
(b) Suppose $m = 2$, $\beta_{11} = \beta_{22} > \beta_{12} > 0 = \beta_{21}$; investigate the solution.

2.2   Suppose that the classification of a population by its disease state (susceptible, infective, removal) is extended by interpolating a *latency* state between susceptible and infectious, with the numbers $w(t)$ in this class at time t satisfying the differential equations $\dot{x} = -\beta xy$, $\dot{w} = \beta xy - \delta w$, $\dot{y} = \delta w - \gamma y$, and $\dot{z} = \gamma y$. Show that the final size in such an epidemic model coincides with the general epidemic model at equation (2.3.6), and is independent of δ.

2.3   Use a latency state as in Exercise 2.2 in a model for a simple epidemic, so that the equations of the model consist of the first two equations (for $\dot{x}$ and $\dot{w}$) and $\dot{y} = \delta w$ in place of the other two equations. Investigate whether any solution, parametric or otherwise, is available to describe the time evolution of such a model.

2.4   In the general epidemic in a stratified population described by the d.e.s at (2.4.1)–(2.4.3), suppose that the rates $\beta_{ij} = \beta_j$ and $\gamma_j = \gamma$ (all j). Show that the solution curve of the d.e.s satisfies

$$[x_i(t)/x_i(0)]^{1/\beta_i} = [x_1(t)/x_1(0)]^{1/\beta_1} \quad \text{(all } i),$$

and hence that
$$z_j^\infty = y_{j0} + x_{j0}(1 - e^{-\beta_j Z/\gamma}),$$

where $Z \equiv \sum_{j=1}^m z_j^\infty$ is the unique positive root of

$$Z = \sum_{j=1}^m [y_{j0} + x_{j0}(1 - e^{-\beta_j Z/\gamma})].$$

Prove that the dominant eigenvalue of Theorem 2.2(ii) is given by $\lambda_{\max} = \sum_{j=1}^m x_{j0}\beta_j/\gamma$.
[Ball (1985) calls such a process a Gart epidemic after the work of Gart (1968, 1972).]

2.5   Show that the quantities z_∞ and $z_{-\infty}$ illustrated in Figure 2.5 can be determined iteratively as $\lim_{n \to \infty} z^{(n)}$ and $\lim_{n \to \infty} z^{(-n-1)}$ respectively, where

$$z^{(n+1)} = y_0 + x_0[1 - \exp(-z^{(n)}/\rho)],$$
$$z^{(-n-1)} = -\rho \ln[1 + (y_0 - z^{(-n)})/x_0],$$

and $z^{(0)} = 0$ and $n = 0, 1, \ldots$. For a stratified population, the first of these equations has the analogue (2.4.9). Investigate the relations

$$z_j^{(-n-1)} = -[\mathbf{B}_\gamma^{-1} \ln[1 + (\mathbf{y}_0 - \mathbf{z}^{(-n)})/\mathbf{x}_0]]_j,$$

where $\ln[\cdot]$ here denotes a vector with components $\ln[1 + (y_{j0} - z_j^{(-n)})/x_{j0}]$, much as below (2.4.4), as a possible analogue of the equation for $z^{(-n-1)}$. When $z_j^{(-\infty)} = \lim_{n\to\infty} z_j^{(-n)}$ exists and differs from $z_j^{(\infty)} \equiv \lim_{n\to\infty} z_j^{(n)}$, define analogues of i at (2.5.18) by $i_j = [z_j^{(\infty)} + |z_j^{(-\infty)}|]/N_j'$ where $N_j' = x_{j0}\exp(-[\mathbf{B}_\gamma \mathbf{z}^{(-\infty)}]_j)$. As an analogue of z_ρ consider the vector $\mathbf{B}_\gamma^{-1}\ln[\boldsymbol{\rho}]$ where $\ln[\boldsymbol{\rho}]$ is the vector with components $\ln[\gamma_j/\beta_{jj}]$.

2.6 For a simple epidemic model, the analogues of the jth generation removals $z_j(t)$ in a general epidemic model (cf. (2.5.7)), are the jth generation infectives $z_j^s(t)$ who have been in this state for an exponentially distributed time with mean $1/\gamma$, i.e. 'aged infectives'. These $z_j^s(t)$ satisfy the d.e. $\dot{z}_j^s = \gamma(y_j^s - z_j^s)$ where quantities with superscript s refer to the simple epidemic. Show that the analogue m^s of the function m at (2.5.8) equals M^s/z^s, where $M^s = \sum_j j z_j^s$, illustrated in Figure 2.8, satisfies the d.e.

$$\frac{\mathrm{d}M^s}{\mathrm{d}t} = -\gamma M^s + \frac{\gamma y^s}{I}\ln\frac{y^s}{I}.$$

2.7 The following is a prescription for using continuous time methods to track the generation-wise evolution of an epidemic process when the latency period is large relative to the infectious period, and successive generations of infectives are non-overlapping. Introduce functions $\{X_n(\cdot), Y_n(\cdot) : n = 0, 1, \ldots\}$ satisfying the d.e.s

$$\dot{X}_n(t_n) = -\beta X_n(t_n)Y_n(t_n) \quad \text{and} \quad \dot{Y}_n(t_n) = -\gamma Y_n(t_n) \quad (t \geq 0),$$

together with boundary conditions $X_0(0) = N$, $Y_0(0) = I$ and, for $n = 0, 1, \ldots$,

$$X_{n+1}(0) = X_n(\infty), \qquad Y_{n+1}(0) = X_n(0) - X_n(\infty) = X_n(0) - X_{n+1}(0).$$

In this formulation, 'time' t_n runs from 0 to ∞ while the number of nth generation infectives declines from $Y_n(0)$ to zero; at the same time, the first generation latent infectives are increasing, and the number of susceptibles declines from $X_n(0)$ to $X_n(\infty)$ through the growth of such infectives. At $t_n = \infty$ a new time axis t_{n+1} starts at 0 and the process iterates. The d.e. for Y_n has solution $Y_n(t_n) = Y_n(0)e^{-\gamma t_n}$ and so

$$\ln[X_n(t_n)/X_n(0)] = -[\beta Y_n(0)/\gamma](1 - e^{-\gamma t_n}) \to -\beta Y_n(0)/\gamma \quad (t_n \to \infty).$$

(a) Show that $X_\infty \equiv \lim_{n\to\infty} X_n(t_n)$ exists and satisfies equation (2.3.7).
(b) Prove that, if I is allowed to vary, then $\lim_{I\downarrow 0}[Y_1(0)/Y_0(0)] = \beta N/\gamma = R_0$ as in Figure 2.8 and in Section 3.5.
(c) Compare $Y_0(0) + \cdots + Y_n(0)$ numerically with $Z_0(\infty) + \cdots + Z_n(\infty)$, using the solution of the generation-wise evolution results in Section 2.5, for some suitable β/γ, N and I.

(d) Interpret the sequence $\{Z_n(\infty)\}$ in the context of a discrete time general epidemic model (cf. discussion at end of Section 2.8 and Chapter 4).

2.8 In the carrier model described by the d.e.s at (2.6.1), suppose that a (small) proportion α of the susceptibles infected become carriers, so that the second of the equations is now

$$\frac{dw}{dt} = -\gamma w + \alpha\beta xw = \frac{\gamma}{\beta}\frac{d\ln x}{dt} - \alpha\frac{dx}{dt},$$

with x and w related by $w = w_0 + \alpha(x_0 - x) - \rho\ln(x_0/x)$. Deduce that the number of susceptibles x_∞ surviving the epidemic is the unique solution of the equation

$$\alpha(x_0 - x_\infty) + w_0 = \rho\ln(x_0/x_\infty), \qquad x_0 > x_\infty > 0.$$

[Observe that with this modification, the carrier model is similar to the general epidemic model.]

2.9 Suppose that outbreaks of an epidemic take place in a given region (or village) each year. Consider how to combine data from several years so as to display features of the evolution of the disease; how could these data be used to estimate parameters of a suitable model? As a possible model, assume the same population size for different years and the same parameters β and γ in the case of the general epidemic of Section 2.3 or its discrete analogue (cf. En'ko's work in Dietz (1988), En'ko (transl. 1989), and Exercise 1.3 above).

3

Stochastic Models in Continuous Time

In this chapter and the next, perhaps the most important of this book, we describe the evolution of an epidemic as a stochastic process. Such a stochastic approach is essential when the number of members of the population subject to the epidemic is relatively small. While deterministic methods may be adequate to characterize the spread of an epidemic in a large population, they are not satisfactory for smaller populations, in particular those of family size.

We shall use the tools of non-negative integer-valued Markov processes in continuous or discrete time, retaining much of the approach of the previous chapter in the dissection of the population. However, we no longer use continuous functions to approximate the evolution of the epidemic; rather, we consider a closed population of individuals, each of whom is classified as either a susceptible, an infective or (except for the 'simple' epidemic of Section 3.1) a removal. This S–I–R classification[1] is possible because we regard the epochs where individuals change their classification as randomly determined points in continuous time, or as fixed points in discrete time. For mathematical convenience but with sufficient simplistic realism, we assume that the processes involved are Markovian. The reader is presumed to have some familiarity with the elements of Markov processes on countable state space, as for example in Bailey (1964), Cox & Miller (1965), Karlin & Taylor

---

[1] Waltman (see Waltman and Hoppensteadt (1970, 1971)) introduced this notation to designate both the possible disease states of an individual, and the possible progression of disease in an individual; here, it denotes susceptible → infected → removed. A simple epidemic as in Chapter 2 or the first two sections below is an S–I epidemic. For an S–I–S disease like malaria, a simple model envisages that an individual is either susceptible, infectious or (after recovery) susceptible again. Superinfection is not allowed in this simplest version in which individuals are either infected to the same extent, or susceptible; a variant of this model would allow superinfection. Hethcote (1994) surveys deterministic models more extensively.

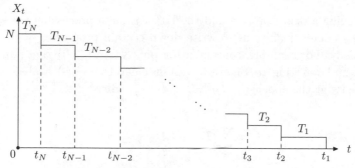

Figure 3.1. The death process $\{X(t) : t \geq 0\}$.

(1975, 1984), Bartlett (1978) or Ross (1983). In this chapter we concentrate on Markov models of epidemics in continuous time.

3.1 The simple stochastic epidemic in continuous time

A *simple stochastic (Markovian) epidemic* model in continuous time is one in which the population consists only of susceptibles and infectives; once a susceptible is infected, it becomes an infective and remains in that state indefinitely. Thus, the main features of the simple deterministic epidemic in continuous time also hold for the simple stochastic epidemic we now describe.

We suppose that the total population is closed, so that

$$X(t) + Y(t) = N + I \quad \text{(all } t \geq 0) \tag{3.1.1}$$

where $X(t)$ and $Y(t)$ denote the numbers of susceptibles and infectives at time t, with initial conditions $(X, Y)(0) = (N, I)$ where $I \geq 1$. We assume that $\{(X, Y)(t) : t \geq 0\}$ is a homogeneous Markov chain in continuous time, with state space the non-negative integers in $\mathbf{Z}^2$ satisfying (3.1.1) and $N \geq X(t) \geq 0$. The only non-zero transition probabilities occur for $0 \leq i \leq N$, $j = N + I - i$ and are

$$\Pr\{(X,Y)(t+\delta t) = (i-1, j+1) \mid (X,Y)(t) = (i,j)\} = \beta ij\delta t + o(\delta t),$$
$$\Pr\{(X,Y)(t+\delta t) = (i,j) \mid (X,Y)(t) = (i,j)\} = 1 - \beta ij\delta t - o(\delta t),$$
$$\tag{3.1.2}$$

with $(X, Y)(t) = (0, N + I)$ being an absorbing state; $\beta > 0$ is the pairwise infection parameter.

Because of (3.1.1), such a Markov chain is in fact one-dimensional on that part of $\mathbf{Z}$ satisfying $N \geq X(t) \geq 0$, or equivalently, $I \leq Y(t) \leq N + I$, the former being a death process and the latter a birth process on the integers concerned. This enables us to write down certain properties of the model fairly easily. For example, concentrating on $\{X(t) : t \geq 0\}$ as a pure death process and referring to Figure 3.1, it is clear that $X(\cdot)$ evolves by unit decrements at the epochs $t_N, t_{N-1}, \ldots, t_1$ say, where

$$t_j = \sum_{i=j}^{N} T_i \qquad (1 \leq j \leq N), \tag{3.1.3}$$

and the T_i are independent exponentially distributed random variables for which $\mathrm{E}T_i = 1/[\beta i(N + I - i)]$. Consequently

$$\mathrm{E}t_j = \frac{1}{\beta} \sum_{i=j}^{N} \frac{1}{i(N + I - i)} = \frac{1}{\beta(N+I)} \left[\sum_{i=j}^{N} \frac{1}{i} + \sum_{i'=0}^{N-j} \frac{1}{I + i'} \right]$$

$$= \frac{1}{\beta(N+I)} \times \begin{cases} \ln \dfrac{N(N+I-1)}{I-1} + \gamma_{N,I,1} & (j = 1, I \geq 2), \\[2mm] 2\ln N + 2\gamma_N & (j = 1, I = 1), \\[2mm] \ln \dfrac{N(N+I-j)}{(j-1)(I-1)} + \gamma_{N,I,j} & \text{otherwise.} \end{cases} \tag{3.1.4}$$

Here $\gamma_{N,I,j} = \gamma_N - \gamma_{I-1} + \gamma_{N+I-j} - \gamma_{j-1}$ with the sequence $\{\gamma_j\}$ defined by

$$\gamma_0 = 0, \qquad \gamma_j = \sum_{i=1}^{j} \frac{1}{i} - \ln j \quad (j = 1, 2, \ldots), \tag{3.1.5}$$

and γ_j converges as $j \to \infty$ to Euler's constant $\gamma_\infty = 0.577\,216\ldots$ Equation (3.1.4) shows that the mean time $\mathrm{E}t_j$ until the number of susceptibles is reduced to $j - 1$ $(j = N, \ldots, 1)$ can be approximated by the inverse of the logistic rate (see Exercise 3.1); Williams (1965) and Bartholomew (1973, Chapter 9) give further comparisons. See Exercise 3.2 for $\mathrm{var}\,t_1$ when $I = 1$.

3.1.1   Analysis of the Markov chain

We now analyse the Markov chain $\{X(t) : t \geq 0\}$ by the usual methods, given that the only non-zero transition probabilities, for $1 \leq i \leq N$, are

$$\Pr\{X(t + \delta t) = i - 1 \mid X(t) = i\} = \beta i(N + I - i)\delta t + o(\delta t),$$
$$\Pr\{X(t + \delta t) = i \mid X(t) = i\} = 1 - \beta i(N + I - i)\delta t - o(\delta t),$$

with $X(t) = 0$ being the absorbing state. Then the forward Kolmogorov equations for the state probabilities $p_i(t) = \Pr\{X(t) = i \mid X(0) = N\}$, $(0 \le i \le N)$, are

$$\dot{p}_N = -\beta N I p_N(t),$$

$$\dot{p}_i = -\beta i (N + I - i) p_i(t) + \beta(i+1)(N + I - i - 1)p_{i+1}(t)$$
$$(1 \le i \le N - 1), \qquad (3.1.6)$$

$$\dot{p}_0 = \beta(N + I - 1)p_1(t),$$

where $\dot{p} = \dfrac{\mathrm{d}p}{\mathrm{d}t}$. In matrix terms, for $P(t) = (p_N(t), \ldots, p_0(t))'$, $\dot{P} \equiv \dfrac{\mathrm{d}P(t)}{\mathrm{d}t}$ equals

$$-\beta \begin{pmatrix} NI & \cdot & \cdot & \cdots & \cdot \\ -NI & (N-1)(I+1) & \cdot & \cdots & \cdot \\ \cdot & -(N-1)(I+1) & (N-2)(I+2) & \cdots & \cdot \\ \vdots & \vdots & & \ddots & \vdots \\ \cdot & \cdot & \cdots & -1(N+I-1) & 0 \end{pmatrix} \begin{pmatrix} p_N(t) \\ p_{N-1}(t) \\ p_{N-2}(t) \\ \vdots \\ p_0(t) \end{pmatrix}$$

so that

$$\dot{P} = -\beta A P(t). \qquad (3.1.7)$$

Here the square matrix A of order $N + 1$ is the difference of two matrices, one diagonal and the other subdiagonal:

$$A = \operatorname{diag}(NI, (N-1)(I+1), \ldots, 1(I + N - 1), 0)$$
$$- \operatorname{subdiag}(NI, (N-1)(I+1), \ldots, 1(I + N - 1)).$$

Note that both the diagonal and subdiagonal matrices may have repeated elements, as in Example 3.1.1 worked out shortly.

The solution of this matrix equation (3.1.7) is known to be

$$P(t) = e^{-\beta A t} P(0), \qquad P(0) = (1, 0, \cdots, 0)' \equiv e_{N+1}, \qquad (3.1.7')$$

but explicit results may not be easy to derive by this method. A much simpler approach is through the Laplace transforms $\hat{p}_i(\theta) = \int_0^\infty e^{-\theta t} p_i(t)\,\mathrm{d}t$, $\operatorname{Re}(\theta) > 0$, $0 \le i \le N$ which, applied to equations (3.1.7), yield

$$\int_0^\infty e^{-\theta t} \frac{\mathrm{d}p_N}{\mathrm{d}t}\,\mathrm{d}t = \theta \hat{p}_N(\theta) - 1 = -\beta N I \hat{p}_N(\theta),$$

$$\int_0^\infty e^{-\theta t} \frac{\mathrm{d}p_i}{\mathrm{d}t}\,\mathrm{d}t = \theta \hat{p}_i(\theta) = -\beta i (N + I - i)\hat{p}_i(\theta)$$
$$+ \beta(i+1)(N + I - i - 1)\hat{p}_{i+1}(\theta), \quad (1 \le i \le N - 1),$$

$$\int_0^\infty e^{-\theta t} \frac{\mathrm{d}p_0}{\mathrm{d}t}\,\mathrm{d}t = \theta \hat{p}_0(\theta) = \beta(N + I - 1)\hat{p}_1(\theta). \qquad (3.1.8)$$

We can express equations (3.1.8) in matrix terms as

$$(\theta I_{N+1} + \beta A)\hat{P} = e_{N+1} \tag{3.1.9}$$

where I_{N+1} is the unit matrix of order $N + 1$, e_{N+1} is the $(N + 1)$-vector defined at (3.1.7′) and $\hat{P}$ is the vector of Laplace transforms $\hat{p}_i(\theta)$ of the elements $p_i(t)$ of P. Equivalently,

$$\hat{p}_N(\theta) = \frac{1}{\theta + \beta NI},$$
$$\hat{p}_i(\theta) = \frac{\beta(i + 1)(N + I - i - 1)}{\theta + \beta i(N + I - i)}\hat{p}_{i+1}(\theta) \qquad (1 \leq i \leq N - 1), \tag{3.1.10}$$
$$\hat{p}_0(\theta) = \frac{\beta(N + I - 1)}{\theta}\hat{p}_1(\theta).$$

We can solve for $\hat{p}_i(\theta)$ recursively, starting with $\hat{p}_N(\theta)$ to obtain the result

$$\hat{p}_i(\theta) = \prod_{j=i}^{N} \frac{\beta(j + 1)(N + I - j - 1)}{\theta + \beta j(N + I - j)} \qquad (0 \leq i \leq N - 1),$$

where some factors $\theta + \beta j(N + I - j)$ appear twice for $\hat{p}_i(\theta)$ with $i < \frac{1}{2}(N + I)$.

Example 3.1.1. To illustrate the procedure, suppose that $(N, I) = (4, 1)$, $\beta = 1$. Then

$$\hat{p}_4(\theta) = \frac{1}{\theta + 4}, \qquad \hat{p}_3(\theta) = \frac{4}{(\theta + 4)(\theta + 6)}, \qquad \hat{p}_2(\theta) = \frac{(4)(6)}{(\theta + 4)(\theta + 6)^2},$$
$$\hat{p}_1(\theta) = \frac{(4)(6^2)}{(\theta + 4)^2(\theta + 6)^2}, \qquad \hat{p}_0(\theta) = \frac{(4^2)(6^2)}{(\theta + 4)^2(\theta + 6)^2\theta}.$$

Note the double factors in $\hat{p}_j(\theta)$ for $j = 0, 1, 2$. Inverting these Laplace transforms shows that for all $0 \leq t \leq \infty$,

$$\begin{aligned}
p_4(t) &= e^{-4t}, & p_3(t) &= 2(e^{-4t} - e^{-6t}), \\
p_2(t) &= 6(e^{-4t} - e^{-6t} - 2te^{-6t}), \\
p_1(t) &= 36\big(-e^{-4t} + te^{-4t} + e^{-6t} + te^{-6t}\big), \\
p_0(t) &= 1 + 27e^{-4t} - 36te^{-4t} - 28e^{-6t} - 24te^{-6t}.
\end{aligned} \tag{3.1.11}$$

For details of similar calculations see Bailey (1963; 1975, Chapter 5).

3.1.2 A simplifying device

It will be obvious that the fact that some of the eigenvalues $\lambda_j = j(N+I-j)$ $(0 \le j \le N)$ of the matrix A in (3.1.7) are repeated, increases the complexity of the solutions for $p_j(t)$. In the case of Example 3.1.1 where

$$A = \mathrm{diag}(4, 6, 6, 4, 0) - \mathrm{subdiag}(4, 6, 6, 4)$$

the solutions $p_j(t)$ involve both e^{-4t}, e^{-6t} and $t\mathrm{e}^{-4t}$, $t\mathrm{e}^{-6t}$. Suppose the initial number of susceptibles is not an integer N but the quantity $N_\epsilon = N + \epsilon$ where $0 < \epsilon < 1$; make $X(t) = \epsilon$ an absorbing state for the termination of the epidemic. Then the matrix A becomes

$$A_\epsilon \equiv \mathrm{diag}(4+\epsilon, 6+2\epsilon, 6+3\epsilon, 4+4\epsilon, 0) - \mathrm{subdiag}(4+\epsilon, 6+2\epsilon, 6+3\epsilon, 4+4\epsilon).$$
$$(3.1.12)$$

The eigenvalues are now all distinct, so there is a solution of the form

$$p_j^\epsilon(t) = a_j\mathrm{e}^{-(4+\epsilon)t} + b_j\mathrm{e}^{-(3+\epsilon)2t} + c_j\mathrm{e}^{-(2+\epsilon)3t} + d_j\mathrm{e}^{-(1+\epsilon)4t},$$

where for simplicity j denotes the state $X(t) = j + \epsilon$. Elementary calculations starting from $\dot{P}_\epsilon(t) = -A_\epsilon P_\epsilon(t)$, with $P_\epsilon(\cdot)$ much as at (3.1.7), lead to

$$p_4^\epsilon(t) = \mathrm{e}^{-(4+\epsilon)t}, \qquad p_3^\epsilon(t) = \frac{4+\epsilon}{2+\epsilon}\left(\mathrm{e}^{-(4+\epsilon)t} - \mathrm{e}^{-(6+2\epsilon)t}\right),$$

$$p_2^\epsilon(t) = \frac{(6+2\epsilon)(4+\epsilon)}{2+\epsilon}\left[\frac{\mathrm{e}^{-(4+\epsilon)t} - \mathrm{e}^{-(6+3\epsilon)t}}{2+2\epsilon} + \frac{\mathrm{e}^{-(6+3\epsilon)t} - \mathrm{e}^{-(6+2\epsilon)t}}{\epsilon}\right],$$

$$p_1^\epsilon(t) = \frac{(6+3\epsilon)(6+2\epsilon)(4+\epsilon)}{2+\epsilon}\left[\frac{\mathrm{e}^{-(4+\epsilon)t} - \mathrm{e}^{-(4+4\epsilon)t}}{(2+2\epsilon)3\epsilon} + \frac{\mathrm{e}^{-(6+3\epsilon)t} - \mathrm{e}^{-(4+4\epsilon)t}}{(2+2\epsilon)(2-\epsilon)}\right.$$
$$\left. + \frac{\mathrm{e}^{-(6+2\epsilon)t} - \mathrm{e}^{-(4+4\epsilon)t}}{\epsilon(2-2\epsilon)} + \frac{\mathrm{e}^{-(4+4\epsilon)t} - \mathrm{e}^{-(6+3\epsilon)t}}{\epsilon(2-\epsilon)}\right],$$

$$p_0^\epsilon(t) = 1 - p_1^\epsilon(t) - \cdots - p_4^\epsilon(t). \qquad (3.1.13)$$

Recovery of the solutions at (3.1.11) for $\epsilon = 0$ is a straightforward matter of taking limits. By inspection, as $\epsilon \to 0$, $p_4^\epsilon(t) \to \mathrm{e}^{-4t}$ and $p_3^\epsilon(t) \to 2(\mathrm{e}^{-4t} - \mathrm{e}^{-6t})$. In the case of $p_2^\epsilon(t)$, taking limits for the last term yields

$$\lim_{\epsilon \to 0} \mathrm{e}^{-6t}(\mathrm{e}^{-3\epsilon t} - \mathrm{e}^{-2\epsilon t})/\epsilon = -t\mathrm{e}^{-6t}$$

so that

$$p_2^\epsilon(t) \to 12\left(\tfrac{1}{2}(\mathrm{e}^{-4t} - \mathrm{e}^{-6t}) - t\mathrm{e}^{-6t}\right).$$

Similarly we can check that $p_1^\epsilon(t) \to p_1(t)$ as at (3.1.11), and then appeal to $p_0^\epsilon(t)$ as at (3.1.13) to complete this derivation of the full solution (3.1.11).

We use this simplifying device later when considering the probability generating function method in Section 3.2. The solution (3.1.13) for small ϵ can be considered as a close approximation to the exact solution (3.1.11).

3.1.3   Distribution of the duration time

A quantity of some importance mentioned earlier is the duration time t_1 of the epidemic (see Figure 3.1); it equals the sum

$$t_1 = T_1 + \cdots + T_N = \sum_{j=1}^{N} T_j \tag{3.1.14}$$

of N independent exponential variables, each with its own parameter

$$\lambda_j = \beta j(N + I - j) \qquad (j = 1, \ldots, N).$$

The Laplace–Stieltjes transform[2] of T_j equals

$$\mathrm{E}(\mathrm{e}^{-\theta T_j}) = \frac{\lambda_j}{\theta + \lambda_j} = \left(1 + \frac{\theta}{\lambda_j}\right)^{-1} = \left(1 + \frac{\theta}{\beta j(N + I - j)}\right)^{-1}$$

so that if t_1 has the p.d.f. $f_1(t)$, then

$$\mathrm{E}(\mathrm{e}^{-\theta t_1}) = \int_0^\infty \mathrm{e}^{-\theta t} f_1(t)\, \mathrm{d}t = \prod_{j=1}^{N} \left(1 + \frac{\theta}{\beta j(N + I - j)}\right)^{-1}. \tag{3.1.15}$$

This p.d.f. is related to the state probabilities $p_j(\cdot)$ at (3.1.7) by

$$f_1(t)\, \mathrm{d}t = p_1(t)\, \beta(N + I - 1)\, \mathrm{d}t, \tag{3.1.16}$$

so for example when $N = 4$, $I = 1$ and $\beta = 1$ as in Example 3.1.1,

$$f_1(t) = 4 \times 36[-\mathrm{e}^{-4t} + t\mathrm{e}^{-4t} + (1 + t)\mathrm{e}^{-6t}],$$

and thus t_1 has the distribution function

$$F_1(t) = 1 + \mathrm{e}^{-4t}(27 - 36t) - \mathrm{e}^{-6t}(28 + 24t). \tag{3.1.17}$$

Kendall (1957) used the transform at (3.1.15) to obtain the limit distribution of t_1 in the case $\beta = 1$, $I = 1$, $N \to \infty$. Using the transformation

$$W = (N + 1)t_1 - 2\ln N, \tag{3.1.18}$$

---

[2]We distinguish between the *Laplace–Stieltjes transform* $\mathrm{E}(\mathrm{e}^{-\theta X}) = \int_0^\infty \mathrm{e}^{-\theta x}\, \mathrm{d}F(x)$ of a random variable X with distribution function $F(\cdot)$, and the *Laplace transform* $\int_0^\infty \mathrm{e}^{-\theta t} p(t)\, \mathrm{d}t$ of an integrable function $p(\cdot)$. They coincide when F has a p.d.f. $f(\cdot)$.

it follows from (3.1.15) that, with $f(\cdot)$ denoting the p.d.f. for W,

$$E(e^{-\theta W}) = \int_0^\infty e^{-\theta w} f(w)\,dw = N^{2\theta} \prod_{j=1}^N \left(1 + \frac{(N+1)\theta}{j(N+1-j)}\right)^{-1}$$

$$= N^{2\theta} \prod_{j=1}^N \left(1 + \frac{\theta}{j} + \frac{\theta}{N+1-j}\right)^{-1} \qquad (3.1.19)$$

$$\approx N^{2\theta} \prod_{j=1}^N \left[1 + \frac{\theta}{j}\right]^{-1} \left[1 + \frac{\theta}{N+1-j}\right]^{-1} \qquad (N \text{ large}),$$

$$= \left[N^\theta \prod_{j=1}^N \left(1 + \frac{\theta}{j}\right)^{-1}\right]^2 \to [\Gamma(1+\theta)]^2 \qquad (N \to \infty); \quad (3.1.20)$$

here Euler's formula $\Gamma(1+z) = z\Gamma(z) = \lim_{N\to\infty} N^z \prod_{j=1}^N [1+(z/j)]^{-1}$ (e.g. Whittaker and Watson, 1927, p. 237) justifies taking the limit. Inversion of the Laplace transform $[\Gamma(1+\theta)]^2$ leads to

$$f(w) = 2e^{-w} K_0\big(2e^{-w/2}\big), \qquad (3.1.21)$$

where $K_0(\cdot)$ is the modified Bessel function of the second kind of order zero (see Exercise 3.3).

This limit distribution for t_1 is interesting as an example of a sum of independent non-identically distributed r.v.s having a non-Gaussian limit distribution. This is not surprising, for the components in the sum at (3.1.14) are certainly not uniformly asymptotically negligible. These components can be grouped into three phases, so that the sum t_1 consists of a starting phase of the epidemic where the first few $T_1, T_2, \ldots$ have means that are $O(1/N)$, then a middle phase consisting of most of the N r.v.s T_i, when i is not close to either 1 or N, with means that are $O(1/N^2)$, and an ending phase with the last few $T_N, T_{N-1}, \ldots$ when the means are again $O(1/N)$. Daley, Gani and Yakowitz (2000) use this three-phase decomposition of t_1. An analogue for the general epidemic is indicated in Exercise 3.13.

3.2 Probability generating function methods for Markov chains

An alternative way of studying a Markov chain $\{X(t) : t \geq 0\}$ on the non-negative integers as state space, is through the analysis of the probability generating function (p.g.f.)

$$\varphi(z,t) \equiv E\big(z^{X(t)}\big) = \sum_{j=0}^N \Pr\{X(t) = j \mid X(0)\} z^j \qquad (|z| \leq 1), \quad (3.2.1)$$

where $0 \leq X(t) \leq N$. It is usually possible to obtain a partial differential equation (p.d.e.) for $\varphi(z,t)$ from the Kolmogorov equations for the probabilities for $X(t)$, at least when the transition rates are simple polynomial functions of the non-negative integers as is often the case in models of population processes. In some cases the p.d.e. admits an explicit solution. We consider the Markov chain for the simple epidemic of Section 3.1 to illustrate the method; we shall use the technique again in Sections 3.3 and 3.6.

We use the forward Kolmogorov equations (3.1.6) for the probabilities of $X(t)$ taking values in $0, \ldots, N$, but first simplify them by changing the time scale so that the new time $t' = \beta t$. Then since

$$\frac{\mathrm{d}}{\mathrm{d}t} = \frac{\mathrm{d}}{\mathrm{d}t'}\frac{\mathrm{d}t'}{\mathrm{d}t} = \beta\frac{\mathrm{d}}{\mathrm{d}t'}, \tag{3.2.2}$$

equations (3.1.6) are replaced by the same relations with $\beta = 1$ and t' in place of t. For convenience below, we write $t = t'$. Now multiply the equation for $\mathrm{d}p_j/\mathrm{d}t$ by z^j and sum over j. Writing

$$\varphi(z,t) = \sum_{j=0}^{N} p_j(t)z^j, \quad \text{with} \quad \varphi(z,0) = z^N \quad \text{and} \quad \frac{\partial\varphi(z,t)}{\partial t} = \sum_{j=0}^{N} \frac{\mathrm{d}p_j(t)}{\mathrm{d}t}z^j,$$

this gives

$$\frac{\partial\varphi(z,t)}{\partial t} = \sum_{j=0}^{N} z^j\left[-j(N+I)p_j + j^2 p_j + (j+1)(N+I)p_{j+1} - (j+1)^2 p_{j+1}\right],$$

where $p_{N+1} \equiv 0$. Simplifying the sums yields

$$\frac{\partial\varphi(z,t)}{\partial t} = z(z-1)\frac{\partial^2\varphi(z,t)}{\partial z^2} - (z-1)(N+I-1)\frac{\partial\varphi(z,t)}{\partial z}. \tag{3.2.3}$$

If we differentiate (3.2.3) with respect to z and let $z \uparrow 1$, we deduce that

$$\frac{\mathrm{d}\,\mathrm{E}X(t)}{\mathrm{d}t} = \mathrm{E}\big(X(t)[(X(t)-1)]\big) - (N+I-1)\mathrm{E}X(t), \tag{3.2.4}$$

so with $\xi_t = \mathrm{E}X(t)$,

$$\dot{\xi}_t = -\xi_t(N+I-\xi_t) + \mathrm{var}\,X(t).$$

Recall from (2.1.1) that for the deterministic model of a simple epidemic, with the change of time scale used here, the function $x(t)$ denoting the number of susceptibles at time t satisfies

$$\dot{x} = -x(N+I-x).$$

Consequently, since $x(0) = \xi_0 = X(0)$, $\mathrm{E}X(t) \approx x(t)$ so long as $\mathrm{var}\, X(t)$ is small relative to $x(N+I-x)$. But, it should be noted that the deterministic results do not necessarily approximate the mean of the stochastic model well for all t.

We can solve the second-order p.d.e. at (3.2.3) by the standard method of separation of variables. This means writing $\varphi(z,t) = Z(z)T(t)$ for some functions Z and T, in which case (3.2.3) becomes

$$\frac{\dot{T}}{T} = z(z-1)\frac{Z''}{Z} - (z-1)(N+I-1)\frac{Z'}{Z} = -\lambda \quad \text{say,} \tag{3.2.5}$$

where

$$Z' = \frac{\mathrm{d}Z(z)}{\mathrm{d}z}, \qquad Z'' = \frac{\mathrm{d}^2 Z(z)}{\mathrm{d}z^2}, \qquad \dot{T} = \frac{\mathrm{d}T(t)}{\mathrm{d}t}$$

and λ is a constant. The simpler relation at (3.2.5) gives $\dot{T} = -\lambda T$, so that $T = \mathrm{e}^{-\lambda t}$. However we know from Section 3.1.2 that this result will be correct only if the initial number of susceptibles N is replaced by $N_\epsilon = N+\epsilon$ ($0 < \epsilon < 1$) in the eigenvalues of the matrix A of (3.1.7). Assume this is done: then from the rest of (3.2.5),

$$z(1-z)Z'' - (1-z)(N_\epsilon + I - 1)Z' - \lambda Z = 0. \tag{3.2.6}$$

This is a hypergeometric differential equation of the general form

$$z(1-z)Z'' + [c - (a+b+1)z]Z' - abZ = 0,$$

where $c = 1 - (N_\epsilon + I)$, $a + b = -(N_\epsilon + I)$, $ab = \lambda$. A suitable solution of (3.2.6) is known to be the hypergeometric function

$$Z(z) = F(a,b;\,c;\,z) \equiv 1 + \sum_{k=1}^{\infty} \frac{\Gamma(a+k)\,\Gamma(b+k)\,\Gamma(c)\,z^k}{\Gamma(a)\,\Gamma(b)\,\Gamma(c+k)\,k!}.$$

The eigenvalues λ_j must be such that $F(a,b;c;z)$ is a polynomial in z of degree not greater than N, which means that a or b must be a negative integer such that $a \mid b = -(N_\epsilon + I)$ is satisfied. Thus the λ_j must be of the form

$$\lambda_j = j(N_\epsilon + I - j) \qquad (0 \le j \le N), \tag{3.2.7}$$

with $a = -j$ say and $b = -(N_\epsilon + I - j)$. It follows that

$$\varphi(z,t) = \sum_{j=0}^{N} \alpha_j \mathrm{e}^{-j(N_\epsilon + I - j)t} F(-j, j - N_\epsilon - I; 1 - N_\epsilon - I;\, z), \tag{3.2.8}$$

where the coefficients α_j can be obtained from the initial condition

$$\varphi(z,0) = z^N = \sum_{j=0}^{N} \alpha_j F(-j, j - N_\epsilon - I; 1 - N_\epsilon - I; z)$$

and certain orthogonality conditions satisfied by the functions $F(\cdot, \cdot; \cdot; z)$. If we now let $\epsilon \to 0$, so $N_\epsilon \to N$, we recover the exact solution to (3.2.4). Bailey (1963) gives full details of this solution in the case $I = 1$.

Clearly, while this result may be satisfying analytically, it is not easy to use in practice. Nevertheless p.g.f. methods can be useful, especially in condensing equations from which summary information like moments can be deduced.

3.3   The general stochastic epidemic

We consider next an S–I–R model in which the total population $N + I$ is subdivided into $X(t)$ susceptibles, $Y(t)$ infectives and $Z(t)$ immunes or removals, with $(X, Y, Z)(0) = (N, I, 0)$ and

$$X(t) + Y(t) + Z(t) = N + I \qquad \text{(all } t \geq 0\text{)}. \tag{3.3.1}$$

We assume that $\{(X, Y)(t) : t \geq 0\}$ is a bivariate Markov process; (3.3.1) ensures that $Z(t) = N + I - X(t) - Y(t)$ is known when $(X, Y)(t)$ is known. We again assume that there is homogeneous mixing so that in the time interval $(t, t + \delta t)$ infections occur at rate $\beta i j \delta t$ and removals at rate $\gamma j \delta t$, yielding for the infinitesimal transition probabilities

$$\Pr\{(X, Y)(t + \delta t) = (i - 1, j + 1) \mid (X, Y)(t) = (i, j)\} = \beta i j \delta t + o(\delta t),$$
$$\Pr\{(X, Y)(t + \delta t) = (i, j - 1) \mid (X, Y)(t) = (i, j)\} = \gamma j \delta t + o(\delta t),$$
$$\Pr\{(X, Y)(t + \delta t) = (i, j) \mid (X, Y)(t) = (i, j)\} = 1 - (\beta i + \gamma) j \delta t - o(\delta t),$$

where β is the (pairwise) infection parameter and γ the removal parameter. Then if we write the state probabilities as

$$p_{ij}(t) = \Pr\{(X, Y)(t) = (i, j) \mid (X, Y)(0) = (N, I)\}, \tag{3.3.2}$$

we can readily derive the Kolmogorov forward equations in the form

$$\frac{dp_{NI}(t)}{dt} = -I(\beta N + \gamma)p_{NI},$$
$$\frac{dp_{ij}(t)}{dt} = \beta(i + 1)(j - 1)p_{i+1,j-1} - j(\beta i + \gamma)p_{ij} + \gamma(j + 1)p_{i,j+1} \tag{3.3.3}$$
$$(0 \leq i + j \leq N + I, 0 \leq i \leq N, 0 \leq j \leq N + I),$$

subject to the initial conditions $p_{NI}(0) = 1$, $p_{ij}(0) = 0$ otherwise. Note for later use that the distribution $\{P_n\}$ of the ultimate size of the epidemic, meaning, the distribution of the number of initial susceptibles ultimately infected, is given by

$$P_n = \Pr\{\lim_{t \to \infty} (X, Y)(t) = (N - n, 0) \mid (X, Y)(0) = (N, I)\} = p_{N-n,0}(\infty).$$

This distribution is computed most efficiently, in terms of time, numerical precision and range of values of $N + I$, via an embedded jump process: see Section 3.4.2 and Figure 3.2.

Some slight simplification is achieved if we define $t' = \beta t$ so that $\mathrm{d}/\mathrm{d}t = \beta \, \mathrm{d}/\mathrm{d}t'$ much as before at (3.2.2). With $\rho = \gamma/\beta$ as the *relative removal rate*, the equations (3.3.3) become (again writing $t = t'$ for convenience)

$$\frac{\mathrm{d}p_{NI}(t)}{\mathrm{d}t} = -I(N + \rho)p_{NI},$$

$$\frac{\mathrm{d}p_{ij}(t)}{\mathrm{d}t} = (i+1)(j-1)p_{i+1,j-1} - j(i+\rho)p_{ij} + \rho(j+1)p_{i,j+1} \qquad (3.3.4)$$

$$(0 \le i + j \le N + I, 0 \le i \le N, 0 \le j \le N + I),$$

subject to the same initial condition $p_{NI}(0) = 1$. We could now attempt to solve these equations recursively, starting with $p_{NI}(t) = \mathrm{e}^{-(N+\rho)It}$. Such a procedure is tedious (see Exercise 3.4), and it is preferable to use a systematic approach such as one based on a mixture of Laplace transform and p.g.f. methods. Such solutions were offered around the same time by Gani (1965, 1967), Siskind (1965) and Sakino (1968): we outline Gani's solution of 1967.

It is worth remarking that these solutions are possible here, essentially because the processes concerned are Markov chains with well-ordered sample paths. The states (i, j) for $\{(X, Y)(t) : t \ge 0\}$ have an hierarchical structure, with the value of X declining by single units, and the value of Y increasing or decreasing by single units also. The process is 'strictly evolutionary': once a state is visited and left, it cannot be revisited, so, each state (i, j) is entered either once or not at all. The forward Kolmogorov equations (3.3.3) relate the derivative of any given state probability, to state probabilities for that state and the states immediately preceding it along any well-ordered sample path. See also Section 3.4.2 and Exercises 3.6 and 3.7.

3.3.1   Solution by the p.g.f. method

Multiply the respective equations in (3.3.4) by $z^i w^j$ and sum them over i and j. Then for the p.g.f. $\varphi(z, w; t)$ of the bivariate Markov process $\{(X, Y)(t) : t \geq 0\}$ defined by the sum

$$\sum_{0 \leq i \leq N} \sum_{0 \leq j \leq N+I-i} p_{ij}(t) z^i w^j = \mathrm{E}(z^{X(t)} w^{Y(t)} \mid (X, Y)(0) = (N, I)),$$

we obtain the p.d.e.

$$\frac{\partial \varphi}{\partial t} = w(w - z) \frac{\partial^2 \varphi}{\partial z \, \partial w} + \rho(1 - w) \frac{\partial \varphi}{\partial w} \tag{3.3.5}$$

with $\varphi(z, w; 0) = z^N w^I$. Differentiation of (3.3.5) with respect to z or w followed by putting $z = w = 1$ yields (in the original time scale)

$$\begin{aligned}
\frac{\mathrm{d}\,\mathrm{E}[X(t)]}{\mathrm{d}t} &= -\beta \mathrm{E}[X(t)]\, \mathrm{E}[Y(t)] - \beta \operatorname{cov}(X(t), Y(t)), \\
\frac{\mathrm{d}\,\mathrm{E}[Y(t)]}{\mathrm{d}t} &= \beta \mathrm{E}[X(t)]\, \mathrm{E}[Y(t)] - \gamma \mathrm{E}[Y(t)] + \beta \operatorname{cov}(X(t), Y(t)),
\end{aligned} \tag{3.3.6}$$

respectively. Neglecting the covariance terms and putting $(x(t), y(t)) = (\mathrm{E}X(t), \mathrm{E}Y(t))$ yields the d.e.s. of the deterministic model of Section 2.3.

Equation (3.3.5) is more simply studied in terms of its Laplace transform

$$\begin{aligned}
\hat{\varphi}(z, w; \theta) &= \int_0^\infty \mathrm{e}^{-\theta t} \varphi(z, w; t) \, \mathrm{d}t \quad (\operatorname{Re}(\theta) \geq 0) \\
&= \sum_{0 \leq i \leq N} \sum_{0 \leq j \leq N+I-i} z^i w^j \hat{p}_{ij}(\theta) \equiv \sum_{0 \leq i \leq N} z^i \hat{f}_i(w; \theta),
\end{aligned} \tag{3.3.7}$$

where

$$\hat{f}_i(w; \theta) = \sum_{j=0}^{N+I-i} w^j \hat{p}_{ij}(\theta), \qquad \hat{p}_{ij}(\theta) = \int_0^\infty \mathrm{e}^{-\theta t} p_{ij}(t) \, \mathrm{d}t.$$

Taking Laplace transforms of (3.3.5) yields

$$\theta \hat{\varphi}(z, w; \theta) - z^i w^j = w(w - z) \frac{\partial^2 \hat{\varphi}}{\partial z \, \partial w} + \rho(1 - w) \frac{\partial \hat{\varphi}}{\partial w}.$$

Substituting for $\varphi(z, w; \theta)$ from (3.3.7), we deduce the set of equations

$$\begin{aligned}
\theta \hat{f}_N &= w^I - [(N + \rho)w - \rho] \frac{\partial \hat{f}_N}{\partial w}, \\
\theta \hat{f}_i &= w^2(i + 1) \frac{\partial \hat{f}_{i+1}}{\partial w} - [(i + \rho) - \rho] \frac{\partial \hat{f}_i}{\partial w} \quad (0 \leq i \leq N - 1).
\end{aligned} \tag{3.3.8}$$

These equations can expressed succinctly in matrix form as

$$\mathbf{A}\frac{\partial \mathbf{F}}{\partial w} + \theta \mathbf{F} = w^I \mathbf{e}_{N+1}, \tag{3.3.9}$$

where $\mathbf{F} = (\hat{f}_N \ \hat{f}_{N-1} \ \cdots \ \hat{f}_0)'$ and $\mathbf{e}_{N+1}$ is the $(N+1)$-row vector with 1 in its first row and zeros elsewhere, as at (3.1.9). With $\mathbf{I}_{N+1}$ denoting the unit matrix of order $N+1$, the square matrix $\mathbf{A} = \mathbf{A}(w)$ of order $N+1$ equals

$$-\rho(1-w)\mathbf{I}_{N+1} + w \operatorname{diag}(N, N-1, \ldots, 1, 0) - w^2 \operatorname{subdiag}(N, N-1, \ldots, 1)$$
$$= -\rho \mathbf{I}_{N+1} + w\mathbf{A}'(0) + \tfrac{1}{2}w^2\mathbf{A}''(0). \tag{3.3.10}$$

Since each component of the vector $\mathbf{F}$ is a finite series in w, $\mathbf{F}$ has a finite Taylor series expansion

$$\mathbf{F}(w; \theta) = \sum_{j=0}^{N+I} \frac{w^j}{j!} \mathbf{F}^{(j)}(0; \theta), \tag{3.3.11}$$

where $\mathbf{F}^{(j)}(0; \theta)$ is the jth partial derivative of $\mathbf{F}(w; \theta)$ with respect to w at $w = 0$. Then setting $w = 0$ in (3.3.9) we have for $I \geq 1$

$$\mathbf{A}(0)\frac{\partial \mathbf{F}(0; \theta)}{\partial w} + \theta \mathbf{F}(0; \theta) = 0$$

or

$$\mathbf{F}'(0; \theta) = (\theta/\rho)\mathbf{F}(0; \theta). \tag{3.3.12}$$

Differentiating (3.3.9) with respect to w yields

$$[\mathbf{A}'(w) + \theta \mathbf{I}_{N+1}]\mathbf{F}'(w; \theta) + \mathbf{A}(w)\mathbf{F}''(w; \theta) = Iw^{I-1}\mathbf{e}_{N+1}; \tag{3.3.13}$$

setting $w = 0$ and rearranging gives

$$\mathbf{F}''(0; \theta) = \frac{1}{\rho}\big([\mathbf{A}'(0) + \theta \mathbf{I}_{N+1}]\mathbf{F}'(0; \theta) - I\delta_{1I}\mathbf{e}_{N+1}\big), \tag{3.3.14}$$

where δ_{1I} is the Kronecker delta and $\mathbf{A}'(0) = \operatorname{diag}(N, N-1, \ldots, 0) + \rho \mathbf{I}_{N+1}$. Differentiating (3.3.13) leads to

$$\mathbf{A}''(w)\mathbf{F}'(w; \theta) + [2\mathbf{A}'(w) + \theta \mathbf{I}_{N+1}]\mathbf{F}''(w; \theta) + \mathbf{A}(w)\mathbf{F}'''(w; \theta)$$
$$= I(I-1)w^{I-2}\mathbf{e}_{N+1}, \tag{3.3.15}$$

so setting $w = 0$ and rearranging as before, we have

$$\mathbf{F}'''(0;\theta) = \frac{1}{\rho}\left[[2\mathbf{A}'(0) + \theta\mathbf{I}_{N+1}]\mathbf{F}''(0;\theta) + \mathbf{A}''(0)\mathbf{F}'(0;\theta) - \frac{I!\,\delta_{2I}}{(I-2)!}\mathbf{e}_{N+1}\right].$$

$$(3.3.16)$$

In general, further differentiation of (3.3.15) with respect to w followed by setting $w = 0$ and rearranging, shows that $\mathbf{F}^{(j+1)}(0;\theta)$ equals

$$\frac{1}{\rho}\left[[j\mathbf{A}'(0) + \theta\mathbf{I}_{N+1}]\mathbf{F}^{(j)}(0;\theta) + \binom{j}{2}\mathbf{A}''(0)\mathbf{F}^{(j-1)}(0;\theta) - \frac{I!\,\delta_{jI}}{(I-j)!}\mathbf{e}_{N+1}\right].$$

$$(3.3.17)$$

These equations yield a first-order recurrence relation when expressed in the matrix form

$$\rho\begin{pmatrix} \mathbf{F}^{(j+1)}(0;\theta) \\ \mathbf{F}^{(j)}(0;\theta) \end{pmatrix}$$
$$= \begin{pmatrix} j\mathbf{A}'(0) + \theta\mathbf{I}_{N+1} & \binom{j}{2}\mathbf{A}''(0) \\ \rho\mathbf{I}_{N+1} & 0 \end{pmatrix}\begin{pmatrix} \mathbf{F}^{(j)}(0;\theta) \\ \mathbf{F}^{(j-1)}(0;\theta) \end{pmatrix} - \frac{I!\,\delta_{jI}}{(I-j)!}\begin{pmatrix} \mathbf{e}_{N+1} \\ 0 \end{pmatrix};$$

$$(3.3.18)$$

this relation is valid for $j = 0, 1, \ldots, N + I$ when we define $\mathbf{F}^{(0)}(0;\theta) = \mathbf{F}(0;\theta)$, $\mathbf{F}^{(-1)}(0;\theta) = 0$.

We see that for $j = 0, \ldots, I - 1$,

$$\begin{pmatrix} \mathbf{F}^{(j+1)}(0;\theta) \\ \mathbf{F}^{(j)}(0;\theta) \end{pmatrix} = \prod_{i=0}^{j}\begin{pmatrix} \dfrac{i\mathbf{A}'(0) + \theta\mathbf{I}_{N+1}}{\rho} & \dfrac{1}{\rho}\binom{i}{2}\mathbf{A}''(0) \\ \mathbf{I}_{N+1} & 0 \end{pmatrix}\begin{pmatrix} \mathbf{F}(0;\theta) \\ 0 \end{pmatrix}$$

$$= \prod_{i=0}^{j}\mathbf{B}_i\begin{pmatrix} \mathbf{F}(0;\theta) \\ 0 \end{pmatrix} = \mathbf{B}_j\cdots\mathbf{B}_1\mathbf{B}_0\begin{pmatrix} \mathbf{F}(0;\theta) \\ 0 \end{pmatrix}, \quad (3.3.19)$$

where for $k \leq j$ we define the product $\prod_{i=k}^{j}\mathbf{B}_i = \mathbf{B}_j\mathbf{B}_{j-1}\ldots\mathbf{B}_{k+1}\mathbf{B}_k$. For $j = I$, however, we have

$$\begin{pmatrix} \mathbf{F}^{(I+1)}(0;\theta) \\ \mathbf{F}^{(I)}(0;\theta) \end{pmatrix} = \prod_{i=0}^{I}\mathbf{B}_i\begin{pmatrix} \mathbf{F}(0;\theta) \\ 0 \end{pmatrix} - \frac{I!}{\rho}\begin{pmatrix} \mathbf{e}_{N+1} \\ 0 \end{pmatrix}, \quad (3.3.19')$$

and for $j = I + 1, \ldots, I + N$,

$$\begin{pmatrix} \mathbf{F}^{(j+1)}(0;\theta) \\ \mathbf{F}^{(j)}(0;\theta) \end{pmatrix} = \prod_{i=0}^{j}\mathbf{B}_i\begin{pmatrix} \mathbf{F}(0;\theta) \\ 0 \end{pmatrix} - \frac{I!}{\rho}\prod_{i=I+1}^{j}\mathbf{B}_i\begin{pmatrix} \mathbf{e}_{N+1} \\ 0 \end{pmatrix}. \quad (3.3.20)$$

Since $\mathbf{F}^{(N+I+1)}(0; \theta) = 0$, it follows that

$$
\begin{pmatrix} \mathbf{F}^{(N+I+1)}(0;\theta) \\ \mathbf{F}^{(N+I)}(0;\theta) \end{pmatrix}
$$

$$
= \prod_{i=0}^{N+I} \mathbf{B}_i \begin{pmatrix} \mathbf{F}(0;\theta) \\ 0 \end{pmatrix} - \frac{I!}{\rho} \prod_{i=I+1}^{N+I} \mathbf{B}_i \begin{pmatrix} \mathbf{e}_{N+1} \\ 0 \end{pmatrix} = \begin{pmatrix} 0 \\ \mathbf{F}^{(N+I)}(0;\theta) \end{pmatrix}.
$$

Hence,

$$
\left[\prod_{i=0}^{N+I} \mathbf{B}_i \right]_{N+1} \mathbf{F}(0;\theta) = \frac{I!}{\rho} \left[\prod_{i=I+1}^{N+I} \mathbf{B}_i \right]_{N+1} \mathbf{e}_{N+1},
$$

where $[\cdot]_{N+1}$ denotes the truncated $(N+1)$-square matrix consisting of the first $N+1$ rows and columns of its argument. Now from (3.3.18), because $j\mathbf{A}'(0) + \theta\mathbf{I}_{N+1}$ is a diagonal matrix and $\mathbf{A}''(0)$ is a subdiagonal matrix, both with non-zero elements, any product $\prod_{i=0}^{j} \mathbf{B}_i$ is a lower triangular matrix with non-zero eigenvalues for $\mathrm{Re}(\theta) > 0$. Hence its inverse exists, and thus

$$
\mathbf{F}(0;\theta) = \frac{I!}{\rho} \left[\left[\Pi_{i=0}^{N+I} \mathbf{B}_i \right]_{N+1} \right]^{-1} \left[\Pi_{i=I+1}^{N+I} \mathbf{B}_i \right]_{N+1} \mathbf{e}_{N+1}. \tag{3.3.21}
$$

Thus, a complete solution of the general stochastic epidemic, in the sense of describing the Laplace transforms of the state probabilities of $(X(t), Y(t))$ for finite $t > 0$, is given by

$$
\begin{pmatrix} \mathbf{F}(w;\theta) \\ \int_0^w \mathbf{F}(v;\theta)\,dv \end{pmatrix} = \sum_{j=0}^{N+I+1} \frac{w^j}{j!} \begin{pmatrix} \mathbf{F}^{(j)}(0;\theta) \\ \mathbf{F}^{(j-1)}(0;\theta) \end{pmatrix} \tag{3.3.22}
$$

$$
= \sum_{j=0}^{N+I+1} \frac{w^j}{j!} \left[\Pi_{i=0}^{j-1} \mathbf{B}_i \right] \begin{pmatrix} \mathbf{F}(0;\theta) \\ 0 \end{pmatrix} - \sum_{j=I+1}^{N+I+1} \frac{w^j I!}{j!\rho} \left[\Pi_{i=I+1}^{j-1} \mathbf{B}_i \right] \begin{pmatrix} \mathbf{e}_{N+1} \\ 0 \end{pmatrix},
$$

with $\mathbf{B}_i$ as defined at (3.3.18) and $\mathbf{F}(0;\theta)$ given by (3.3.21).

Example 3.3.1. Gani (1967) illustrates this solution for the simplest case $(N, I) = (1, 1)$, from which it is clear that the solution is not easily calculated in practice for larger N or I. First we have

$$
\mathbf{A}'(0) = \begin{pmatrix} 1+\rho & 0 \\ 0 & \rho \end{pmatrix}, \qquad \mathbf{A}''(0) = \begin{pmatrix} 0 & 0 \\ -2 & 0 \end{pmatrix}.
$$

The matrices $\mathbf{B}_i$ are given by

$$\rho\mathbf{B}_0 = \begin{pmatrix} \theta & 0 & 0 & 0 \\ 0 & \theta & 0 & 0 \\ \rho & 0 & 0 & 0 \\ 0 & \rho & 0 & 0 \end{pmatrix}, \qquad \rho\mathbf{B}_1 = \begin{pmatrix} 1+\rho+\theta & 0 & 0 & 0 \\ 0 & \rho+\theta & 0 & 0 \\ \rho & 0 & 0 & 0 \\ 0 & \rho & 0 & 0 \end{pmatrix},$$

$$\rho\mathbf{B}_2 = \begin{pmatrix} 2(1+\rho)+\theta & 0 & 0 & 0 \\ 0 & 2\rho+\theta & -2 & 0 \\ \rho & 0 & 0 & 0 \\ 0 & \rho & 0 & 0 \end{pmatrix},$$

so the required products are

$$\rho^2\mathbf{B}_1\mathbf{B}_0 = \begin{pmatrix} \theta(1+\rho+\theta) & 0 & 0 & 0 \\ 0 & \theta(\rho+\theta) & 0 & 0 \\ \rho\theta & 0 & 0 & 0 \\ 0 & \rho\theta & 0 & 0 \end{pmatrix},$$

$$\rho^3\mathbf{B}_2\mathbf{B}_1\mathbf{B}_0 = \begin{pmatrix} \theta(1+\rho+\theta)(2+2\rho+\theta) & 0 & 0 & 0 \\ -2\rho\theta & \theta(\rho+\theta)(2\rho+\theta) & 0 & 0 \\ \rho\theta(1+\rho+\theta) & 0 & 0 & 0 \\ 0 & \rho\theta(\rho+\theta) & 0 & 0 \end{pmatrix}.$$

According to (3.3.21) this yields

$$\mathbf{F}(0;\theta) = \left[\mathbf{B}_2\mathbf{B}_1\mathbf{B}_0\right]_2^{-1}\left[\rho^{-1}\mathbf{B}_2\right]_2\mathbf{e}_{N+1}$$

$$= \frac{\rho}{\theta^2(1+\rho+\theta)(2+2\rho+\theta)(\rho+\theta)(2\rho+\theta)} \times$$

$$\begin{pmatrix} \theta(\rho+\theta)(2\rho+\theta) & 0 \\ 2\rho\theta & \theta(1+\rho+\theta)(2+2\rho+\theta) \end{pmatrix} \begin{pmatrix} 2+2\rho+\theta \\ 0 \end{pmatrix}$$

$$= \left(\frac{\rho}{\theta(1+\rho+\theta)} \quad \frac{2\rho^2}{\theta(\rho+\theta)(2\rho+\theta)(1+\rho+\theta)} \right)'. \tag{3.3.23}$$

The full solution to the 2-person epidemic may now be obtained from (3.3.22) as the upper left 2×2 matrix in

$$\left(\mathbf{I}_2 + w\mathbf{B}_0 + \tfrac{1}{2}w^2\mathbf{B}_1\mathbf{B}_0\right) \begin{pmatrix} \mathbf{F}(0;\theta) \\ 0 \end{pmatrix},$$

so $\mathbf{F}(w;\theta)$ equals

$$\begin{pmatrix} 1+\dfrac{w\theta}{\rho} & 0 \\ 0 & 1+\dfrac{w\theta}{\rho}+\dfrac{w^2\theta(\rho+\theta)}{2\rho^2} \end{pmatrix} \begin{pmatrix} \dfrac{\rho}{\theta(1+\rho+\theta)} \\ \dfrac{2\rho^2}{\theta(\rho+\theta)(2\rho+\theta)(1+\rho+\theta)} \end{pmatrix}.$$

$$\tag{3.3.24}$$

This Laplace transform solution is more than enough to indicate that the form of the time-dependent solution to the problem of describing the evolution of a general stochastic epidemic is algebraically formidable, at least with pen and paper (see also Exercise 3.4). Fortunately a composite picture of such stochastic development is possible; we concentrate on the ultimate behaviour of the epidemic process, first with the analogue of the Kermack–McKendrick threshold theorem, and then with a description of the ultimate size of the epidemic.

3.3.2 Whittle's threshold theorem for the general stochastic epidemic

One may well ask whether there is a stochastic threshold theorem similar in nature to the Kermack–McKendrick theorem for the deterministic general epidemic (part (ii) of Theorem 2.1). We start by considering the case, first published by Bartlett in 1955 (around equations (19) and (20) of §4.4 of the first edition of Bartlett, 1978), in which the susceptible population N is very large, so that

$$\Pr\{(X,Y)(t+\delta t) = (i-1, j+1) \mid (X,Y)(t) = (i,j)\} \approx Nj\delta t + o(\delta t)$$

instead of the exact $ij\delta t + o(\delta t)$, and

$$\Pr\{(X,Y)(t+\delta t) = (i, j-1) \mid (X,Y)(t) = (i,j)\} = \rho j\delta t + o(\delta t).$$

We write $\tilde{Y}(t)$ for the marginal process of the number of infectives that satisfies these approximate relations exactly, observing that such a $\{\tilde{Y}(t) : t \geq 0\}$, with $\tilde{Y}(0) = I$, is a birth-and-death process with rate parameters N for births and ρ for deaths. The p.g.f. of $\tilde{Y}$ is given by

$$\varphi(z;t) = \begin{cases} \left[\dfrac{\rho e^{(N-\rho)t}(z-1) - (Nz - \rho)}{N e^{(N-\rho)t}(z-1) - (Nz - \rho)} \right]^I & \text{if } N \neq \rho, \\[3ex] \left[\dfrac{1 - (\rho t - 1)(z-1)}{1 - \rho t(z-1)} \right]^I & \text{if } N = \rho. \end{cases} \tag{3.3.25}$$

Note that the result for $N = \rho$ can be readily derived from that for $N \neq \rho$ by setting $N = \rho + \epsilon$ in this case and letting $\epsilon \to 0$. We are interested in the probability of extinction of $\tilde{Y}(t)$, i.e. in $\lim_{t\to\infty} \Pr\{\tilde{Y}(t) = 0\} = \lim_{t\to\infty} \varphi(0,t)$. From the first of equations (3.3.25) we see that the behaviour differs between $N > \rho$ and $N < \rho$, namely

$$\lim_{t\to\infty} \varphi(0,t) = \begin{cases} \lim\limits_{t\to\infty} \left[\dfrac{\rho - \rho e^{-(N-\rho)t}}{N - \rho e^{-(N-\rho)t}} \right]^I = \left[\dfrac{\rho}{N} \right]^I < 1 & (N > \rho), \\[3ex] \lim\limits_{t\to\infty} \left[\dfrac{\rho - \rho e^{(N-\rho)t}}{\rho - N e^{(N-\rho)t}} \right]^I = 1 & (N < \rho). \end{cases} \tag{3.3.26}$$

When $N = \rho$ the second equation in (3.3.25) yields the limit 1, which is equal to the limit of either of the expressions in (3.3.26). Thus, for $N \leq \rho$, $\lim_{t\to\infty} \Pr\{\tilde{Y}(t) = 0\} = 1$ so that the epidemic outbreak is likely to be small. On the other hand, for $N > \rho$, the limit is positive but < 1, so that the outbreak may be either small or large. Whittle (1955) gave a more precise analysis of Bartlett's approximation; the essential step is to bound the number of infectives $Y(t)$ in the actual epidemic process between two birth-and-death processes like $\tilde{Y}(t)$.

For any ζ in $(0,1)$ we can ask whether the *intensity* of the epidemic, meaning the proportion of susceptibles who are ever infected, exceeds ζ. To this end define

$$\pi(\zeta) = \lim_{t\to\infty} \Pr\{X(0) - X(t) \leq N\zeta\} = \sum_{n=0}^{[N\zeta]} P_n \qquad (3.3.27)$$

with P_n the probability that the final size of the epidemic is n, as given below (3.3.3). We can bound the component $Y(t)$ in the epidemic process $\{(X,Y)(t) : t \geq 0\}$ by $\tilde{Y}(t)$ in two bivariate processes

$$\{\tilde{Y}(t),\ U(t) = I + X(0) - X(t) : t \geq 0\},$$

where $\tilde{Y}(\cdot)$ is a birth-and-death process with birth parameter either $\lambda_1 = N$, as in (3.3.25), or $\lambda_2 = N(1 - \zeta)$, and with death parameter $\mu_1 = \mu_2 = \rho$. Note that $U(t)$ counts all the individuals who have ever been infected up to time t, including the initial I infectives. Write

$$p_{jk}(t) = \Pr\{(Y,U)(t) = (j,k) \mid (Y,U)(0) = (I,I)\},$$

and

$$\varphi(z,w;t) = \sum_{j,k} p_{jk}(t) z^j w^k.$$

Now the forward Kolmogorov equations for the birth-and-death process with general birth parameter λ are

$$\frac{\mathrm{d}p_{jk}}{\mathrm{d}t} = \lambda(j-1)p_{j-1,k-1} - (\lambda+\rho)jp_{jk} + \rho(j+1)p_{j+1,k},$$

$$(0 \leq j \leq N+I,\ I \leq k \leq N+I),$$

defining $p_{jk} = 0$ when (j,k) lies outside the permissible range. This leads to the p.d.e.

$$\frac{\partial\varphi}{\partial t} = \left[\lambda z^2 w + (\lambda+\rho)z + \rho\right]\frac{\partial\varphi}{\partial z}, \qquad (3.3.28)$$

with the initial condition $\varphi(z, w; 0) = z^N w^I$. Equation (3.3.28) can be solved by classical methods. The characteristic equations for Lagrange's method yield

$$\frac{d\varphi}{0} = \frac{dt}{1} = \frac{dz}{\lambda z^2 w + (\lambda + \rho)z + \rho} = \frac{dw}{0}.$$

Denote the two roots of the quadratic equation $\lambda z^2 w + (\lambda + \rho)z + \rho = 0$ in z by $\eta_1(w)$, $\eta_2(w)$; then

$$\eta_{1,2}(w) = \frac{\lambda + \rho \pm \sqrt{(\lambda + \rho)^2 - 4\rho\lambda w}}{2\lambda w}, \qquad (3.3.29)$$

where for $0 < w \le 1$, $\eta_1 > \eta_2 > 0$. The general solution is thus of the form

$$\varphi(z, w; t) = g\left(\frac{z - \eta_2}{\eta_1 - z} e^{-\lambda z(\eta_1 - \eta_2)t}, w\right),$$

where g is a function which can be found from the initial condition

$$g\left(\frac{z - \eta_2}{\eta_1 - z}, w\right) = z^N w^I.$$

Write $\xi = \dfrac{z - \eta_2}{\eta_1 - z}$, so that $z = \dfrac{\eta_1 \xi + \eta_2}{\xi + 1}$, implying that

$$g(\xi, w) = \left[\frac{\eta_1 \xi + \eta_2}{\xi + 1}\right]^I w^I.$$

It then follows that

$$\varphi(z, w; t) = w^I \left[\frac{\eta_1(z - \eta_2)e^{-\lambda z(\eta_1 - \eta_2)t} + \eta_2(\eta_1 - z)}{(z - \eta_2)e^{-\lambda z(\eta_1 - \eta_2)t} + (\eta_1 - z)}\right]^I. \qquad (3.3.30)$$

As $t \to \infty$, the asymptotic distribution of the total number of individuals $U(t)$ ultimately infected is given by

$$\lim_{t \to \infty} \varphi(1, w; t) = w^I \eta_2^I(w) = \left[\frac{\lambda + \rho}{2\lambda}\right]^I \left(1 - \sqrt{1 - \kappa w}\right)^I, \qquad (3.3.31)$$

where $\kappa = 4\lambda\rho/(\lambda + \rho)^2$. We now expand this relation, using Lagrange's expansion for the function $\psi(s) = s^I$, where $s(w) = 1 - \sqrt{1 - \kappa w}$ can conveniently be given as the root $s(\kappa)$ of $s^2 - 2s + \kappa w = 0$ that satisfies $\lim_{w \to 0} s(w) = 0$. Note that

$$w = \frac{s(2 - s)}{\kappa} = \frac{s}{\kappa/(2 - s)};$$

thus using the formula

$$\psi\big(s(w)\big) = \sum_{n=1}^{\infty} \frac{w^n}{n!} \left[\frac{d^{n-1}}{ds^{n-1}} \left[I s^{I-1} \left(\frac{\kappa}{2-s} \right)^n \right] \right]_{s=0}$$

for Lagrange's expansion, we see that this leads to

$$P_n(\lambda) = \lim_{t \to \infty} \Pr\{U(t) = I + n\} = \lim_{t \to \infty} \Pr\{X(0) - X(t) = n\}$$

$$= \begin{cases} I \dfrac{(2n + I - 1)!}{n!\,(n+I)!} \dfrac{\lambda^n \rho^{n+I}}{(\lambda + \rho)^{2n+I}} & (0 \le n \le N - 1), \\ 1 - \sum_{m=0}^{N-1} P_m(\lambda) & (n = N), \end{cases} \tag{3.3.32}$$

where $\{P_n(\lambda)\}$ is the probability distribution for the total number of initial susceptibles ultimately infected, for a specific birth parameter λ.

Now we know from (3.3.31) that for $N \to \infty$,

$$\lim_{t \to \infty} \varphi(1, 1; t) = \sum_{n=0}^{\infty} P_n(\lambda) = \begin{cases} \left(\dfrac{\rho}{\lambda} \right)^I & (\rho < \lambda), \\ 1 & (\rho \ge \lambda), \end{cases} \tag{3.3.33}$$

so that

$$\sum_{n=0}^{\infty} P_n(\lambda) = \left[\min \left(\frac{\rho}{\lambda}, 1 \right) \right]^I. \tag{3.3.34}$$

Thus for N large enough, in the case of an epidemic of intensity ζ, with bounding values $\lambda_1 = N \ge X(t) \ge \lambda_2 = N(1 - \zeta)$ for the birth parameters of the birth-and-death processes involved, we have approximately

$$\sum_{n=0}^{[N\zeta]} P_n(\lambda_1) \le \sum_{n=0}^{[N\zeta]} P_n \le \sum_{n=0}^{[N\zeta]} P_n(\lambda_2),$$

or equivalently

$$\left[\min \left(\frac{\rho}{N}, 1 \right) \right]^I \le \pi(\zeta) \le \left[\min \left(\frac{\rho}{N(1 - \zeta)}, 1 \right) \right]^I. \tag{3.3.35}$$

We can draw the following conclusions from this result.

Theorem 3.1 (Whittle's Threshold Theorem). *Consider a general epidemic process with initial numbers of susceptibles N and infectives I, and relative removal rate ρ. For any ζ in $(0, 1)$, let $\pi(\zeta)$ denote the probability that at most $[N\zeta]$ of the susceptibles are ultimately infected i.e. that the intensity of the epidemic does not exceed ζ.*

(i) If $\rho < N(1 - \zeta)$, then

$$\left(\frac{\rho}{N}\right)^I \leq \pi(\zeta) \leq \left(\frac{\rho}{N(1 - \zeta)}\right)^I.$$

(ii) If $N(1 - \zeta) \leq \rho < N$, then

$$\left(\frac{\rho}{N}\right)^I \leq \pi(\zeta) \leq 1.$$

In both these cases there is a probability approximately equal to $1 - (\rho/N)^I$ that the epidemic achieves an intensity $> \zeta$ for small ζ.
(iii) If $\rho \geq N$, then $\pi(\zeta) = 1$, and the probability that the epidemic achieves an intensity greater than any predetermined ζ in $(0, 1)$, is zero.

3.4   The ultimate size of the general stochastic epidemic

Various approaches have been used to find the distribution $\{P_n\}$ of the ultimate size of an epidemic, where in the notation used in and below (3.3.2–3),

$$P_n = \lim_{t \to \infty} p_{N-n,0}(t) \tag{3.4.1}$$

is the probability that n of the initial susceptibles become infected at some stage during the epidemic. When there are no more infectives, there are therefore $n + I$ removals including the I initial infectives. In this section we indicate two methods of finding this distribution, one as an illustration of the p.g.f. technique of Section 3.3, the other using an embedded random walk technique that is much superior numerically, in terms of speed, numerical accuracy and population size that can be conveniently handled. This method is essentially due to Foster (1955). We give a third method, based on another embedded Markov chain, in Section 4.5, while other methods have been used by Bailey (1953) and Williams (1971), as outlined in Bailey (1975).

3.4.1   The total size distribution using the p.g.f. method

For a Markov process on countable state space in continuous time, the limiting probability π_i that the process is in state i can be computed from the Laplace transform $\hat{p}_i(\theta)$ of the probability $p_i(t)$ that the process is in i at time t. The Abelian property

$$\pi_i = \lim_{t \to \infty} p_i(t) = \lim_{\theta \to 0} \theta \hat{p}_i(\theta),$$

where $\hat{p}_i(\theta) = \int_0^\infty e^{-\theta t} p_i(t)\,dt$, yields this probability π_i. In terms of the generating function $\hat{f}_i(w, \theta)$ of transforms defined at (3.3.7), this means that, since for all i, $\lim_{t\to\infty} p_{ij}(t) = 0$ for $j \neq 0$. then

$$P_n = \lim_{\theta \to 0} \theta \hat{p}_{N-n,0}(\theta) = \lim_{\theta \to 0} \theta \hat{f}_{N-n}(0, \theta).$$

Thus

$$\mathbf{P} = \begin{pmatrix} P_0 \\ P_1 \\ \vdots \\ P_N \end{pmatrix} = \lim_{\theta \to 0} \theta \begin{pmatrix} \hat{f}_N(0, \theta) \\ \hat{f}_{N-1}(0, \theta) \\ \vdots \\ \hat{f}_0(0, \theta) \end{pmatrix} = \lim_{\theta \to 0} \theta F(0, \theta), \tag{3.4.2}$$

where $F(0, \theta)$ is given by (3.3.21). From that equation, recalling that

$$B_0 = \begin{pmatrix} \theta I/\rho & 0 \\ I & 0 \end{pmatrix},$$

we see that

$$\left[\prod_{i=1}^{N+I} B_i \right]_{N+1} \theta F(0, \theta) = I! \left[\prod_{i=I+1}^{I+N} B_i \right]_{N+1} e_{N+1},$$

whence, taking the limit as $\theta \to 0$, we find

$$\left[\prod_{i=1}^{I+N} \begin{pmatrix} iA'(0)/\rho & \binom{i}{2}A''(0)/\rho \\ I & 0 \end{pmatrix} \right]_{N+1} \lim_{\theta \to 0} \theta F(0, \theta)$$
$$= I! \left[\prod_{i=I+1}^{I+N} \begin{pmatrix} iA'(0)/\rho & \binom{i}{2}A''(0)/\rho \\ I & 0 \end{pmatrix} \right]_{N+1} e_{N+1}. \tag{3.4.3}$$

Thus, $\mathbf{P} = \lim_{\theta \to 0} \theta F(0, \theta)$ equals the right-hand side here pre-multiplied by the inverse of the matrix product on the left-hand side, where as noted above (3.3.21), this matrix product is non-singular, with a unique inverse. The following example indicates what is involved in using this matrix result in practice.

Example 3.4.1. We compute the distribution of the ultimate size of the epidemic in the case $(N, I) = (3, 1)$ with $\rho = 1$. Setting

$$\frac{A'(0)}{\rho} = A = \begin{pmatrix} 4 & & \\ & 3 & \\ & & 2 \\ & & & 1 \end{pmatrix}, \qquad \frac{A''(0)}{\rho} = -2\Delta = -2 \begin{pmatrix} 0 & & \\ 3 & 0 & \\ & 2 & 0 \\ & & 1 & 0 \end{pmatrix},$$

the products appearing in (3.4.3) on the right- and left-hand sides are, respectively,

$$\left[\begin{pmatrix} 4A & -12\Delta \\ I & 0 \end{pmatrix} \begin{pmatrix} 3A & -6\Delta \\ I & 0 \end{pmatrix} \begin{pmatrix} 2A & -2\Delta \\ I & 0 \end{pmatrix} \right]_4$$
$$= 24(A^3 - A\Delta - \Delta A),$$

$$\left[\begin{pmatrix} 4A & -12\Delta \\ I & 0 \end{pmatrix} \begin{pmatrix} 3A & -6\Delta \\ I & 0 \end{pmatrix} \begin{pmatrix} 2A & -2\Delta \\ I & 0 \end{pmatrix} \begin{pmatrix} A & 0 \\ I & 0 \end{pmatrix} \right]_4$$
$$= 24(A^4 - A\Delta A - \Delta A^2 - A^2\Delta + \Delta^2).$$

Hence, after some calculation,

$$\mathbf{P} = \begin{pmatrix} 256 & & & \\ -111 & 81 & & \\ 6 & -38 & 16 & \\ 0 & 2 & -7 & 1 \end{pmatrix}^{-1} \begin{pmatrix} 64 \\ -21 \\ 0 \\ 0 \end{pmatrix} = \begin{pmatrix} 0.2500 \\ 0.0833 \\ 0.1042 \\ 0.5625 \end{pmatrix}.$$

Observe the presence here of both positive and negative terms. In larger matrices this is a source of numerical instability, assuming that there is the capacity to handle the larger size (e.g. square matrices that are $O(100)$).

3.4.2 Embedded jump processes

We commented below (3.4.3) that properties like the size[3] of the general stochastic epidemic are most readily studied from a practical point of view by using an embedded jump chain technique. Aspects of this technique can be found for example in Todorovic (1992, §8.7); we rehearse here, for the sake of notation and general convenience, some properties of these processes.

Processes are often modelled as Markov chains because these incorporate in a simple manner dependence from one time point to another. This is true for phenomena in both continuous time (as in the earlier part of this chapter) and discrete time (as in the next chapter). In the case of continuous time, a further class of Markov chains can arise as embedded processes. By concentrating on the jump points or other epochs of a continuous time process which does not necessarily have a Markovian structure, we may derive a discrete time process which is Markovian (see Section 4.5 for an example). For a Markov process in continuous time on a countable state space,

---

[3]The 'total size' of an epidemic usually includes the initial I infectives, whereas the 'size' (or, 'ultimate size') of an epidemic usually designates the number of initial susceptibles that are (ultimately) infected.

the natural process to consider is the one embedded at the jump epochs of the process. Except for certain pathological cases which do not arise in the models we have considered, the continuous time and embedded jump processes both have the same long-term behaviour, such as the development of major and minor epidemics, and the ultimate size of the epidemic. This section reviews briefly some results of this kind. The particular usefulness of embedded jump processes is that they are well-suited to numerical work.

To make these ideas explicit, we use $\{X(t) : t \geq 0\}$ in this subsection to denote a Markov process in continuous time on the countable state space $\mathcal{X} \equiv \{i, j, \ldots\}$ having time-homogeneous transition probabilities with rates (q_{ij}). We assume that X is determined by its initial state and the rates q_{ij} $(j \neq i)$ and $q_i \equiv \sum_{i \neq j} q_{ij} = -q_{ii}$ $(i, j \in \mathcal{X})$. One dichotomous classification of states is that any state i is either absorbing or non-absorbing, depending on whether $q_i = 0$ or $q_i > 0$.

Given a sample path for X for which $X(0) = i$, the time $T_i \equiv \inf\{t > 0 : X(t) \neq i\}$ is well-defined, finite or infinite, with $T_i < \infty$ a.s. if and only if $q_i > 0$, i.e. i is non-absorbing. Then T_i is an exponentially distributed r.v. with mean $1/q_i$. Indeed, supposing without loss of generality[4] that the sample paths are right-continuous with left-limits, these paths can be described by a sequence of intervals of lengths $T^{(n)}$, with epochs t_n determined by the partial sums

$$t_0 = 0, \qquad t_{n+1} = T^{(0)} + \cdots + T^{(n)} = t_n + T^{(n)} \quad (n = 0, 1, \ldots). \quad (3.4.4)$$

For these,

$$X(t) = i_n \qquad (t_n \leq t < t_{n+1}, \quad n = 0, 1, \ldots), \qquad (3.4.5)$$

for some sequence of states $i_0, i_1, \ldots$, it being understood that if any such i_n is an absorbing state the associated interval length $T^{(n)}$ is infinite and $t_r = \infty$ for all $r \geq n + 1$. We can now define the embedded jump chain by

$$\{X_n\} \equiv \{X(t_n + 0) : t_n < \infty\}, \qquad (3.4.6)$$

with one-step transition probabilities for non-absorbing states i

$$p_{ij} \equiv \Pr\{X_{n+1} = j \mid X_n = i\} = \frac{q_{ij}}{q_i}. \qquad (3.4.7)$$

Also, for all sample paths for which $X_n = i_n$, it follows from the strong Markov property that $T^{(n)}$, when finite, is exponentially distributed with mean $1/q_{i_n}$.

---

[4]To be more precise mathematically, suppose that the process is separable, etc.

Markov chains with well-ordered sample paths are easily studied using this formalism. Define $\pi_{ij} = \Pr\{X(t) = j \text{ for some } t \mid X(0) = i\}$. Then the forward Chapman–Kolmogorov equations for the jump chain give the relations

$$\pi_{ik} = p_{ik} + \sum_{j \neq k: p_{jk} > 0} \pi_{ij} p_{jk}. \tag{3.4.8}$$

In this equation, all quantities on the right-hand side are positive; this is the reason the equation is the basis of a relatively stable numerical procedure for the computation of the probability

$$P_{ik} = \Pr\{\lim_{t \to \infty} X(t) = k \mid X(0) = i\} \tag{3.4.9}$$

of reaching the absorbing state k, starting from the state i.

We can also study first passage time r.v.s like

$$t_{ik} \equiv \inf\{t > 0 : X(t) = k; X(u) = k \text{ for some } u > 0 \mid X(0) = i\}. \tag{3.4.10}$$

The well-ordered property of sample paths, i.e. their strictly evolutionary nature, means that, given a sample path from i to k that passes through some intermediate state j, which will necessarily exist if the one-step transition probability $p_{ik} = 0$, then

$$t_{ik} = t_{ij} + t_{jk}. \tag{3.4.11}$$

Define

$$\tau_{ik} = \mathrm{E}(t_{ik} \mid X(0) = i, X(u) = k \text{ for some } u > 0). \tag{3.4.12}$$

Taking expectations over appropriate sample paths in (3.4.11) and using the same forward decomposition as in (3.4.8) gives

$$\pi_{ik}\tau_{ik} = \sum_{j:p_{jk}>0} (\pi_{ij}\tau_{ij}p_{jk} + \pi_{ij}p_{jk}\tau_{jk}) = \sum_{j:p_{jk}>0} \pi_{ij}p_{jk}(\tau_{ij} + 1/q_j). \tag{3.4.13}$$

More complex relations for higher moments can be developed similarly (see Exercise 3.8).

3.4.3 The total size distribution using the embedded jump chain

It follows from the development of the general stochastic epidemic model in Section 3.3.1 that an embedded Markov chain which is conveniently denoted

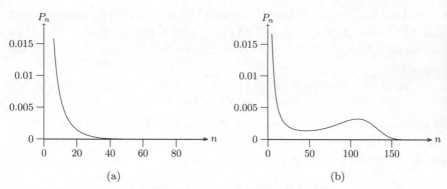

(a)   (b)

Figure 3.2. Final size distributions of epidemics with $\rho = 150$ and
(a) $(N, I) = (100, 1)$, (b) $(N, I) = (200, 1)$.

by $\{(X_n, Y_n) : n = 0, 1, \ldots\}$ takes place on the finite region $\mathcal{X}_{NI}$ of the two-dimensional integer lattice defined by

$$\mathcal{X}_{NI} \equiv \{(i, j) : i = 0, 1, \ldots, N; \ j = 0, 1, \ldots, I + N - i\}.$$

For $(i, j) \in \mathcal{X}_{NI}$, the only non-zero one-step transition probabilities are given by

$$p_{(i,j),(i-1,j+1)} = \frac{\beta i j}{\beta i j + \gamma j} = \frac{i}{i + \rho} = p_i,$$

$$p_{(i,j),(i,j-1)} = \frac{\gamma j}{\beta i j + \gamma j} = \frac{\rho}{i + \rho} = 1 - p_i. \tag{3.4.14}$$

Consequently, writing $p_{(i,j)} = \Pr\{(X_n, Y_n) = (i, j)$ for some $n \mid (X_0, Y_0) = (N, I)\}$, it follows from (3.4.8) that

$$p_{(i,j)} = \begin{cases} p_{(i+1,j-1)} p_{i+1} + p_{(i,j+1)}(1 - p_i) & (j \geq 2), \\ p_{(i,j+1)}(1 - p_i) & (j = 0, 1), \end{cases} \tag{3.4.15}$$

where on the right-hand side we set $p_{(i,j)} = 0$ if $(i, j) \notin \mathcal{X}_{NI}$. In particular,

$$p_{(i,0)} = \Pr\{\text{epidemic is of size } N - i\} = \lim_{t \to \infty} p_{i0}(t) = P_{N-i} \tag{3.4.16}$$

with $p_{i0}(t)$ and P_n as defined in (3.4.1).

Figure 3.2 illustrates most of the distributions of the size of general stochastic epidemics for which $\rho = 150$ and $(N, I) = (100, 1)$ for (a) and $(200, 1)$ for (b), illustrating sub- and super-critical behaviour respectively. Some probability masses near the origin are off the scale used; in case (a) their values at 0, \ldots, 5 are 0.600, 0.145, 0.070, 0.042, 0.029, 0.021, and in case (b) at 0, \ldots, 4 they are 0.429, 0.106, 0.052, 0.032, 0.022 respectively.

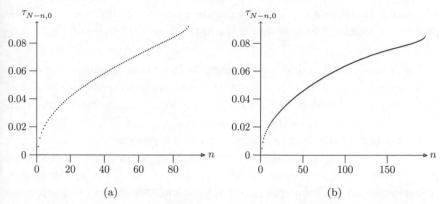

Figure 3.3. Conditional mean durations of epidemics with $\rho = 150$ and (a) $(N, I) = (100, 1)$, (b) $(N, I) = (200, 1)$. Abscissae give the number of susceptibles infected. The means were not computed for large n for which $P_n = p_{N-n,0} < 10^{-9}$. Cf. Exercise 3.13 and Daley et al. (1999).

We have also computed the conditional mean durations of these epidemics with $\beta = 1$ for those final sizes for which the probabilities exceed 10^{-9}. In the notation of (3.4.12), we have found $\tau_{i0} \equiv \tau_{(N,I),(i,0)}$ for those i for which $p_{(i,0)} > 10^{-9}$. These conditional means satisfy the recurrence relations, for $(i, j) \in \mathcal{X}_{NI}$, starting from $\tau_{NI} = 0$,

$$p_{(i,j)}\tau_{ij} = p_{(i+1,j-1)}p_{i+1}(\tau_{i+1,j-1} + \mu_{i+1,j-1})$$
$$+ p_{(i,j+1)}(1 - p_i)(\tau_{i,j+1} + \mu_{i,j+1}) \qquad (j \geq 2),$$

and

$$\tau_{ij} = \tau_{i,j+1} + \mu_{i,j+1} \qquad \begin{cases} (j = 0, 1 \text{ for } i = 0, \dots, N-1, \\ j = 0, \dots, I-1 \text{ for } i = N), \end{cases}$$

where $\mu_{ij} = 1/[j(\rho + i)] \equiv 1/q_{(i,j)}$ for the state (i, j) in the notation of (3.4.13). They are illustrated in Figure 3.3 for the same two epidemics as in the previous figure.

3.4.4 Behaviour of the general stochastic epidemic model: a composite picture

We now draw together these and other results to describe in general terms how the general stochastic epidemic model behaves, and point out some of its weaknesses.

First the Threshold Theorem distinguishes between sub- and super-critical conditions. In the case of a sub-critical epidemic, the numbers of infectives and removals behave roughly like live and dead individuals in a sub-critical birth-and-death process. This is borne out principally by Whittle's

Threshold Theorem 3.1. Both the duration and final size of the epidemic process are roughly the same as for the approximating birth-and-death process.

The super-critical case is more involved. Here it is possible that only a minor epidemic occurs, with probability approximately $(\rho/N)^I$. The size of such a minor outbreak is similar to that of a super-critical birth-and-death process conditional on extinction. From the work of Waugh (1958), this is exactly that of a sub-critical birth-and-death process whose linear birth (death) rates are the linear death (birth) rates of the original super-critical process respectively. Otherwise, the early behaviour of the epidemic process is similar to that of a super-critical birth-and-death process conditional on non-extinction, until the number of infectives represents an appreciable proportion of the initial number of susceptibles. If the deterministic model of the epidemic is any guide, the evolution of the epidemic process through a number of generations of infectives is still similar to the birth-and-death process (see Figures 2.7 and 2.8 and Exercise 3.5), until the number of susceptibles approaches the borderline value ρ between sub- and super-criticality. At this stage, in terms of numbers of susceptibles and infectives, the process follows approximately the solution of the deterministic epidemic model (with $\mathrm{E}\,X(t) \approx x(t)$ etc., much as for the simple epidemic; cf. Exercise 3.1). The 'imprecision' of the approximation, which in model terms incorporates both the stochastic lag and variability about the mean behaviour ($\approx$ deterministic solution), is approximately normally distributed if N and $\rho < N$ are both sufficiently large. This leads (Barbour, 1972, 1974) to the ultimate number of susceptibles being approximately normally distributed about the mean $\mathrm{E}\,X(\infty) \approx N\theta$, where $N\theta$ is the number of susceptibles surviving the deterministic epidemic, with a variance that can be computed using Kendall's 'Principle of Diffusion of Arbitrary Constants' (cf. Daley and Kendall, 1965, and Section 5.4 below).

If it happens that $R_0 = N/\rho$ is somewhat larger than 1 (e.g. 3 or more), then, conditional on the occurrence of a major outbreak, the number of susceptibles surviving the epidemic is approximately Poisson distributed, still with mean $N\theta$ where θ is now much closer to 0 (cf. Daniels, 1967). This number can be regarded as representing those individuals having a 'small' chance of avoiding infection. If $N\theta$ is itself not close to 0, then the closeness of a Poisson distribution to normality ties together this result with the previous paragraph. Sellke (1983) proved Daniels's result by considering a sequence of general epidemic models with parameters (N_k, I_k, ρ_k). These parameters are such that as $k \to \infty$, all three diverge to ∞ in such a way that

$N_k e^{-(N_k + I_k)/\rho_k} \to M$, say, for some finite positive M. Then the number of susceptibles $X_k(\infty)$ ultimately surviving the epidemic is shown to converge in distribution to the Poisson with mean M.

This ultimate size distribution is considered in more detail for the different cases of N and ρ in Nagaev and Startsev (1970) (see also Nagaev, 1971) using the embedded jump chain. The most general formulation of such results may be found in Reinert (1995).

In the limit theorem setting for these results, the duration of the epidemic may ultimately be exceedingly short; this indicates a need for rescaling time or else reviewing the conditions under which the model may apply. When one considers the observation of measles epidemics in large cities as reviewed in detail by Bartlett (1960), it becomes clear that the time- and generation-dependent evolution of the models need modification if they are to reflect this aspect more realistically. Fortunately, both the stratification models of the next section, and the chain binomial models of the next chapter, offer avenues for overcoming the drawbacks of the overly simple S–I–R model.

3.5 The general stochastic epidemic in a stratified population

This section starts by describing a continuous time Markov process model that extends the ideas of Section 3.3 to a stratified population, consistent with the deterministic setting of Section 2.4. In that setting we discussed what criterion should be used to distinguish a major from a minor outbreak; in the stochastic setting two further factors need to be considered, namely the discreteness of the population, and the stochastic modelling of the infection and removal processes. These factors lead us to a digression on the notion of the Basic Reproduction Ratio of an epidemic model. We conclude the section with an example of a stochastic model for an epidemic taking place in a community of households, a problem to which we return in Chapter 7.

A stochastic analogue[5] of the general deterministic epidemic of Section 2.4 assumes that a finite population of susceptibles is stratified into m groups of sizes $\mathbf{N} = (N_1, \ldots, N_m)'$, where as in Section 2.4, vector notation is convenient. At time $t = 0$ suppose a single infective is added to

---

[5]Daley and Kendall (1965) remark that the 'natural' formulation of a population process at the micro-level is discrete and (more than likely) stochastic. From this point of view, a discrete stochastic model is the prototype of which the deterministic model, with both continuous state space and deterministic (non-stochastic) evolution, is the analogue or approximation. As Barbour (1994) puts it, a deterministic model 'only has a meaning as an approximation to some underlying jump process'. Anderson and May (1991) consider deterministic models almost exclusively.

stratum i. At time $t \geq 0$ the jth group consists of $X_j(t)$ susceptibles, $Y_j(t)$ infectives and $Z_j(t) = N_j + \delta_{ij} - X_j(t) - Y_j(t)$ removals, so that $(X_j, Y_j, Z_j)(0) = (N_j, \delta_{ij}, 0)$, $(j = 1, \ldots, m)$, with δ_{ij} the Kronecker delta. We use a continuous time Markov process to model the infection and removal mechanisms, analogous to that used earlier in this Chapter. As in Section 2.4, β_{ij} denotes the pairwise rate for an infective in i to infect a susceptible in j, and γ_j the removal rate per infective in j. In vector notation, the property of constant sizes of the several strata is expressible as

$$\mathbf{X}(t) + \mathbf{Y}(t) + \mathbf{Z}(t) = \mathbf{N} + \mathbf{1}_i \qquad \text{(all } t\text{)}, \tag{3.5.1}$$

and the initial condition is that $(\mathbf{X}, \mathbf{Y}, \mathbf{Z})(0) = (\mathbf{N}, \mathbf{1}_i, \mathbf{0})$, where the m-row vector $\mathbf{1}_i$ has 1 as its ith component and all other elements zero.

The process $\{(\mathbf{X}, \mathbf{Y}, \mathbf{Z})(t) : t \geq 0\}$ takes place on a finite state space, so it is completely specified as a continuous time Markov process when its initial state and infinitesimal transition probabilities are given. We know $(\mathbf{X}, \mathbf{Y}, \mathbf{Z})(0)$ already, and the constraint (3.5.1) means that it is enough to describe $(\mathbf{X}, \mathbf{Y})(t)$. We assume that for the strata $i = 1, \ldots, m$, with $\mathbf{x}$ and $\mathbf{y}$ denoting m-vectors of non-negative integer-valued components,

$$\Pr\{(\mathbf{X}, \mathbf{Y})(t + \delta t) = (\mathbf{x} - \mathbf{1}_j, \mathbf{y} + \mathbf{1}_j) \mid (\mathbf{X}, \mathbf{Y})(t) = (\mathbf{x}, \mathbf{y})\}$$
$$= x_j \left(\textstyle\sum_{i=1}^{m} \beta_{ij} y_i \right) \delta t + o(\delta t) = x_j (\mathbf{y}'\mathbf{B})_j \delta t + o(\delta t) \quad (x_j \geq 1),$$
$$\Pr\{(\mathbf{X}, \mathbf{Y})(t + \delta t) = (\mathbf{x}, \mathbf{y} - \mathbf{1}_j) \mid (\mathbf{X}, \mathbf{Y})(t) = (\mathbf{x}, \mathbf{y})\}$$
$$= \gamma_j y_j \delta t + o(\delta t) \quad (y_j \geq 1),$$
$$\Pr\{(\mathbf{X}, \mathbf{Y})(t + \delta t) = (\mathbf{x}, \mathbf{y}) \mid (\mathbf{X}, \mathbf{Y})(t) = (\mathbf{x}, \mathbf{y})\}$$
$$= 1 - \textstyle\sum_{j=1}^{m} [x_j (\mathbf{y}'\mathbf{B})_j + \gamma_j y_j] \delta t - o(\delta t),$$
$$\tag{3.5.2}$$

where $\mathbf{B} = (\beta_{ij})$. We can now write down the forward Kolmogorov equations, but they are too unwieldy to give an explicit solution, whether in the time or transform domain. We have described this model here because (a) it is easily studied via simulation techniques, (b) it is general enough to capture inhomogeneity, and (c) it provides an adequate setting to discuss the basic threshold phenomenon.

We first consider a method of approximating the behaviour of the process, entirely consistent with Whittle's approach in Section 3.2. This approach effectively keeps the size of the susceptible population fixed during the early stage of the epidemic, so that the only changes occurring in the population are in the numbers of infectives $\tilde{Y}$ say. In the m-strata context we therefore approximate the process by a multi-type linear birth-and-death process

$\tilde{\mathbf{Y}}(t)$, in which at time t there are $\tilde{Y}_j(t)$ $(j = 1, \ldots, m)$ j-type individuals, for whom the birth and death rates are respectively $\sum_{i=1}^{m} \beta_{ij} \tilde{Y}_i(t) N_j$ and $\gamma_j \tilde{Y}_j$; provided no N_j is small these birth rates differ little from $\sum_{i=1}^{m} \beta_{ij} \tilde{Y}_i(t) X_j(t)$ for t small enough (cf. (3.5.2)). This process $\tilde{\mathbf{Y}}(t)$ is an irreducible multi-type Markovian branching process in continuous time. For such processes it is known (e.g. Athreya and Ney, 1972, §V.7.5) that the vector $\mathbf{q}$ whose ith element

$$q_i = \Pr\{\lim_{t \to \infty} \tilde{Y}_j(t) = 0 \mid \tilde{\mathbf{Y}}(0) = \mathbf{1}_i\} \tag{3.5.3}$$

gives the probability of ultimate extinction, is the least positive solution of the equations

$$\sum_{j=1}^{m} \beta_{ij} N_j q_i q_j + \gamma_i = \left(\sum_{j=1}^{m} \beta_{ij} N_j + \gamma_i\right) q_i \qquad (i = 1, \ldots, m). \tag{3.5.4}$$

Now $q_i = 1$ (all i) is always a solution, but need not be the least positive one. Also, the process is irreducible if and only if the matrix $\mathbf{B}$ is primitive, meaning that for some integer n, which is at most equal to m, $\mathbf{B}^n$ has its (i, j)th element positive. Because of irreducibility, either $q_i < 1$ (all i) or else $q_i = 1$ (all i), and the former holds if and only if

$$\mathbf{B} \operatorname{diag}(\mathbf{N}) - \operatorname{diag}(\boldsymbol{\gamma}) \tag{3.5.5}$$

has a real positive eigenvalue; this is equivalent (see Exercise 3.9) to $R > 1$ where R is the largest eigenvalue of the non-negative matrix

$$\mathbf{M}_1 \equiv \operatorname{diag}(\boldsymbol{\gamma}^{-1}) \mathbf{B} \operatorname{diag}(\mathbf{N}). \tag{3.5.6}$$

In the one-dimensional case equation (3.5.6) gives $R = \beta N / \gamma = N / \rho \equiv R_0$, and the condition $R > 1$ is exactly the condition in Whittle's Threshold Theorem 3.1 for a major outbreak. Thus, we have indeed generalized that result to the m-strata context.

For birth-and-death processes, as for branching processes and random walks, conditions for behaviour like extinction or return to the origin, are typically given both probabilistically and in terms of first moments. Application of the latter method to epidemics makes use of the *Basic Reproduction Ratio*. This is defined for epidemics in homogeneous populations as 'the average number of persons directly infected by an infectious case during its entire infectious period, after entering a totally susceptible population' (Giesecke, 1994, p. 111). This definition formalizes the notion that a major epidemic will occur when, in the earlier stages of an outbreak of a disease, each infective on average produces more than one further infective.

In particular, in the simplest case $(I = 1)$ of the general epidemic model of Section 3.2, the initial infective is placed in a population of N susceptibles where it mixes homogeneously during its infectious period T, with T exponentially distributed with mean $1/\gamma$. Then the number among the N initial susceptibles contacted (and therefore, potentially infected), is a binomial r.v. $\mathrm{Bin}(N, 1 - e^{-\beta T})$. Unconditionally therefore, if susceptibles are affected only by the initial infective until its removal, the mean number of new infectives directly contacted by the initial infective equals

$$NE(1 - e^{-\beta T}) = \frac{\beta N}{\beta + \gamma} = \frac{N}{1 + \rho} \approx \frac{\beta N}{\gamma} = \frac{N}{\rho} = R_0, \qquad (3.5.7)$$

where R_0 is as below (3.5.6), and the approximation is valid when $\rho \gg 1$, i.e. $\beta \ll \gamma$. While this condition is stated in terms of ρ rather than N, the case of super-criticality (i.e. $R_0 > 1$) then implies that $N \gg 1$. The analogy of the criticality condition, that $R_0 <$ or > 1, with that for Galton–Watson branching processes, is immediate.

To apply this idea to the m-strata context, we refer to the initial infective, in stratum i say, as a zero generation i-stratum infective. Let m_{ij} denote the expected numbers of first generation j-stratum infectives $(j = 1, \ldots, m)$ to which it gives rise. We ask whether these various first generation infectives in different strata, if each is placed in the same environment of N susceptibles as the initial infective, would produce on average a larger number of second generation infectives, and so on. Now the expected number of k-stratum second generation infectives produced by an initial i-stratum infective, *on the assumption that each first generation infective is placed in the same initial population of N susceptibles*, equals $\sum_{j=1}^{m} m_{ij}m_{jk}$, i.e. the (i, k)th component of the matrix $\mathbf{M}^2$ where $\mathbf{M} = (m_{ij})$. Continuing this process, the expected numbers of j-stratum infectives after r generations, for r not too large, equals the (i, j)th element of the matrix $\mathbf{M}^r$. Since $\mathbf{M}$ is a non-negative matrix (indeed, it is primitive because $\mathbf{B}$ is primitive), Perron–Frobenius theory implies that each column of $\mathbf{M}^r$ is like $R_0^r \mathbf{v}$ for large r, where R_0 is the largest eigenvalue of $\mathbf{M}$ and $\mathbf{v}$ is the right-eigenvector corresponding to R_0. It follows that the expected number of infectives after r generations either dies away to 0 when $R_0 < 1$, or else grows exponentially for a while when $R_0 > 1$, reflecting the possibility of a major outbreak.

To identify $\mathbf{M}$, note that an i-stratum infective is infectious for an exponentially distributed time T_i with mean $1/\gamma_i$. If the N susceptibles were not otherwise subject to infection during this period T_i, the number of j-stratum infectives produced would be a binomial r.v. $\mathrm{Bin}(N_j, 1 - e^{-\beta_{ij} T_i})$. Hence, unconditionally, the expected number m_{ij} of first generation j-stratum infectives produced by an i-stratum infective is given by

$$m_{ij} = N_j \mathrm{E}(1 - e^{-\beta_{ij} T_i}) = N_j \left(1 - \frac{\gamma_i}{\gamma_i + \beta_{ij}}\right) \approx \frac{\beta_{ij} N_j}{\gamma_i}, \qquad (3.5.8)$$

the approximation again being valid for $\beta_{ij} \ll \gamma_i$. The matrix $\mathbf{M}$ is

$$\mathbf{M} = \left(\frac{\beta_{ij} N_j}{\beta_{ij} + \gamma_i}\right) \approx \left(\frac{\beta_{ij} N_j}{\gamma_i}\right) = \mathrm{diag}(\boldsymbol{\gamma}^{-1}) \mathbf{B} \, \mathrm{diag}(\mathbf{N}) = \mathbf{M}_1, \qquad (3.5.9)$$

with $\mathbf{M}_1$ as at (3.5.6). It follows that $R_0 \approx R$, and we should call R_0 the *Basic Reproduction Ratio* for the epidemic. This terminology is that of Diekmann, Heesterbeek and Metz (1990) who noted that it is a dimensionless quantity (hence, *ratio* rather than *rate* or *number*), which measures 'reproductiveness'. The discussion concerning Examples 3.5.1–2 supports our contention that this moment-based definition for R_0 is more appropriate than R, defined in more probabilistic terms around (3.5.6). We summarize our discussion thus far.

Theorem 3.2. *A stochastic epidemic in a stratified population such that no component of $\mathbf{N}$ is small, with infection rates β_{ij} and removal rates γ_j as for (3.5.2), exhibits sub- or super-critical behaviour (i.e. only minor outbreaks occur, or major outbreaks may occur) according as the Basic Reproduction Ratio R_0 is $<$ or > 1, where R_0 is the eigenvalue of largest modulus of $\mathbf{M} = (m_{ij})$.*

The birth-and-death continuous time approximation, leading to $\mathbf{M}_1$, and the generation-wise approach leading to $\mathbf{M}$, give similar but not exactly identical conditions for distinguishing between sub- and super-criticality. Under the first approach the matrix $\mathbf{M}_1$ is computed after a single jump of the process whereas contributions to the matrix $\mathbf{M}$ arise from both this single jump and possibly several subsequent jumps. Because of this, approximations based on $\mathbf{M}$ are better than those based on $\mathbf{M}_1$.

Stochastic analysis of the model defined by (3.5.2), such as the computation of the ultimate size of an epidemic, is complicated by the dimensionality of the state space needed to provide a Markovian description of the process. Clearly, one possible description is the $(2m)$-dimensional process $(\mathbf{X}, \mathbf{Y})(t)$. If the size of m is appreciable, this may be too large for exact computation. When the parameters β_{ij} and γ have a simple structure, the analysis can be correspondingly simplified, as in the following Examples.

Example 3.5.1 *(m interacting communities).* Consider a population which consists of m communities of N_i individuals $(i = 1, \ldots, m)$, all of whom are susceptible to a disease which, if introduced, spreads by pairwise contact at rates $\beta_{ii} = \beta_H$ (all i) and $\beta_{ij} = \beta_C$ (all (i, j) with $i \neq j$), where $\beta_H \geq \beta_C$ (typically, $\beta_H \gg \beta_C$). Removal of infectives occurs at a common rate γ per infective. Suppose that a single infective is introduced into the ith community. Using the approximations at (3.5.9), the Basic Reproduction Ratio that gives us a threshold criterion is the largest eigenvalue of the $m \times m$ matrix $\mathbf{M}_1$ with elements

$$
m_{jk} = \begin{cases} \beta_H N_k/\gamma & (k = j), \\ \beta_C N_k/\gamma & (k \neq j). \end{cases} \tag{3.5.10}
$$

Thus, R_0 is the largest positive root of the characteristic equation $f(\lambda) = 0$ where

$$
f(\lambda) = \det \begin{pmatrix} \beta_H N_1/\gamma - \lambda & \beta_C N_2/\gamma & \cdots & \beta_C N_m/\gamma \\ \beta_C N_1/\gamma & \beta_H N_2/\gamma - \lambda & \cdots & \beta_C N_m/\gamma \\ \vdots & \vdots & \ddots & \vdots \\ \beta_C N_1/\gamma & \beta_C N_2/\gamma & \cdots & \beta_H N_m/\gamma - \lambda \end{pmatrix}
$$

$$
= \det \begin{pmatrix} \beta_H \tilde{N}_1 - \lambda & \beta_C \tilde{N}_2 & \beta_C \tilde{N}_3 & \cdots & \beta_C \tilde{N}_m \\ -\beta_{HC} \tilde{N}_1 + \lambda & \beta_{HC} \tilde{N}_2 - \lambda & 0 & \cdots & 0 \\ -\beta_{HC} \tilde{N}_1 + \lambda & 0 & \beta_{HC} \tilde{N}_3 - \lambda & \cdots & 0 \\ \vdots & \vdots & \vdots & \ddots & \vdots \\ -\beta_{HC} \tilde{N}_1 + \lambda & 0 & 0 & \cdots & \beta_{HC} \tilde{N}_m - \lambda \end{pmatrix},
$$

with $\tilde{N}_j = N_j/\gamma$ and $\beta_{HC} = \beta_H - \beta_C$. Expanding the determinant,

$$
f(\lambda) = (\beta_H \tilde{N}_1 - \lambda) \prod_{i=2}^{m} (\beta_{HC} \tilde{N}_i - \lambda) + \beta_C \tilde{N}_2 (\beta_{HC} \tilde{N}_1 - \lambda) \prod_{i=3}^{m} (\beta_{HC} \tilde{N}_i - \lambda)
$$

$$
+ \cdots + \beta_C \tilde{N}_m (\beta_{HC} \tilde{N}_1 - \lambda) \prod_{i=2}^{m-1} (\beta_{HC} \tilde{N}_i - \lambda)
$$

$$
= \left(\prod_{i=1}^{m} (\beta_{HC} \tilde{N}_i - \lambda) \right) \left[\frac{\beta_H \tilde{N}_1 - \lambda}{\beta_{HC} \tilde{N}_1 - \lambda} + \sum_{i=2}^{m} \frac{\beta_C \tilde{N}_i}{\beta_{HC} \tilde{N}_i - \lambda} \right]
$$

$$
= \left(\prod_{i=1}^{m} (\beta_{HC} \tilde{N}_i - \lambda) \right) \left[1 + \sum_{i=1}^{m} \frac{\beta_C \tilde{N}_i}{\beta_{HC} \tilde{N}_i - \lambda} \right]. \tag{3.5.11}
$$

This expression is a polynomial of degree m in λ; we require the largest λ solving $f(\lambda) = 0$. By inspection we see that the m-fold product is finite and non-zero for $\lambda > \max_i \beta_{HC} \tilde{N}_i$, so any zero of the second factor in that region is a candidate for R_0. Now this second factor is strictly increasing in λ for $\max_i \beta_{HC} \tilde{N}_i < \lambda < \infty$, ranging from $-\infty$ at the left-hand end of this semi-infinite interval to $+1$ at $+\infty$, so

$$1 + \sum_{i=1}^{m} \frac{\beta_C \tilde{N}_i}{\beta_{HC} \tilde{N}_i - \lambda} \tag{3.5.12}$$

has exactly one zero there. Therefore R_0 equals this zero, i.e.

$$1 = \sum_{i=1}^{m} \frac{\beta_C \tilde{N}_i}{R_0 - \beta_{HC} \tilde{N}_i} \quad \text{where} \quad R_0 > \beta_{HC} \max_i \tilde{N}_i. \tag{3.5.13}$$

Each term on the right-hand side of (3.5.13) is increasing and convex in $\tilde{N}_i$, so by Jensen's inequality

$$1 \geq \frac{m \beta_C \overline{N}/\gamma}{R_0 - \beta_{HC} \overline{N}/\gamma}, \tag{3.5.14}$$

where $\overline{N} = \sum_{i=1}^{m} N_i/m$; equality holds if and only if either $\beta_H = \beta_C$ or $\tilde{N}_i = \tilde{N}_1$ (all i). Hence, when $\gamma \gg \beta_H \geq \beta_C$,

$$R_0 \geq [\beta_H + (m-1)\beta_C]\overline{N}/\gamma, \tag{3.5.15}$$

with equality holding as for (3.5.14).

When the β_{ij} and γ_j have the structure of this Example but without the condition $\gamma \gg \max(\beta_C, \beta_H)$, the approximation given in (3.5.8) should not be used. In place of $f(\lambda) = \det(\mathbf{M}_1 - \lambda I)$, we must instead identify R_0 with the largest root of $\det(\mathbf{M} - \lambda I) = 0$. Exercise 3.10 details the changes to (3.5.13–15) that then ensue. For example, if $\beta_H = 1 = \gamma$, $\beta_C = 0.001$, $m = 101$ and all $N_i = N_1$, (3.5.15) used as an approximation gives $R_0 \approx 1.1N_1$ whereas the analysis in Exercise 3.10 gives $R_0 = 0.600N_1$.

We also emphasize that the discussion and example above are based on the assumption that *all* components N_j of $\mathbf{N}$ are 'large'. To illustrate what may happen when this assumption is false, suppose that $\beta_H = 100$, $\beta_C = 0.0001$, and the other parameters are those just considered. Using Exercise 3.10 yields $R_0 \approx 1.0001N_1$, which we interpret as N_1 new infectives within the household containing the initial infective, with only a small expected number of infectives in other households. Because the household sizes are small, the disease must be propagated *outside* the household of the initial infective for a major outbreak to occur. The expected number of such outside contacts is at most about $0.01N_1$ per infective per generation, as against about N_1 infectives produced within the household of any such infective. So in two generations there may be up to about $0.01N_1^2$ outside infectives produced per initial infective, corresponding to $0.1N_1$ new infectives per generation. Consequently, until N_1 is about 10 or more, no major outbreak can be expected (see also Exercise 3.11), contrary to the interpretation that follows from Theorem 3.2 when $R_0 > 1$ which holds for all $N_1 \geq 2$. This contradiction stems from assuming that all N_j are large. Fortunately we can rework the analysis on the basis of distinguishing newly infected individuals, not by the stratum or household to which they belong, but by the number of susceptible individuals in the same household who remain susceptible after the initial infective is removed, before the influence of any secondary infectives.

Example 3.5.2 (*A community of m households*). Assume the model of the previous example, where the strata are now households. Suppose a given infective is initially in a household with i susceptibles, and call it an i-type infective. Assume that the initial infective is infectious for a time T, and that during this infectious period, only the initial infective can make susceptibles infectious. At the end of this infectious period, identify each of the individuals now infected by the number j of susceptibles remaining in its household. Then the probability that j susceptibles remain in the household of the initial infective at the end of the random time T is $P_{ij}(\beta_H)$, where

$$P_{ij}(\beta) = \left[\prod_{r=j+1}^{i} \frac{r\beta}{r\beta + \gamma} \right] \frac{\gamma}{j\beta + \gamma} \qquad (3.5.16)$$

(see Exercise 3.11). For any other household where there are initially i susceptibles, the probability that j susceptibles remain after the random time T is $P_{ij}(\beta_C)$. Regard the household of the initial infective as being additional to the initial population of $\mathbf{N}$ susceptibles as described; then the expected number m_{ij} of j-type infectives produced by this initial i-type infective is given by

$$m_{ij} = (i-j)_+ P_{ij}(\beta_H) + \sum_{r=1}^{m} (N_r - j)_+ P_{N_r j}(\beta_C) \equiv (i-j)_+ p_{ij}^H + m_j \quad (3.5.17)$$

say. Define $\mathbf{M} = (m_{ij})$. Then using the same argument as above (3.5.8), the expected number of second generation k-type infectives (i.e. infectives in households with k susceptibles) equals the (i,k)th element of $\mathbf{M}^2$. We conclude that, with $n' = \max_{1 \leq r \leq m}(N_r - 1)$, the Basic Reproduction Ratio R_0 for the process is the largest eigenvalue of the $(n'+1) \times (n'+1)$ matrix

$$
\mathbf{M} = \begin{pmatrix}
m_0 & m_1 & m_2 & \cdots & m_{n'} \\
p_{10}^H + m_0 & m_1 & m_2 & \cdots & m_{n'} \\
2p_{20}^H + m_0 & p_{21}^H + m_1 & m_2 & \cdots & m_{n'} \\
\vdots & \vdots & \vdots & \ddots & \vdots \\
i'p_{n'0}^H + m_0 & (n'-1)p_{n'1}^H + m_1 & (n'-2)p_{n'2}^H + m_2 & \cdots & m_{n'}
\end{pmatrix}.
$$
$$(3.5.18)$$

Explicit computation of this eigenvalue does not appear possible in general. We can compute the limiting value of R_0 when $\beta_H \gg \gamma$ because then $p_{ij}^H \approx \delta_{j0}$ and R_0 is the largest root of $f_c(\lambda) = 0$, where

$$
f_c(\lambda) = \det \begin{pmatrix}
m_0 - \lambda & m_1 & m_2 & \cdots & m_{n'} \\
1 + m_0 & m_1 - \lambda & m_2 & \cdots & m_{n'} \\
2 + m_0 & m_1 & m_2 - \lambda & \cdots & m_{n'} \\
\vdots & \vdots & \vdots & \ddots & \vdots \\
n' + m_0 & m_1 & m_2 & \cdots & m_{n'} - \lambda
\end{pmatrix}
$$

$$
= \det \begin{pmatrix}
m_0 - \lambda & m_1 & m_2 & \cdots & m_{n'} \\
1 + \lambda & -\lambda & 0 & \cdots & 0 \\
2 + \lambda & 0 & -\lambda & \cdots & 0 \\
\vdots & \vdots & \vdots & \ddots & \vdots \\
n' + \lambda & 0 & 0 & \cdots & -\lambda
\end{pmatrix}
$$

$$
= (-\lambda)^{n'-1}\left(\lambda^2 - \lambda \sum_{j=0}^{n'} m_j - \sum_{j=1}^{n'} j m_j\right)
$$

$$
\equiv (-\lambda)^{n'-1}(\lambda^2 - \lambda A - B), \qquad \text{say.} \tag{3.5.19}
$$

Thus, when $\beta_H \gg \gamma$,

$$
R_0 \approx \tfrac{1}{2}\left(A + \sqrt{A^2 + 4B}\right). \tag{3.5.20}
$$

The expressions for A and B implied by (3.5.19) reduce to

$$
A = \frac{\sum_{i=1}^m N_i \beta_C}{\gamma + \beta_C}, \qquad B = \frac{\sum_{i=1}^m N_i(N_i - 1)\beta_C \gamma}{(\gamma + \beta_C)(\gamma + 2\beta_C)}, \tag{3.5.21}
$$

because

$$
A = \sum_{j=1}^{n'} m_j = \sum_{i=1}^m \sum_{j=0}^{n'} (N_i - j)_+ P_{N_i j}(\beta_C),
$$

where terms in the inner summation are zero for $j \geq N_i$, and the inner sum equals the expected number of infectives in a given household of N_i

susceptibles produced by a single infective outside the household. Introduce N_i identically distributed indicator r.v.s I_k ($k = 1, \ldots, N_i$) to denote that the kth susceptible in the household is infected. Then $\mathrm{E}I_k$ is just the probability that this kth individual is infected before the initial infective becomes a removal, so $\mathrm{E}I_k = \beta_C/(\gamma + \beta_C)$, and the expression for A follows. Similarly,

$$B = \sum_{i=1}^{m} \sum_{j=1}^{n'} j(N_i - j)_+ P_{N_i j}(\beta_C),$$

in which the inner sum is expressible in terms of the same indicator r.v.s as

$$\mathrm{E}\left[\sum_{k'=1}^{N_i} (1 - I_{k'}') \sum_{k=1}^{N_i} I_k \right] = N_i^2 \mathrm{E}(I_k) - N_i \mathrm{E}(I_k I_k) - N_i(N_i - 1)\mathrm{E}(I_{k'} I_k)$$

where $k \neq k'$. Using properties of exponential r.v.s, we see that $\mathrm{E}(I_{k'} I_k) = 2\beta_C \beta_C/[(\gamma + 2\beta_C)(\gamma + \beta_C)]$. Collecting terms together then leads to (3.5.21).

To illustrate the relevance of the assumption that $\beta_H \gg \gamma$, suppose that $\beta_H = 1 = \gamma$, $\beta_C = 0.001$, $m = 100$, $N_i = N_1 = 3$ (cf. the example in the text below (3.5.15) where we should have $R_0 = 1.8$ from Exercise 3.10). Then from (3.5.18), $\det(\mathbf{M} - \lambda I) = 0$ is a cubic equation, with largest root $R_0 = 0.7864$, whereas the approximation at (3.5.20) which depends on $\beta_H \gg \gamma$, gives $R_0 \approx 0.9369$. The same approximate R_0 holds on changing β_H to 3, but the corresponding exact root 0.8992 is closer to it, and closer still ($R_0 = 0.9318$) for $\beta_H = 9$. See Ball, Mollison and Scalia-Tomba (1997) for related work.

3.6   The carrier-borne epidemic

Suppose that a population of $X(t)$ susceptibles of initial size n is being infected by $W(t)$ carriers of a disease with $W(0) = b$, who are themselves immune to infection but subject to a pure death process. Any infected susceptible is directly removed from the population. Then the stochastic process $X(t)$ is subject to the influence of the process $W(t)$ which is independent of $X(t)$.

Let the death process $\{W(t) : t \geq 0\}$ be a homogeneous Markov chain in continuous time with death rate γ; then we know that its p.g.f. is

$$\mathrm{E}(v^{W(t)}) = (ve^{-\gamma t} + 1 - e^{-\gamma t})^b \qquad (|v| \leq 1), \qquad (3.6.1)$$

so that

$$\Pr\{W(t) = k \mid W(0) = b\} = \binom{b}{k}e^{-\gamma kt}(1 - e^{-\gamma t})^{b-k},$$

and

$$E[W(t) \mid W(0) = b] = be^{-\gamma t} = w(t)$$

where $w(t)$ is as in the deterministic carrier model of Section 2.6.

To analyse the process $\{X(t) : t \geq 0\}$, assume that $\{(X, W)(t) : t \geq 0\}$ is a bivariate Markov chain with transition probabilities

$$\Pr\{(X, W)(t + \delta t) = (i - 1, k) \mid (X, W)(t) = (i, k)\} = \beta ik\, \delta t + o(\delta t),$$
$$\Pr\{(X, W)(t + \delta t) = (i, k - 1) \mid (X, W)(t) = (i, k)\} = \gamma k\, \delta t + o(\delta t),$$
$$\Pr\{(X, W)(t + \delta t) = (i, k) \mid (X, W)(t) = (i, k)\} = 1 - (\beta i + \gamma)k\, \delta t - o(\delta t).$$

The forward Kolmogorov equations for the process are given for $0 \leq i \leq n$, $0 \leq k \leq b$, by

$$\frac{\mathrm{d}p_{ik}}{\mathrm{d}t} = \beta(i + 1)kp_{i+1,k} - (\beta i + \gamma)kp_{ik} + \gamma(k + 1)p_{i,k+1}$$

subject to the initial condition $p_{nb}(0) = 1$, where

$$p_{ik}(t) = \Pr\{(X, W)(t) = (i, k) \mid (X, W)(0) = (n, b)\},$$

and $p_{n+1,k} = p_{i,b+1} = 0$ when either i or k lies outside its respective range. Use the same transformation $t' = \beta t$ as at (3.2.2), and set $\rho = \gamma/\beta$. Then for $0 \leq i \leq n$, $0 \leq k \leq b$, the forward Kolmogorov equations become

$$\frac{\mathrm{d}p_{ik}}{\mathrm{d}t'} = (i + 1)kp_{i+1,k} - (i + \rho)kp_{ik} + \rho(k + 1)p_{i,k+1} \qquad (3.6.2)$$

with the initial condition $p_{nb}(0) = 1$. For convenience, we use t below for this new t'.

We discuss two methods for solving this equation: the first is the p.g.f. method discussed earlier, while the second is based on a method of Puri (1975) for a Markov process developing under the influence of another process. Such a process could be described as a doubly stochastic Markov process by analogy with the previously named doubly stochastic Poisson process.

Referring to (3.6.2) we derive for the p.g.f.

$$\varphi(z,v,t) \equiv \mathrm{E}(z^{X(t)}v^{W(t)}) = \sum_{0 \le i \le n, 0 \le k \le b} p_{ik}(t)z^i v^k \quad (0 \le z, v \le 1),$$

the p.d.e.

$$\frac{\partial \varphi}{\partial t} = (1-z)v\frac{\partial^2 \varphi}{\partial z\,\partial v} + \rho(1-v)\frac{\partial \varphi}{\partial v}, \tag{3.6.3}$$

subject to the initial condition $\varphi(z,v,0) = z^n v^b$.

To solve this equation, assume that $\varphi(z,v,t) = Z(z)V(v)T(t)$ and use the standard method of separation of variables. Then from (3.6.3) we have, writing $\dot{T} = dT/dt$, $Z' = dZ/dz$ and $V' = dV/dv$,

$$\frac{\dot{T}}{T} = (1-z)v\frac{Z'}{Z}\frac{V'}{V} + \rho(1-v)\frac{V'}{V} = -\lambda \tag{3.6.4}$$

so that $T = e^{-\lambda t}$ directly. We also see that

$$(1-z)\frac{Z'}{Z} = -\frac{\rho(1-v)}{v} - \frac{\lambda V}{vV'} = -j, \tag{3.6.5}$$

where j is a quantity that we discuss shortly. These relations lead to

$$\frac{Z'}{Z} = \frac{-j}{1-z}, \qquad \frac{V'}{V} = \frac{\lambda}{v(j+\rho)-\rho},$$

so that, apart from constants,

$$Z = (1-z)^j, \qquad V = \left(v - \frac{\rho}{j+\rho}\right)^{\lambda/(j+\rho)}.$$

Now we know that $\varphi(z,v,t)$ must be a polynomial in z and v, of degree n in z and b in v. Hence j must be an integer in the range $0 \le j \le n$, and so too must $0 \le \lambda/(j+\rho) \le b$. Corresponding to a particular value of j, the eigenvalue λ_j will be

$$\lambda_j = k(j+\rho) \quad (k = 0, 1, \ldots, b).$$

It follows that

$$\varphi(z,v,t) = \sum_{j=0}^{n}\sum_{k=0}^{b} c_{jk}e^{-k(j+\rho)t}(1-z)^j\left(v - \frac{\rho}{j+\rho}\right)^k, \tag{3.6.6}$$

where we now need to find the values of the coefficients c_{jk}. We do this by setting $t = 0$, when

$$\varphi(z, v, 0) = z^n v^b = \sum_{j=0}^{n} \sum_{k=0}^{b} c_{jk}(1-z)^j \left(v - \frac{\rho}{j+\rho}\right)^k.$$

Writing $\zeta = 1 - z$, $\eta = v - \rho/(j+\rho)$, this reduces to

$$(1-\zeta)^n \left(\eta + \frac{\rho}{j+\rho}\right)^b = \sum_{j=0}^{n} \sum_{k=0}^{b} c_{jk}\zeta^j \eta^k,$$

whence c_{jk}, being the coefficient of $\zeta^j \eta^k$ in the expansion of the left-hand side, can be identified as

$$c_{jk} = (-1)^j \binom{n}{j} \left(\frac{\rho}{j+\rho}\right)^{bk} \binom{b}{k}, \tag{3.6.7}$$

and

$$\varphi(z, v, t) = \sum_{j=0}^{n} (z-1)^j \binom{n}{j} \sum_{k=0}^{b} \left(\frac{\rho}{j+\rho}\right)^{b-k} \binom{b}{k} e^{-k(j+\rho)t} \left(v - \frac{\rho}{j+\rho}\right)^k$$

$$= \sum_{j=0}^{n} (z-1)^j \binom{n}{j} \left[\frac{\rho}{j+\rho} + \left(v - \frac{\rho}{j+\rho}\right)e^{-(j+\rho)t}\right]^b. \tag{3.6.8}$$

It is easily checked that for $z = 1$ we recover $\varphi(1, v, t) = \left[1 + (v-1)e^{-\rho t}\right]^b$, i.e. the p.g.f. (3.4.1) of the pure death process $W(t)$, following the change in time parameter at (3.2.2).

The joint distribution of $(X, W)(t)$ for any $t \geq 0$ can be found by expanding (3.6.8). Perhaps more important is the distribution of $X(t)$ whose p.g.f. equals

$$\varphi(z, 1, t) = \sum_{i=0}^{n} (z-1)^i \binom{n}{i} \left[\frac{\rho}{i+\rho} + \frac{i}{i+\rho} e^{-(i+\rho)t}\right]^b. \tag{3.6.9}$$

It follows that

$$p_i.(t) \equiv \Pr\{X(t) = i \mid X(0) = n\} = \sum_{j=i}^{n} (-1)^{j-i} \binom{n}{j} \binom{j}{i} \left[\frac{\rho + je^{-(j+\rho)t}}{\rho+j}\right]^b$$

$$= \binom{n}{i} \sum_{j=i}^{n} (-1)^{j-i} \binom{n-i}{j-i} \left[\frac{\rho + je^{-(j+\rho)t}}{\rho+j}\right]^b, \tag{3.6.10}$$

and

$$E[X(t)] = \frac{\partial \varphi(z,1,t)}{\partial z}\bigg|_{z=1} = n\left(\frac{\rho + e^{-(\rho+1)t}}{\rho+1}\right)^b. \qquad (3.6.11)$$

For the deterministic model of Section 2.6 the analogous function is $x(t)$, given at (2.5.4). Rewrite it, after changing the time-parameter to make it consistent with the notation used in this section, as

$$x(t) = n\left[\exp\left(-\frac{1-e^{-\rho t}}{\rho}\right)\right]^b.$$

Then

$$\lim_{t\to\infty} x(t) = ne^{-b/\rho} < n\left(1+\frac{1}{\rho}\right)^{-b} = \lim_{t\to\infty} E[X(t)],$$

where the inequality, a trivial consequence of $e^{1/\rho} > 1 + 1/\rho$, shows that the expected ultimate size of the stochastic epidemic is smaller than the ultimate size of the deterministic epidemic. More precisely, we can show that $\lim_{t\to\infty} (E[X(t)] - x(t)]) \approx b/2\rho^2$, which is $o(1)$ for small to moderate integers b and somewhat larger integers ρ. See Exercise 3.12 for more detail.

As in the case of earlier models, we are interested in the number of initial susceptibles that are ultimately infected. For this, we can readily obtain the probabilities $P_k \equiv \lim_{t\to\infty} p_{n-k,\cdot}(t)$ of the size k of the epidemic from (3.6.10), namely

$$P_k = \binom{n}{k} \sum_{j=n-k}^{n} (-1)^{j-n+k} \binom{k}{j-n+k} \left(\frac{\rho}{\rho+j}\right)^b$$

$$= \binom{n}{k} \sum_{i=0}^{k} (-1)^i \binom{k}{i} \left[\frac{\rho}{\rho+i+n-k}\right]^b \qquad (0 \le k \le n). \qquad (3.6.12)$$

Let T be the duration of the epidemic and F its d.f. Then $F(t) = \Pr\{\text{no further infection after } t\}$ is given by

$$F(t) = p_{0\cdot}(t) + p_{\cdot 0}(t) - p_{00}(t),$$

where the terms on the right-hand side can be determined algebraically from (3.6.10), (3.6.1) and (3.6.8), respectively. Hence,

$$F(t) = \sum_{j=0}^{n} (-1)^j \binom{n}{j} \left(\left[\frac{\rho+je^{-(j+\rho)t}}{\rho+j}\right]^b - \left[\frac{\rho(1-e^{-(j+\rho)t})}{\rho+j}\right]^b\right) + (1-e^{-\rho t})^b.$$

$$(3.6.13)$$

In the particular case $b = 1$ this expression simplifies and yields for example

$$E(T \mid W(0) = 1) = \int_0^\infty [1 - F(u)] \, du = \frac{1}{\rho} - \sum_{j=0}^n \binom{n}{j} \frac{(-1)^j}{\rho + j}$$

$$= \int_0^\infty \left[e^{-\rho t} - \sum_{j=0}^n (-1)^j \binom{n}{j} e^{-(j+\rho)t} \right] dt$$

$$= \frac{1}{\rho} - \int_0^\infty e^{-\rho t}(1 - e^{-t})^n \, dt = \frac{1}{\rho} - \int_0^1 v^{\rho-1}(1 - v)^n \, dv$$

$$= \frac{1}{\rho}\left[1 - \frac{n!}{(\rho + 1)\cdots(\rho + n)} \right]$$

(Bailey, 1975, p. 196). For integers $b \geq 2$, the complete beta integral here is replaced by one or more incomplete beta integrals that can no longer be simplified.

The following, alternative approach, due to Puri (1975), relies on the observation that, conditional on $W(\cdot)$, $X(t)$ is itself a pure death process with the random, time-varying death-rate parameter $\beta W(\cdot)$. This implies (e.g. Kendall, 1948) that

$$E\big(z^{X(t)} \mid \{W(u) : 0 \leq u < t\}\big) = \big(ze^{-\widetilde{W}(t)} + 1 - e^{-\widetilde{W}(t)}\big)^n, \qquad (3.6.14)$$

where $\widetilde{W}(t) = \int_0^t W(u) \, du$, the initial condition $(X, W)(0) = (n, b)$ being understood. Expanding (3.6.14) and taking expectations yields the p.g.f.

$$E(z^{X(t)}) = \sum_{j=0}^n \binom{n}{j}(z - 1)^j E\big(e^{-j\widetilde{W}(t)}\big). \qquad (3.6.15)$$

The problem now is to evaluate the expectations on the right-hand side. This can be done via the joint Laplace transform of the bivariate Markovian process $(W(t), \widetilde{W}(t))$,

$$\hat{\Pi}(v, \theta, t) \equiv E(v^{W(t)} e^{-\theta \widetilde{W}(t)}) \qquad (|v| \leq 1, \ \mathrm{Re}(\theta) \geq 0),$$

for which the corresponding probability terms are

$$q_{bk}(u, t) = \Pr\{W(t) = k, \widetilde{W}(t) \leq u \mid W(0) = b\}.$$

The forward Kolmogorov equations for these functions q_{bk} are easily derived because $\{W(t) : t \geq 0\}$ is a pure death process: we find

$$\frac{\partial q_{bk}(u, t)}{\partial t} + k\frac{\partial q_{bk}(u, t)}{\partial u} = -\rho k q_{bk} + \rho(k + 1)q_{b,k+1}, \qquad (3.6.16)$$

with $q_{kk}(u, 0) = 1$ (all $u > 0$). Now

$$\hat{\Pi}(v, \theta, t) = \int_0^\infty e^{-\theta u} \frac{\partial \Pi(v, u, t)}{\partial u} \, du,$$

subject to $\hat{\Pi}(v, \theta, 0) = v^b$. Taking Laplace transforms, equations (3.6.16) become

$$\frac{1}{\theta} \frac{\partial \hat{\Pi}}{\partial t} + v \frac{\partial \hat{\Pi}}{\partial v} = -\frac{\rho}{\theta} v \frac{\partial \hat{\Pi}}{\partial v} + \frac{\rho}{\theta} \frac{\partial \hat{\Pi}}{\partial v}$$

or

$$\frac{\partial \hat{\Pi}}{\partial t} = [(\theta + \rho)v - \rho] \frac{\partial \hat{\Pi}}{\partial v}. \tag{3.6.17}$$

This equation can be solved by using Lagrange's method: write

$$\frac{dt}{1} = \frac{dv}{(\theta + \rho)v - \rho} = \frac{d\theta}{0} = \frac{d\hat{\Pi}}{0},$$

whence

$$\ln\left((\theta + v)\rho - \rho\right) = (\theta + \rho)t + A, \qquad \hat{\Pi} = B,$$

where A and B are constants. It follows that

$$\hat{\Pi}(v, \theta, t) = f\left(e^{-(\theta+v)t}[(\theta + \rho)v - \rho]\right), \tag{3.6.18}$$

subject to $\hat{\Pi}(v, \theta, 0) = v^b$, i.e. $v^b = f([\theta + \rho]v - \rho)$, so

$$f(\xi) = \left(\frac{\xi + \rho}{\theta + \rho}\right)^b.$$

This gives

$$\hat{\Pi}(v, \theta, t) = \left(ve^{-(\theta+\rho)t} + \frac{\rho(1 - e^{-(\theta+\rho)t})}{\theta + \rho}\right)^b. \tag{3.6.19}$$

Setting $\theta = j$ for $j = 0, \ldots, n$ and combining the resulting expressions as in (3.6.15), we recover (3.6.8).

Other examples exploiting this method can be found in Puri (1975).

3.7 Exercises and Complements to Chapter 3

3.1 The analogue of t_j at (3.1.3) in the deterministic simple epidemic is the solution t'_j of the equation (cf. (2.1.2)) $x(t'_j) = j - 1$, equivalently, $y(t'_j) = N + I + 1 - j$. Show that

$$t'_j = \frac{1}{\beta(N + I)} \ln \frac{N(N + I + 1 - j)}{I(j - 1)},$$

and hence deduce that when $I \geq 2$,

$$\mathrm{E}t_j - t'_j = \frac{1}{\beta(N+I)} \ln[(1 + (N + I - 1 + j)^{-1})(1 - I^{-1})] - \gamma_{N,I,j}$$

where $\gamma_{N,I,j}$ is defined below (3.1.4). This quantity is negative, and is sometimes called the *stochastic lag*. An alternative derivation entails the use of the approximation $\sum_{i=j}^{N} i^{-1} \approx \int_{j-\frac{1}{2}}^{N+\frac{1}{2}} u^{-1}\,du$.

3.2 Show that in the special case of a simple stochastic epidemic starting with one infective introduced into a population of N susceptibles, the first two moments $\mathrm{E}t_1$ and $\mathrm{var}\,t_1$ of the duration t_1 of the process in Section 3.1 are related by

$$\mathrm{var}\,t_1 = \frac{1}{\beta^2(N+1)^2} \sum_{i=1}^{N} \left[\frac{1}{i} + \frac{1}{N+1-i}\right]^2 = \frac{2\beta\,\mathrm{E}t_1 + \frac{1}{3}\pi^2 + O(N^{-1})}{\beta^2(N+1)^2}.$$

Observe that $\mathrm{var}\,t_1/(\mathrm{E}t_1)^2 = [1/(N \ln N)](1 + o(1))$ for large N.

3.3 (a) Check that for real s, the gamma function

$$\Gamma(1 - is) = \int_0^{\infty} e^{-y} y^{-is}\,dy = \int_{-\infty}^{\infty} e^{isx} \exp(-x - e^{-x})\,dx,$$

is the characteristic function of the extreme value distribution with p.d.f. $\exp(-x - e^{-x})$. Hence deduce that the asymptotic distribution of W at (3.1.18), having for its Laplace–Stieltjes transform the product of two gamma functions, is the convolution of two extreme value density functions:

$$\Pr\{W \in (w, w + dw)\} = \int_{-\infty}^{\infty} \exp(-v - e^{-v}) \exp[-(w - v) - e^{-(w-v)}]\,dv\,dw,$$

which reduces to the density at (3.1.21) (Kendall, 1957).

(b) To explain why the extreme value distribution occurs in the limit distribution for the duration t_1 of the simple stochastic epidemic of Section 3.1, take N even, $N = 2M$ say, with $I = 1$ and show that t_1 is expressible as the sum $U_1 + U_2$ of i.i.d. r.v.s $U_k =_d \sum_{i=1}^{M} S_i/[i(2M + 1 - i)]$ $(k = 1, 2)$, where $S_1, S_2, \ldots$ are i.i.d. unit exponential r.v.s. Deduce that each U_k lies between U'/M and $U'/(2M)$, where U' is the r.v. $U' \equiv \sum_{i=1}^{M} S_i/i$. Show that $U' =_d \max_{i=1}^{M}\{S_i\}$, and that $(M + 1)U_k - \ln M$ and $(M + 1)U' - \ln M$ both converge weakly to the same limit r.v. with the extreme value density of (a). (See Kendall's paper for details.)

3.4 (See also Example 3.3.1.) For the general stochastic epidemic model of Section 3.3 starting from $(N, I) = (1, 1)$, and assuming that $\beta \neq \gamma, 2\gamma$, use direct d.e. solution methods to solve the equations $\dot{p}_{11} = -(\beta + \gamma)p_{11}$, $\dot{p}_{10} = \gamma p_{11}$, $\dot{p}_{02} = \beta p_{11} - 2\gamma p_{02}$, $\dot{p}_{01} = 2\gamma p_{02} - \gamma p_{01}$, $\dot{p}_{00} = \gamma p_{01}$. For example, show that

$$p_{10}(t) = \frac{\gamma(1 - e^{-(\beta+\gamma)t})}{\beta + \gamma}, \qquad p_{00}(t) = \frac{\beta}{\beta + \gamma} - e^{-\gamma t}\left[2 - \frac{\beta e^{-\gamma t}}{\beta - \gamma} + \frac{2\gamma^2 e^{-\beta t}}{\beta^2 - \gamma^2}\right].$$

3.5 (Cf. Section 3.3.2 and Figure 2.4.) In a linear birth-and-death process $\{Y(t) : t \geq 0\}$ with birth and death rates λ and μ per individual, where $\lambda > \mu$ and $Y(0) = I$, suppose that at time t there are $Y_j(t)$ jth generation live descendants of the original I individuals and $Z_j(t)$ jth generation descendants no longer living (cf. Section 2.5). Show that the expected numbers $y_j(t) = EY_j(t)$ and $z_j(t) = EZ_j(t)$ satisfy the system of d.e.s

$$\dot{y}_j = \lambda y_{j-1} - \mu y_j, \qquad \dot{z}_j = \mu y_j \qquad (j = 0, 1, \ldots),$$

provided we set $y_{-1}(t) \equiv 0$. Deduce the solution

$$y_j(t) = I e^{-\mu t}\frac{(\lambda t)^j}{j!}, \qquad z_j(t) = \mu I \int_0^t e^{-\mu u}\frac{(\lambda u)^j}{j!}\,du, \qquad (j = 0, 1, \ldots),$$

so that $m(t)$, the 'average' generation number of the $\{z_j(t)\}$, is given by (cf. Figure 2.4)

$$m(t) = \frac{\lambda t}{1 - e^{-(\lambda-\mu)t}} - \frac{\lambda}{\lambda - \mu}.$$

Waugh (1958) proved that a super-critical linear birth-and-death process conditional on ultimate extinction, behaves like the birth-and-death process with birth and death rates interchanged, and so is sub-critical. Use this result to show that

$$E\left(\sum_j Z_j(u)\mid Y(t) \to 0\ (t \to \infty)\right) = \frac{\lambda I(1 - e^{-(\lambda-\mu)u})}{\lambda - \mu},$$

$$E\left(\sum_j jZ_j(u)\mid Y(t) \to 0\ (t \to \infty)\right) = \frac{\lambda\mu I(1 - e^{-(\lambda-\mu)u}[1 - (\lambda - \mu)u])}{(\lambda - \mu)^2}.$$

Deduce that $\Pr\{Y(t) \to 0\} = (\mu/\lambda)^I$, so that for the non-extinction set $\{Y(t) \to \infty\}$, setting $r = \mu/\lambda$,

$$\frac{E\left[\sum_j jZ_j(u)\mid Y(t) \to \infty\ (t \to \infty)\right]}{E\left[\sum_j Z_j(u)\mid Y(t) \to \infty\ (t \to \infty)\right]}$$

$$= \frac{\lambda}{\lambda - \mu} \cdot \frac{[(\lambda - \mu)u - 1][e^{(\lambda-\mu)u} - r^I e^{-(\lambda-\mu)u}] + 1 - r^I}{e^{(\lambda-\mu)u} - r^{I-1}e^{-(\lambda-\mu)u} - 1 + r^{I-1}}.$$

3.6 For the general stochastic epidemic, show that the first passage time distribution into any state can be constructed as a weighted sum of convolutions of distributions of exponential r.v.s, where the components of the convolutions correspond to the sojourn times in the states visited along the paths and the weights are the respective probabilities of those paths.
[*Remark.* The same result holds true for any continuous time Markov process on countable state space with well-ordered sample paths and bounded transition rates. This algorithmic principle explains why the p.g.f. method is applicable to the simple and general stochastic epidemic models.]

3.7 Show that if j is a non-absorbing state in a Markov process with well-ordered sample paths, then $\pi_{ij} = q_j \int_0^\infty \Pr\{X(u) = j \mid X(0) = i\}\, du$ (cf. (3.4.8)). In particular, for the general stochastic epidemic as in Section 3.4.3,

$$p_{(i,j)} = (i\beta + \gamma)j \int_0^\infty \Pr\{(X,Y)(t) = (i,j) \mid (X,Y)(0) = (N,I)\}\, dt.$$

[*Remark.* This principle, complementary to the previous exercise, underlies the simplicity of the jump-chain algorithm for computing both intermediate and final state probabilities of strictly evolutionary Markov chain models.]

3.8 Using the same notation as at (3.4.10), show that the quantities

$$\tau_{ik}^{(2)} \equiv \mathrm{E}(t_{ik}^2 \mid X(0) = i, X(u) = k \text{ for some } u > 0),$$

starting from $\tau_{ii}^{(2)} = 0$, satisfy the recurrence relation

$$\pi_{ik}\tau_{ik}^{(2)} = \sum_{j:p_{jk}>0} \pi_{ij}p_{jk}(\tau_{ij}^{(2)} + 2\tau_{ij}/q_j + 2/q_j^2).$$

3.9 Let the $m \times m$ non-negative matrix A be primitive, and let the diagonal matrix D have all elements positive, much as in Section 2.4. Use Perron–Frobenius theory (e.g. Seneta, 1981, Chapter 1) as at Lemma 2 of Daley and Gani (1994) to show that
(i) the eigenvalue $\lambda_{\max}$ of $A - D$ that has largest real part, is real;
(ii) the eigenvalue $\mu_{\max}$ of AD^{-1} that has largest modulus, is real and positive;
(iii) $\lambda_{\max} <, = \text{ or } > 0$ according as $\mu_{\max} <, = \text{ or } > 1$, respectively.
Suppose that the pairwise infectious rates β_{ij} of Sections 2.4 and 3.5 have the product form $\beta_{ij} = \beta_i\alpha_j$ so that $\mathbf{B} = (\beta_{ij}) = \boldsymbol{\beta}\boldsymbol{\alpha}'$, where the vectors $\boldsymbol{\beta}$ and $\boldsymbol{\alpha}$ have components β_i denoting the infectivity rate of infectives in stratum i and relative susceptibility of susceptibles in stratum j. Show that when $\mathbf{M}_1$ at (3.5.6) is primitive, its largest eigenvalue is $R = \sum_i N_i\alpha_i\beta_i/\gamma_i$. When is it true that $R \approx R_0$, the Basic Reproduction Ratio for such an epidemic?

3.10 In the context of Example 3.5.1, with the β_{ij} as given there, show that the dominant eigenvalue R_0 of the $m \times m$ matrix $\mathbf{M}$ of (3.5.8), is as at (3.5.12) if we replace $\tilde{N}_i$ by N_i, β_{HC} by $\beta_H/(\beta_H + \gamma) - \beta_C/(\beta_C + \gamma)$ and β_C by $\beta_C/(\beta_C + \gamma)$. Deduce that when $N_j = N_1$ $(j = 2, \ldots, m)$ (cf. (3.5.13)),

$$R_0 = \frac{\{[(m-1)\beta_C + \beta_H]\gamma + m\beta_C\beta_H\}N_1}{(\beta_C + \gamma)(\beta_H + \gamma)}.$$

Check that this is smaller than the case of equality in (3.5.15), which approximates this expression if $\gamma \gg \max(\beta_C, \beta_H)$.

3.11 Derive (3.5.16) using the embedded jump technique of Section 3.4.2. Show that when $\beta \ll \gamma$, $P_{ij}(\beta) \approx (\beta/\gamma)^{i-j}(i!/j!)$. Use (3.5.20) to conclude that in the setting of Example 3.5.2, $R_0 \geq 1$ when $N_1^2 \geq 1/(m\beta_C/\gamma)$; this condition yields $N_1 \geq 4$ when $m = 100$ and $\beta_C = 0.001\gamma$, and $N_1 \geq 10$ when $m = 100$ and $\beta_C = 0.0001\gamma$ (cf. the text preceding Example 3.5.2).

3.12 Use the generating function (3.6.8) to show that for the stochastic carrier epidemic,

$$\mathrm{E}[X(t)W(t)] = \mathrm{E}[X(t)]\,\mathrm{E}[W(t)]\mathrm{e}^{-t}\left[1 - \frac{1 - \mathrm{e}^{-(1+\rho)t}}{1 + \rho}\right],$$

and deduce that $\mathrm{cov}(X(t), W(t)) < 0$ for $0 < t < \infty$. Use (3.6.11) to conclude that $(\mathrm{d}/\mathrm{d}t)\mathrm{E}[X(t)] = -\mathrm{E}[X(t)\,W(t)] > -\mathrm{E}[X(t)]\,\mathrm{E}[W(t)]$. Hence, since $\mathrm{E}[W(t)] = w(t)$ (see below (3.6.1)), conclude that for the deterministic and stochastic carrier models, the inequality

$$\frac{\mathrm{d}}{\mathrm{d}t}(x(t) - \mathrm{E}[X(t)]) < (x(t) - \mathrm{E}[X(t)])w(t)$$

is satisfied. Since $(X, W)(0) = (x, w)(0)$, the right-hand side is zero at $t = 0$ and thus is negative for all sufficiently small positive t, hence negative for all finite positive t, and therefore

$$0 < \mathrm{E}[X(t)] - x(t) \uparrow n[(1 + \rho^{-1})^{-b} - \mathrm{e}^{-b/\rho}] \qquad (0 < t \uparrow \infty).$$

[*Remark.* Alternatively, differentiation shows that when $b = 1$, $\mathrm{E}[X(t)] - x(t)$ is monotonic in t; hence $\mathrm{E}[X(t)] > x(t)$ (all t) for all positive integers b. The covariance inequality is what we should expect intuitively, namely that larger-than-average numbers of carriers should result in smaller-than-average numbers of susceptibles.]

3.13 For a deterministic version of a super-critical general epidemic starting from $(x, y)(0) = (N, 1)$, use Kendall's approach as around equation (2.3.17) to determine an approximate duration time t_∞ by $t_\infty = \inf\{t > 0 : y(t) = 1\}$. Then find $x' = x(\frac{1}{3}t_\infty)$ and $x'' = x(\frac{2}{3}t_\infty)$. Simulate the general stochastic epidemic starting from $(X, Y)_0 = (N, 1)$, and restrict attention to those sample paths for which $X_\infty < x''$. Find empirically the distributions of the phases T', T'' and T''' defined by $T' = \inf\{t : X_t < x'\}$, $T' + T'' = \inf\{t : X_t < x''\}$ and $T' + T'' + T''' = \inf\{t : Y_t = 0\}$.

4

Stochastic Models in Discrete Time

To describe the spread of a disease whose infectious period is relatively short in comparison with the latent period, especially in smaller populations, it is convenient to use a discrete-time model with the latent period as the unit of time. There are two such 'classical' models, one tracing back to Reed and Frost in 1928 (Abbey, 1952) and the other to Greenwood (1931). Both entail sequences of random variables with binomial distributions, hence the term 'chain binomials'. The fact that they are Markov chains was not fully appreciated until the work of Gani and Jerwood (1971).

It should be apparent that in this setting it makes little sense to model a simple epidemic as we did at the start of Chapters 2 and 3; here the 'short' infectious period allows us to identify a class of 'former infectives' that are in fact removed. Any individual that becomes an infective, is thus infectious for exactly one unit of time. However, there can be mathematical reasons for considering such analogues, as for example in Daley and Gani (1999) (see also Section 4.6 below).

It becomes clear in this setting that there are successive generations of infectives. When the initial infectives are infectious around the same time, as is necessarily the case with a single initial infective, successive generations will not overlap in time. The success of the Kermack–McKendrick theory in modelling the spread of epidemics like measles realistically, can be attributed to the fact that there is a considerable number of smaller scale overlapping epidemics.

4.1   The Greenwood and Reed–Frost models

We use a discrete time unit that may be one or more days; when this unit can be viewed as the latent period, it models the time between 'generations' of infectives as in the measles data of En'ko (1889) in Exercise 1.3. Let the

numbers of susceptibles and infectives at time $t = 0, 1, \ldots$ in the population
be X_t and Y_t respectively, with $X_0 = x_0$ and $Y_0 = y_0 \geq 1$. Let p (for
some $p \in (0, 1)$) be the probability of contact between an infective and a
susceptible, the result of the contact being an infection with probability β
for some $\beta \in (0, 1)$. Let $q = 1 - p$ be the probability there is no such contact.
It is convenient to regard this contact as being instantaneous, so that the
infectious period is concentrated at the contact time t, for some integer t.
The probability that there is no infection due to any single infective is

$$1 - p + p(1 - \beta) = 1 - p\beta = \alpha \tag{4.1.1}$$

say; after contact with the susceptibles, the Y_t infectives are identified and
so removed. Note that $X_t + Y_t = X_{t-1}$.

In the simplified Greenwood model (Greenwood, 1931), it is assumed
that the cause of infection is not related to the number of infectives so
that α can be regarded simply as the probability of non-infection. In this
case the number of infectives y_t at time t is determined by x_{t-1} and x_t as
$y_t = x_{t-1} - x_t$, and

$$
\begin{aligned}
p_{(x,y)_t,(x,y)_{t+1}} &\equiv \Pr\{(X,Y)_{t+1} = (x,y)_{t+1} \mid (X,Y)_t = (x,y)_t\} \\
&= \binom{x_t}{x_{t+1}} \alpha^{x_{t+1}} (1-\alpha)^{y_{t+1}} = \binom{x_t}{x_{t+1}} \alpha^{x_{t+1}} (1-\alpha)^{x_t - x_{t+1}}.
\end{aligned} \tag{4.1.2}
$$

Hence, $\{X_t : t = 0, 1, \ldots\}$ is a Markov chain, with $Y_{t+1} = X_t - X_{t+1}$.

In the Reed–Frost model, an individual susceptible at time t is still susceptible at time $t + 1$ only if contact with all Y_t infectives is avoided (more
pointedly, if *infectious* contact is avoided). This event has probability
α^{Y_t}, independently for each of the X_t individuals susceptible at t. Thus
$X_{t+1} = \mathrm{Bin}(X_t, \alpha^{Y_t})$, where $\mathrm{Bin}(n, \pi)$ denotes a r.v. with the binomial
distribution $\{\binom{n}{j} \pi^j (1 - \pi)^{n-j}, j = 0, \ldots, n\}$, and the matrix of one-step
transition probabilities has elements $p_{(x,y)_t,(x,y)_{t+1}}$ given by

$$p_{(x,y)_t,(x,y)_{t+1}} = \binom{x_t}{x_{t+1}} \alpha^{y_t x_{t+1}} (1 - \alpha^{y_t})^{y_{t+1}}. \tag{4.1.3}$$

It follows that a realization $(x,y)_0, (x,y)_1, \ldots, (x,y)_T$ of the epidemic, where
$y_T = 0 < y_{T-1}$, will have a 'chain binomial' probability of products of
the form (4.1.3). Here the y_t infectives behave independently, resulting in
a probability α^{y_t} of non-infection and $x_t = x_{t+1} + y_{t+1}$. The y_{t+1} new
infectives will now mix with the remaining x_{t+1} susceptibles at time $t + 1$

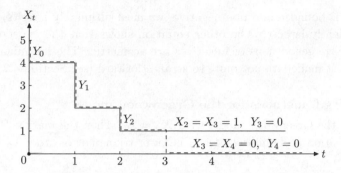

Figure 4.1. Two sample paths of an epidemic in discrete time, ending at $t = 3$ (——) and $t = 4$ (----) respectively.

before being removed, to produce the next generation y_{t+2} of new infectives at $t + 2$. Clearly

$$\{(X, Y)_{t+1} : t = 0, 1, \ldots\}$$

is a bivariate Markov chain with transition probabilities $p_{(x,y)_t,(x,y)_{t+1}}$ of the binomial form (4.1.3).

The least integer t for which $Y_t = 0$, when $X_t = X_{t-1}$ or for which $X_t = 0$, determines the time $T = t$ at which the epidemic terminates. For example, Figure 4.1 (copied from Figure 1.3) shows two possible realizations of a chain binomial process; in one of them, $Y_2 > 0 = Y_3$ so $T = 3$ and in the other, $Y_3 > 0 = Y_4$ so $T = 4$.

The probabilities in the Greenwood and Reed–Frost models are usually different, except for the case of households of two or three individuals with $y_0 = 1$ (see Table 4.2 for households of size four). Bailey (1975, Chapter 14) lists the probabilities for both models for household sizes of up to five individuals (i.e. for $x_0 + y_0 \leq 5$) with different initial y_0. These individually specified probabilities are the basis of Bailey's (1955) and Becker's (1989) work on inference for epidemic models (cf. also Chapter 6 below).

The fact that the numbers of infectives in successive generations of a chain binomial epidemic are determined from a binomial distribution, means that the expectations of these numbers are in principle readily computable. In particular, for a Greenwood model equation (4.1.2) yields $\mathrm{E}[X_{t+1} \mid X_t] = \alpha X_t$, so

$$\begin{aligned} \mathrm{E}[X_t \mid X_0 = x_0] &= \alpha^t x_0, \\ \mathrm{E}[Y_t \mid X_0 = x_0] &= \alpha^{t-1}(1 - \alpha)x_0. \end{aligned} \tag{4.1.4}$$

It follows from the first of these equations that $\mathrm{E}X_t \to 0$ as $t \to \infty$, so since X_t is bounded and non-negative, we must ultimately have $X_t = 0$ for all sufficiently large t. The other equation shows that the expected sizes of successive generations of infectives are geometric. The formulae for the Reed–Frost model are not quite so straightforward (see Section 4.2).

4.1.1 P.g.f. methods for the Greenwood model

Consider the Greenwood model with $X_0 = x_0$. Then the matrix P of one-step transition probabilities (4.1.2) is lower triangular of order $x_0 + 1$ and equals

$$
\begin{pmatrix}
1 & & & \cdots & \\
1-\alpha & \alpha & & \cdots & \\
(1-\alpha)^2 & 2(1-\alpha)\alpha & \alpha^2 & \cdots & \\
\vdots & \vdots & \vdots & \ddots & \vdots \\
(1-\alpha)^{x_0} & x_0(1-\alpha)^{x_0-1}\alpha & \binom{x_0}{2}(1-\alpha)^{x_0-2}\alpha^2 & \cdots & \alpha^{x_0}
\end{pmatrix}. \quad (4.1.5)
$$

We have already noted that when $0 < \alpha < 1$, $X_t = 0$ for sufficiently large t. However, from an epidemiological viewpoint we are interested in the first time T when there are no infectives, and in the number W of susceptibles who have been infected by then. Finding the joint distribution of (W, T) numerically is not difficult. Starting from $p_i^0 \equiv \Pr\{X_0 = i\} = \delta_{x_0 i}$, we have

$$
p_j^t \equiv \Pr\{X_t = j, Y_t > 0\} = \sum_{i=j+1}^{x_0 - (t-1)} p_i^{t-1} p_{ij}, \quad (4.1.6)
$$

where for any integers $t \geq 1$ and $j = 0, \ldots, i$,

$$
p_{ij} = \Pr\{X_{t+1} = j \mid X_t = i, Y_t > 0\} = \binom{i}{j}(1-\alpha)^{i-j}\alpha^j.
$$

Then, using (4.1.6) to calculate p_{i-k}^{n-1} recursively,

$$
\Pr\{(W, T) = (k, n) \mid X_0 = i, Y_0 > 0\} = p_{i-k}^{n-1} p_{i-k, i-k} = p_{i-k}^{n-1}\alpha^{i-k}.
$$

We can also use p.g.f. methods to find the distribution of (W, T) as we now show. Recall that the epidemic stops for the least integer t for which $Y_t = 0$, or equivalently, for the least integer t for which $X_t = X_{t-1}$. Partition the matrix at (4.1.5) as $P = \bar{P} + Q$ where $Q = \operatorname{diag}(1, \alpha, \ldots, \alpha^{x_0})$, so that

$$
\bar{P} = \begin{pmatrix}
0 & & & \cdots & \\
1-\alpha & 0 & & \cdots & \\
(1-\alpha)^2 & 2(1-\alpha)\alpha & 0 & \cdots & \\
\vdots & \vdots & \vdots & \ddots & \vdots \\
(1-\alpha)^{x_0} & x_0(1-\alpha)^{x_0-1}\alpha & \binom{x_0}{2}(1-\alpha)^{x_0-2}\alpha^2 & \cdots & 0
\end{pmatrix} \quad (4.1.7)
$$

is a lower triangular matrix of transition probabilities for transitions that do not allow any repetition, so that they are from some state $\{1, \ldots, x_0\}$ always to a lower state within the same set. Q is the matrix of probabilities for repetition of the state X_t, i.e. for the transition $\{X_{t-1} = i\} \mapsto \{X_t = i\}$ for some state i, and hence $Y_t = 0$. Indeed, we readily see that

$$\Pr\{T = t\} = A' \bar{P}^{t-1} Q E \qquad (t = 1, \ldots, x_0 + 1), \qquad (4.1.8)$$

where $A' = (0, 0, \ldots, 1)$ is the vector of initial probabilities corresponding to $\Pr\{X_0 = x_0\} = 1$, and $E' = (1, 1, \ldots, 1)$ is the unit row vector. The process is allowed to make exactly $t - 1$ downward transitions starting from x_0 through intermediate states to finish at some state $x_0 - (t - 1), \ldots, 0$, without repetition, and then stops at time t when the state $\{X_{t-1} = i\}$ is repeated. The p.g.f. of the distribution is given by

$$\Psi_T(\theta) = A' \left(\sum_{t=1}^{\infty} \bar{P}^{t-1} \theta^{t-1} \right) \theta Q E = A' (I - \theta \bar{P})^{-1} \theta Q E \qquad (4.1.9)$$

where we have used the fact that $\bar{P}^j = 0$ for $j \geq x_0 + 1$.

Example 4.1.1. Consider a Greenwood model for a family of three susceptibles and one initial infective with the transition probability matrix

$$P = \begin{pmatrix} 1 & \cdot & \cdot & \cdot \\ 1 - \alpha & \alpha & \cdot & \cdot \\ (1 - \alpha)^2 & 2(1 - \alpha)\alpha & \alpha^2 & \cdot \\ (1 - \alpha)^3 & 3(1 - \alpha)^2 \alpha & 3(1 - \alpha)\alpha^2 & \alpha^3 \end{pmatrix}.$$

The p.g.f. $\Psi_T(\theta)$ of the duration of the epidemic equals

$$(0, 0, 0, 1)(I - \theta \bar{P})^{-1} \theta \begin{pmatrix} 1 \\ \alpha \\ \alpha^2 \\ \alpha^3 \end{pmatrix} = (0, 0, 0, 1)(I + \theta \bar{P} + \theta^2 \bar{P}^2 + \theta^3 \bar{P}^3) \theta \begin{pmatrix} 1 \\ \alpha \\ \alpha^2 \\ \alpha^3 \end{pmatrix}$$

$$= (0, 0, 0, 1) \left\{ \begin{pmatrix} 1 & \cdot & \cdot & \cdot \\ \cdot & 1 & \cdot & \cdot \\ \cdot & \cdot & 1 & \cdot \\ \cdot & \cdot & \cdot & 1 \end{pmatrix} + \theta \begin{pmatrix} 0 & & \cdot & \cdot \\ 1 - \alpha & 0 & & \cdot \\ (1 - \alpha)^2 & 2\alpha(1 - \alpha) & 0 & \cdot \\ (1 - \alpha)^3 & 3\alpha(1 - \alpha)^2 & 3\alpha^2(1 - \alpha) & 0 \end{pmatrix} \right.$$

$$+ \theta^2 \begin{pmatrix} 0 & & \cdot & \cdot \\ 0 & 0 & & \cdot \\ 2\alpha(1 - \alpha)^2 & 0 & 0 & \cdot \\ 3\alpha(1 + \alpha)(1 - \alpha)^3 & 6\alpha^3(1 - \alpha)^2 & 0 & 0 \end{pmatrix}$$

$$+ \theta^3 \left. \begin{pmatrix} 0 & \cdot & \cdot & \cdot \\ 0 & 0 & \cdot & \cdot \\ 0 & 0 & 0 & \cdot \\ 6\alpha^3(1 - \alpha)^3 & 0 & 0 & 0 \end{pmatrix} \right\} \theta \begin{pmatrix} 1 \\ \alpha \\ \alpha^2 \\ \alpha^3 \end{pmatrix}. \qquad (4.1.10)$$

Hence

$$\Pr\{T=1\} = \alpha^3, \quad \Pr\{T=2\} = (1-\alpha)^3 + 3\alpha^2(1-\alpha)^2 + 3\alpha^4(1-\alpha),$$
$$\Pr\{T=3\} = 3\alpha(1+\alpha)(1-\alpha)^3 + 6\alpha^4(1-\alpha)^2,$$
$$\Pr\{T=4\} = 6\alpha^3(1-\alpha)^3.$$

It is easily checked that these probabilities sum to 1.

To find a p.g.f. for the size W of the epidemic, note that each time that X_t decreases, the number of infectives increases by an equal amount. Thus, in one transition period in which X_t decreases, the matrix $\bar{P}(\varphi)$ of p.g.f.s for the number of new infectives equals

$$
\begin{pmatrix}
0 & \cdot & \cdots & \cdot & \cdot \\
(1-\alpha)\varphi & 0 & \cdots & \cdot & \cdot \\
[(1-\alpha)\varphi]^2 & 2\alpha(1-\alpha)\varphi & \cdots & \cdot & \cdot \\
\vdots & \vdots & \ddots & \vdots & \vdots \\
[(1-\alpha)\varphi]^{x_0} & \binom{x_0}{1}\alpha[(1-\alpha)\varphi]^{x_0-1} & \cdots & \binom{x_0}{1}\alpha^{x_0-1}(1-\alpha)\varphi & 0
\end{pmatrix},
$$

$$\tag{4.1.11}$$

where the nth subdiagonal is the set of the equivalent probabilities in $\bar{P}$ multiplied by φ^n, for $n = 1, \ldots, x_0$. Similarly, $\bar{P}^2(\varphi)$ has elements $\Pr\{X_{t+2} = j \mid X_t = i\}$ multiplied by φ^{i-j} to reflect a total of $i - j$ infectives at times $t + 1$ and $t + 2$. By using the same argument as underlies the relation (4.1.9), it now follows that the joint p.g.f. of (W, T), where W denotes the total size of the epidemic, is given by

$$\Psi_{W,T}(\varphi, \theta) = A'(I - \theta\bar{P}(\varphi))^{-1}\theta QE \qquad (|\varphi| \le 1, |\theta| \le 1). \tag{4.1.12}$$

Example 4.1.2. For the same Greenwood model for a family of three susceptibles as Example 4.1.1, the joint p.g.f. $\Psi_{W,T}(\varphi, \theta)$ equals

$$
(0,0,0,1)\left\{
\begin{pmatrix}
1 & \cdot & \cdot & \cdot \\
\cdot & 1 & \cdot & \cdot \\
\cdot & \cdot & 1 & \cdot \\
\cdot & \cdot & \cdot & 1
\end{pmatrix}
+ \theta
\begin{pmatrix}
0 & \cdot & \cdot & \cdot \\
(1-\alpha)\varphi & 0 & \cdot & \cdot \\
(1-\alpha)^2\varphi^2 & 2\alpha(1-\alpha)\varphi & 0 & \cdot \\
(1-\alpha)^3\varphi^3 & 3\alpha(1-\alpha)^2\varphi^2 & 3\alpha^2(1-\alpha)\varphi & 0
\end{pmatrix}
\right.
$$

$$
+ \theta^2
\begin{pmatrix}
0 & \cdot & \cdot & \cdot \\
0 & 0 & \cdot & \cdot \\
2\alpha(1-\alpha)^2\varphi^2 & 0 & 0 & \cdot \\
3\alpha(1+\alpha)(1-\alpha)^3\varphi^3 & 6\alpha^3(1-\alpha)^2\varphi^2 & 0 & 0
\end{pmatrix}
$$

$$
\left.
+ \theta^3
\begin{pmatrix}
0 & \cdot & \cdot & \cdot \\
0 & 0 & \cdot & \cdot \\
0 & 0 & 0 & \cdot \\
6\alpha^3(1-\alpha)^3\varphi^3 & 0 & 0 & 0
\end{pmatrix}
\right\}
\theta
\begin{pmatrix}
1 \\
\alpha \\
\alpha^2 \\
\alpha^3
\end{pmatrix}.
\tag{4.1.13}
$$

All the joint probabilities $\Pr\{W = w, T = t\}$ for $w = 0, 1, 2, 3$; $t = 1, 2, 3, 4$ can be obtained from $\Psi_{W,T}(\varphi, \theta)$ above; for example for $T = 3$ we obtain

$$\Pr\{W = 3,\ T = 3\} = 3(1 - \alpha)^3 \alpha(1 + \alpha),$$
$$\Pr\{W = 2,\ T = 3\} = 6(1 - \alpha)^2 \alpha^3.$$

If we require only the distribution of the size W of the epidemic, it is clear that

$$\Psi_{W,T}(\varphi, 1) \equiv \Psi_W(\varphi) = A'(I - \bar{P}(\varphi))^{-1} QE$$

$$= (0, 0, 0, 1)(I - \bar{P}(\varphi))^{-1} \begin{pmatrix} 1 \\ \alpha \\ \alpha^2 \\ \alpha^3 \end{pmatrix}$$

$$= \alpha^3 + \varphi[3\alpha^4(1 - \alpha)] + \varphi^2[3\alpha^2(1 + 2\alpha^2)(1 - \alpha)^2]$$
$$+ \varphi^3[(1 - \alpha)^3(1 + 3\alpha + 3\alpha^2 + 6\alpha^3)]. \tag{4.1.14}$$

Thus we obtain the probabilities

$$\Pr\{W = 0\} = \alpha^3, \qquad \Pr\{W = 1\} = 3\alpha^4(1 - \alpha),$$
$$\Pr\{W = 2\} = 3\alpha^2(1 + 2\alpha^2)(1 - \alpha)^2,$$
$$\Pr\{W = 3\} = (1 - \alpha)^3(1 + 3\alpha + 3\alpha^2 + 6\alpha^3).$$

These probabilities add to 1 as they ought.

4.2 Further properties of the Reed–Frost model

In the Reed–Frost model with $X_0 = x_0 \geq y_0 = Y_0$, the matrix of transition probabilities has elements as at (4.1.3). Whereas in the Greenwood model it was enough to know X_t for each time-point, we must now keep track of both X_t and Y_t, or equivalently, since $X_{t-1} = X_t + Y_t$, of $\{(X_t, X_{t-1}) : t = 1, 2, \ldots\}$, which is a Markov chain if we set $X_{-1} = X_0 + Y_0 = x_0 + y_0$. In either specification, the model is a bivariate Markov chain. In what follows we use the formulation in terms of $(X, Y)_t$.

We start by presenting a deterministic analogue of the Reed–Frost model. For such an analogue we refer to equation (4.1.3) with the conditional binomial distribution and readily compute

$$\mathrm{E}[(X, Y)_{t+1} \mid (X, Y)_t = (x, y)_t] = (x_t \alpha^{y_t}, x_t(1 - \alpha^{y_t})). \tag{4.2.1}$$

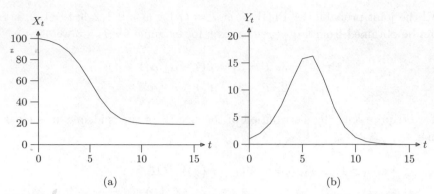

(a)   (b)

Figure 4.2. (a) Susceptibles and (b) infectives in successive generations of deterministic analogues of the Reed–Frost or non-overlapping Kermack–McKendrick epidemic, with $(N, I) = (100, 1)$, $\alpha = e^{-1/\rho} = 0.98$.

These equations, unlike their Greenwood counterparts at (4.1.4), do not lead to an explicit solution, but their recurrent nature makes them amenable to numerical computation, results of which are shown in Figure 4.2. The same figure results from the generation-wise evolution of a deterministic Kermack–McKendrick model with non-overlapping generations described in Exercise 2.7 if we set $\rho = -1/\log\alpha$.

We may write the transition probability matrix for the $p_{(x,y)_t,(x,y)_{t+1}}$ as the partitioned matrix P, of order $(x_0 + 1)^2 \times (x_0 + 1)^2$, given by

$$
P = \begin{pmatrix}
P_{00} & 0 & \cdots & 0 \\
P_{10} & P_{11} & \cdots & P_{1x_0} \\
\vdots & \vdots & \ddots & \vdots \\
P_{x_00} & P_{x_01} & \cdots & P_{x_0x_0}
\end{pmatrix}.
\tag{4.2.2}
$$

Here each submatrix P_{ij} is square, of order $x_0 + 1$, with $P_{ij} = (p_{(k,i),(\ell,j)})$ where we have from (4.1.3), for $k, \ell = 0, \ldots, x_0$, and $j + \ell = k$,

$$
p_{(k,i),(l,j)} = \Pr\{(X, Y)_{t+1} = (l, j) \mid (X, Y)_t = (k, i)\} = \binom{k}{\ell}(1 - \alpha^i)^j \alpha^{i\ell},
$$

and $p_{(k,i),(l,j)} = 0$ otherwise, i.e. P_{ij} records the transition probabilities from $Y_t = i$ to $Y_{t+1} = j$, with values of X_t and X_{t+1} indexing the rows and columns respectively, ranging from 0 to x_0. In particular, $P_{00} = I$, $P_{0j} = 0$ for $j = 1, \ldots, x_0$, and P_{ij} has zero elements except on the jth subdiagonal where one term from each of the binomial distributions for $\mathrm{Bin}(k, \alpha^i)$, for

$j \leq k \leq x_0 + 1 - j$, appears: thus P_{ij} equals

$$
\begin{pmatrix}
0 & 0 & \cdots & 0 & \cdots & 0 \\
0 & 0 & \cdots & 0 & \cdots & 0 \\
\vdots & \vdots & \ddots & \vdots & \ddots & \vdots \\
(1-\alpha^i)^j & 0 & \cdots & 0 & \cdots & 0 \\
0 & (j+1)\alpha^i(1-\alpha^i)^j & \cdots & 0 & \cdots & 0 \\
\vdots & \vdots & \ddots & 0 & \cdots & 0 \\
0 & 0 & \cdots & \binom{x_0}{x_0-j}\alpha^{i(x_0-j)}(1-\alpha^i)^j & \cdots & 0
\end{pmatrix}.
$$

Setting $A' = (0 \cdots 0\ 1\ 0 \cdots 0)$ where the 1 occurs in the place corresponding to $(x,y)_0$, it follows as in the previous section that the duration time T of the epidemic has

$$
\Pr\{T = t\} = A'\bar{P}^{t-1}QE, \qquad E' = (1\ 1 \cdots 1), \tag{4.2.3}
$$

where $P = Q + \bar{P}$ with Q the square matrix of order $(x_0 + 1)^2$ comprising the transition probabilities into the absorbing states $\{(x,0) : x = 0, \ldots, x_0\}$, so Q consists of the first $x_0 + 1$ columns of P in (4.2.2) (i.e. of the $x_0 + 1$ diagonal matrices P_{i0}), and all other elements are zero. Then the non-zero elements of $\bar{P}$ are the one-step transition probabilities into transient states (ℓ, j), these being characterized by having the second component $j > 0$.

As in the previous section, T has p.g.f.

$$
\Psi_T(\theta) = A'(I - \theta\bar{P})^{-1}\theta QE. \tag{4.2.4}
$$

Similarly, the joint p.g.f. of (W, T), where W is the total size of an epidemic and T its duration, is

$$
\Psi_{W,T}(\varphi, \theta) = A'\big(I - \theta\bar{P}(\varphi)\big)^{-1}\theta QE, \tag{4.2.5}
$$

where $\bar{P}(\varphi)$ equals the matrix $\bar{P}$ modified by having the elements in the jth subdiagonal of its component matrix P_{ij} in the partition at (4.2.2), multiplied by φ^j.

It should be clear from this discussion that the principles for the use of the Reed–Frost and Greenwood models are identical, though the Reed–Frost model requires more computation.

Example 4.2.1 *(Measles epidemic data from En'ko (1889)).* For the epidemics listed in Exercise 1.3 we can extract the following data for the successive numbers of infectives in the several generations of the epidemics. En'ko's paper gives sufficiently detailed data to make this possible.

Table 4.1. *Generation sizes in several measles epidemics in St Petersburg Educational Institutions 1865–84*

Epidemic Generation	A	B	C	D	E	F	G	H	I	J	K
0	3	1	2	1	1	1	1	1	1	4	1
1	52	13	28	4	3	4	1	0	70	9	13
2	28	25	14	14	10	5	2	1	45	9	6
3	1	12	1	10	12	3	0	1	2	21	.
4	.	4	.	1	*1	2	.	*2	.	21	.
5	.	.	.	0	.	.	1	.	.	1	.

* Vacation started

Epidemics A–H occurred at the St Petersburg Alexander Institute, I–K at the Educational College for the Daughters of the Nobility. Epidemic G occurred in the Autumn after the Spring outbreak in Epidemic E. For Epidemics A–H excluding G, it is reasonable as a first approximation to assume the same number of initial susceptibles. The numbers and time of onset of the disease in relation to the vacation period suggest that we should exclude H also. The pattern of sizes in successive generations indicate that Epidemics A, C, I and K may be consistent with a Greenwood-type model, and B, D, E, F and J with a Reed–Frost-type model.

We illustrate a type of fitting procedure on Epidemic B. Let the initial number of susceptibles be N; this is unknown, but must be at least as large as 54, the total number of cases after the initial infection. Given the number of infectives y_t in generation t and the number of new cases z_t prior to t (so, $z_0 = 0$ and $z_t = y_1 + \cdots + y_{t-1}$), y_t has expectation $(N - z_t)(1 - \alpha^{y_{t-1}})$. One method of fitting a Reed–Frost model is to minimize the chi-square statistic

$$\chi^2 \equiv \sum_{t=1}^{T-1} \frac{[y_t - (N - z_t)(1 - \alpha^{y_{t-1}})]^2}{(N - z_t)(1 - \alpha^{y_{t-1}})}$$

$$= \sum_{t=1}^{T-1} \left[\frac{y_t^2}{(N - z_t)(1 - \alpha^{y_{t-1}})} + (N - z_t)(1 - \alpha^{y_{t-1}}) - 2y_t \right],$$

where $T = \inf\{t : y_t = 0\}$ as before, with respect to both N and α, subject to the constraint that $\tilde{N} \geq \sum_{t=1}^{T} y_t \equiv \tilde{N}_{\min}$. The minimizing values $\tilde{N}$ and $\tilde{\alpha}$ satisfy the first of the equations

$$\sum_{t=1}^{T} (\tilde{N} - z_t) y_{t-1} \tilde{\alpha}^{y_{t-1}} \left(\left[\frac{y_t}{(\tilde{N} - z_t)(1 - \tilde{\alpha}^{y_{t-1}})} \right]^2 - 1 \right) = 0,$$

$$\sum_{t=1}^{T} (1 - \tilde{\alpha}^{y_{t-1}}) \left(\left[\frac{y_t}{(\tilde{N} - z_t)(1 - \tilde{\alpha}^{y_{t-1}})} \right]^2 - 1 \right) = 0,$$

and the second equation as well if $\tilde{N} > \tilde{N}_{\min}$. We found $(\tilde{N}, \tilde{\alpha}) = (54, 0.794)$. For Epidemic D we found $(\tilde{N}, \tilde{\alpha}) = (29.2, 0.835)$, where now $\tilde{N}_{\min} = 29$.

4.3 Chains with infection probability varying between households

As noted earlier, the chain binomial models we have been describing were the basis of data analyses by Abbey (1952), Bailey (1955) and Becker (1989), among others. One of the deficiencies of the simple models is that the assumption of similar susceptibility to infection for all families is invalid. This deficiency may be countered by allowing the non-infection rate α to vary between households; it is usual to suppose that the non-infection rate α is a random variable following a beta distribution, as this is mathematically and computationally convenient.

Suppose that within a household of x_0 individuals the probability of contact in a unit time period is p and the probability of transmission conditional on a contact is β. It is arguable that both these probabilities should vary between the individuals of a household, but such a level of detail may well make the model intractable. Consider again, as in (4.1.1), the probabilities

$$p\beta \quad \text{(of infection)} \quad \text{and} \quad \alpha = 1 - p\beta \quad \text{(of non-infection)},$$

but assume now that α varies from one household to another: model α as a random variable with a density function $f(\alpha)$. Then for any particular realization of a chain in a household, denoted $(X, Y)_{[0,T]} \equiv \{(X, Y)_t : t = 0, 1, \ldots, T\}$, with the epidemic ending at time T, the probability of the chain can be denoted by

$$P(\alpha) \equiv P((X, Y)_{[0,T]}|\alpha). \tag{4.3.1}$$

Since α varies between households, we need to average $P(\alpha)$ over all possible values of α on $(0, 1)$, yielding

$$\int_{\alpha=0}^{1} P(\alpha) f(\alpha) \, d\alpha. \tag{4.3.2}$$

Below, we assume that the density function $f(\cdot)$ is of the beta function form $(1 - \alpha)^{a-1} \alpha^{b-1} / B(a, b)$ for $a, b > 0$.

We illustrate the procedure for both the Greenwood and Reed–Frost models with transition probabilities as given at (4.1.2) and (4.1.3). In the former case these probabilities are of binomial form

$$p_{ij}(\alpha) = \Pr\{X_{t+1} = j \mid X_t = i\} = \binom{i}{j} (1 - \alpha)^{i-j} \alpha^j \quad (i \geq j).$$

Integrating over all values of α when α has the beta density above, we deduce that for integers i, j and general positive a, b,

$$
\begin{aligned}
\int_0^1 p_{ij}(\alpha) f(\alpha)\, d\alpha &= \int_0^1 \binom{i}{j} \frac{(1-\alpha)^{a+i-j-1}\alpha^{b+j-1}}{B(a,b)}\, d\alpha \\
&= \binom{i}{j} \frac{B(a+i-j, b+j)}{B(a,b)} \\
&= \frac{i!}{j!\,(i-j)!} \cdot \frac{(a+i-j-1)\cdots a\,(b+j-1)\cdots b}{(a+b+i-1)\cdots(a+b)}.
\end{aligned}
\tag{4.3.3}
$$

Thus in a Greenwood chain where we need to record only the values $X_t = x_t$ for $t = 0, \ldots, T$, the probability $P(\alpha)$ of such a realization equals

$$
\begin{aligned}
&\binom{x_0}{x_1}(1-\alpha)^{x_0-x_1}\alpha^{x_1}\cdots\binom{x_{T-1}}{x_T}(1-\alpha)^{x_{T-1}-x_T}\alpha^{x_T} \\
&= \left[\prod_{t=1}^T \binom{x_{t-1}}{x_t}\right](1-\alpha)^{x_0-x_T}\alpha^{\sum_{t=1}^T x_t}.
\end{aligned}
\tag{4.3.4}
$$

It follows that, averaging out over all values of α, we obtain

$$
\int_0^1 P(\alpha) f(\alpha)\, d\alpha = \left[\prod_{t=1}^T \binom{x_{t-1}}{x_t}\right]\frac{B(a+x_0-x_T, b+\sum_{t=1}^T x_t)}{B(a,b)}.
\tag{4.3.5}
$$

In a Reed–Frost model, if the realization has $(X_t, Y_t) = (x_t, y_t)$ for $t = 0, 1, \ldots, T$, then

$$
\begin{aligned}
P(\alpha) &= \prod_{t=1}^T \binom{x_{t-1}}{x_t}\left(1-\alpha^{y_{t-1}}\right)^{x_{t-1}-x_t}\left(\alpha^{y_{t-1}}\right)^{x_t} \\
&= \left[\prod_{t=1}^T \binom{x_{t-1}}{x_t}\left(1-\alpha^{y_{t-1}}\right)^{x_{t-1}-x_t}\right]\alpha^{\sum_{t=1}^T y_{t-1}x_t} \\
&= \left[\prod_{t=1}^T \binom{x_{t-1}}{x_t}\sum_{k=0}^{x_{t-1}-x_t}\binom{x_{t-1}-x_t}{k}(-1)^k\alpha^{ky_{t-1}}\right]\alpha^{\sum_{t=1}^T y_{t-1}x_t}.
\end{aligned}
\tag{4.3.6}
$$

The last expression reduces to a sum of terms of the typical form $\sum_j A_j \alpha^j$; taking its integral over all values of α yields

$$
\begin{aligned}
\sum_j A_j \int_0^1 \frac{(1-\alpha)^{a-1}\alpha^{j+b-1}}{B(a,b)}\, d\alpha &= \sum_j A_j \frac{B(a, j+b)}{B(a,b)} \\
&= \sum_j A_j \frac{(b+j-1)\cdots b}{(a+b+j-1)\cdots(a+b)}.
\end{aligned}
\tag{4.3.7}
$$

Example 4.3.1. Consider both these models for households of four, $x_0 = 3$, starting with a single infective $y_0 = 1$ in the Reed–Frost case. Table 4.2 lists the possible realizations and their probabilities under the two models in terms of a given value of α. Generic values are also given for use later in Section 6.3.2.

Table 4.2. *Epidemics in households of size four with $x_0 = 3$, $y_0 = 1$: possible realizations and their probabilities under two discrete-time models*

	Realization	$\{X\}_{[0,T]}$			Model	
$t =$	0	1	2	3	4	Reed–Frost	Greenwood
$\{X_t\} =$	3	3				α^3	α^3
	3	2	2			$3(1-\alpha)\alpha^4$	$3(1-\alpha)\alpha^4$
	3	2	1	1		$6(1-\alpha)^2\alpha^4$	$6(1-\alpha)^2\alpha^4$
	3	1	1			$3(1-\alpha)^2\alpha^3$	$3(1-\alpha)^2\alpha^2$
	3	2	1	0	0	$6(1-\alpha)^3\alpha^3$	$6(1-\alpha)^3\alpha^3$
	3	2	0	0		$3(1-\alpha)^3\alpha^2$	$3(1-\alpha)^3\alpha^2$
	3	1	0	0		$3(1-\alpha)^3\alpha(1+\alpha)$	$3(1-\alpha)^3\alpha$
	3	0	0			$(1-\alpha)^3$	$(1-\alpha)^3$

Integration over α of any of these probabilities multiplied by the density $f(\alpha)$ is readily effected. Only for the case where $(X_0 \cdots X_3) = (3\ 1\ 0\ 0)$ do they differ between the two models.

In practical applications the parameter values a, b must be estimated from the data, as shown e.g. in Bailey (1975, Chapter 14) and Gani and Mansouri (1987). For this purpose, supposing M households of size four with $x_0 = 3$ and $y_0 = 1$ have been found in a survey, the expected numbers of households with the various patterns of infection are equated to the observed numbers. For example, the expected number of households with the realization (3 1 0 0) equals

$$3M \int_0^1 [(1-\alpha)^3\alpha] \frac{(1-\alpha)^{a-1}\alpha^{b-1}}{B(a,b)} \, d\alpha$$

$$= \frac{3MB(a+3,b+1)}{B(a,b)} = \frac{3M(a+2)(a+1)ab}{(a+b+3)(a+b+2)(a+b+1)(a+b)}$$

for the Greenwood model, and for the Reed–Frost model,

$$3M \int_0^1 [(1-\alpha)^3\alpha + (1-\alpha)^3\alpha^2] \frac{(1-\alpha)^{a-1}\alpha^{b-1}}{B(a,b)} \, d\alpha$$

$$= \frac{3M[B(a+3,b+1) + B(a+3,b+2)]}{B(a,b)}$$

$$= \frac{3M(a+2)(a+1)ab}{(a+b+3)(a+b+2)(a+b+1)(a+b)} \left[1 + \frac{b+1}{a+b+4}\right].$$

If similar integrations for the other possible realizations are carried out, then the parameter values a, b can be estimated by moment fitting techniques or maximum likelihood methods using the data. See Bailey (1975) or Gani and Mansouri (1987) for details.

4.4   Chain binomial models with replacement

There exist situations in which a group that is partially isolated from a larger external population, may lose infectives by emigration, and have them replaced by a mix of infectives and susceptibles immigrating from the external population. This happens, for example, in groups of intravenous drug users (IVDUs) subject to HIV infection, such as those considered by Gani and Yakowitz (1993); here IVDUs who are seropositive leave the group, and are replaced by recruits from an external population.

We model the process, somewhat crudely, by assuming there is a sequence of emigration–immigration episodes at times $t = 0, 1, \ldots$, of relatively short duration in comparison with the length of time between them. Let (X_t, Y_t) denote the numbers of susceptibles and infectives in the group just before the start of the t th such episode; assume that the group is of constant size $N = X_t + Y_t$ (all t). In an emigration–immigration episode, all Y_t infectives are replaced by an equal number of individuals drawn independently and randomly from a much larger population in which each individual is an infective with probability p say ($0 \leq p \leq 1$). Denoting the number of such incoming infectives by Y_t', it follows from the independence assumption that

$$Y_t' =_{\mathrm{d}} \mathrm{Bin}(Y_t, p) = \mathrm{Bin}(N - X_t, p). \qquad (4.4.1)$$

It is of course possible for Y_t' to be zero, in which case the group consists only of susceptibles, and is assumed not to be subject to further infection. Otherwise, $Y_t' > 0$, and in the period until the next emigration–immigration episode, we assume that a binomially distributed number Z_t of the $X_t' \equiv N - Y_t'$ susceptibles become infectives, so $X_{t+1} = X_t' - Z_t$. Under a Greenwood-type model, we assume that

$$X_{t+1} =_{\mathrm{d}} \begin{cases} \mathrm{Bin}(X_t', \alpha) & (X_t' < N), \\ N & (X_t' = N). \end{cases} \qquad (4.4.2)$$

For a Reed–Frost-type model, we assume that the Y_t' infectives mix with the X_t' susceptibles and produce a further $\mathrm{Bin}(X_t', 1 - \alpha^{Y_t'})$ infectives, so that

$$X_{t+1} =_{\mathrm{d}} \mathrm{Bin}(X_t', \alpha^{Y_t'}). \qquad (4.4.3)$$

Since $Y_t' = \text{Bin}(N - X_t, p)$, it follows that under either model, $\{X_t : t = 0, 1, \ldots\}$ is a Markov chain for which N is an absorbing state, because as soon as $Y_t' = 0$ no further infection can then occur among the $X_t' = N$ susceptibles.

For simplicity we consider a Greenwood-type model. The transition probability matrix $R_1 = (r_{ij}^{(1)})$ say from X_t to X_t' is upper triangular with elements

$$r_{ij}^{(1)} = \begin{cases} \binom{N-i}{N-j} p^{N-j} q^{j-i} & j \geq i, \\ 0 & \text{otherwise,} \end{cases} \tag{4.4.4}$$

where $0 \leq p = 1 - q \leq 1$, so that

$$R_1 = \begin{pmatrix} p^N & \binom{N}{N-1}p^{N-1}q & \cdots & \binom{N}{1}pq^{N-1} & q^N \\ \cdot & p^{N-1} & \cdots & \binom{N-1}{1}pq^{N-2} & q^{N-1} \\ \vdots & \vdots & \ddots & \vdots & \vdots \\ \cdot & \cdot & \cdots & p & q \\ \cdot & \cdot & \cdots & \cdot & 1 \end{pmatrix}.$$

If $X_t' < N$, infection now follows as in the Greenwood model. The transition probability matrix $R_2 = (r_{ij}^{(2)})$ say from X_t' to $X_{t+1} = N - Y_t' - Z_t$ is lower triangular and of the form (4.2.1), namely

$$r_{jk}^{(2)} = \begin{cases} \binom{j}{k}(1 - \alpha)^{j-k}\alpha^k & k \leq j < N, \\ \delta_{Nk} & j = N, \\ 0 & \text{otherwise,} \end{cases} \tag{4.4.5}$$

so that, with $\gamma = 1 - \alpha$ as the probability of infection,

$$R_2 = \begin{pmatrix} 1 & \cdot & \cdots & \cdot & \cdot \\ \gamma & \alpha & \cdots & \cdot & \cdot \\ \vdots & \vdots & \ddots & \vdots & \vdots \\ \gamma^{N-1} & \binom{N-1}{1}\gamma^{N-2}\alpha & \cdots & \alpha^{N-1} & \cdot \\ 0 & 0 & \cdots & 0 & 1 \end{pmatrix}.$$

It now follows that transitions from $X_t < N$ to $X_{t+1} < N$ have distributions given by the elements s_{ik} of the matrix $\bar{S} \equiv \bar{R}_1 \bar{R}_2$, where the $N \times N$ matrices $\bar{R}_1$ and $\bar{R}_2$ are derived from R_1 and R_2 by deleting the last row and column. We obtain

$$\begin{aligned} s_{ik} &= \sum_{j=\max(i,k)}^{N-1} \binom{N-i}{N-j} p^{N-j} q^{j-i} \binom{j}{k} \alpha^k \gamma^{j-k} \\ &= \frac{(N-i)!\, p^N}{k!\, q^i} \left(\frac{\alpha}{\gamma}\right)^k \sum_{j=\max(i,k)}^{N-1} \frac{j!}{(j-i)!\,(N-j)!\,(j-k)!} \left(\frac{q\gamma}{p}\right)^j, \end{aligned} \tag{4.4.6}$$

where i, k lie in $\{0, 1, \ldots, N - 1\}$. Note also from (4.4.4) and (4.4.5) that $s_{iN} = q^{N-i}$.

The process $\{X_t\}$ ultimately ends in the absorbing state N, but the time T to absorption (i.e. the duration of the epidemic) need not be small: to get an idea of the expected behaviour of the process we consider $E(X_{t+1} \mid X_t)$. From (4.4.2) we have

$$
\begin{aligned}
E(X_{t+1} \mid Y_t') &= (N - Y_t')\alpha I\{Y_t' > 0\} + N I\{Y_t' = 0\} \\
&= (N - Y_t')\alpha + N(1 - \alpha)I\{Y_t' = 0\},
\end{aligned}
$$

where $I\{\cdot\}$ denotes the indicator r.v. From (4.4.1), $\Pr\{Y_t' = 0 \mid X_t\} = q^{N-X_t}$ and $E(Y_t' \mid X_t) = (N - X_t)p$. Thus

$$
E(X_{t+1} \mid X_t) = [N - (N - X_t)p]\alpha + N(1 - \alpha)q^{N-X_t}, \tag{4.4.7}
$$

or equivalently,

$$
E(Y_{t+1} - Y_t \mid Y_t) = -(1 - p\alpha)Y_t + N(1 - \alpha)(1 - q^{Y_t}). \tag{4.4.8}
$$

The expression on the right-hand side is concave in Y_t, being zero at $Y_t = 0$ and negative at $Y_t = N$ because $1 - p\alpha \geq 1 - \alpha$. So when its slope at $Y_t = 0$ is positive, i.e. when

$$
1 - p\alpha < N(1 - \alpha)\ln(1/q), \tag{4.4.9}
$$

it has a maximum at a point interior to $(0, N)$. Table 4.3 shows the threshold values $N_{p,\alpha} \equiv (1 - p\alpha)/[(1 - \alpha)|\ln(1 - p)|]$ which are such that when the group size $N > N_{p,\alpha}$ there exists a positive value for Y_t such that $E(Y_{t+1} \mid Y_t) = Y_t$, i.e. $\{Y_t\}$ remains stationary (in the mean) and endemicity of infection is likely.

Table 4.3. *Threshold values $N_{p,\alpha}$ of group size for endemicity*

$p =$ / $1 - \alpha$	0.001	0.002	0.003	0.005	0.010	0.020	0.030	0.040	0.050
0.01	99 852.3	49 851.7	33 184.2	19 851.2	9 851.4	4 851.8	3 185.6	2 352.7	1 853.1
0.02	49 926.7	24 926.4	16 592.6	9 926.1	4 926.2	2 426.4	1 593.3	1 176.8	927.0
0.04	24 963.8	12 463.7	8 296.8	4 963.6	2 463.6	1 213.7	797.1	588.9	464.0
0.06	16 642.9	8 309.5	5 531.5	3 309.4	1 642.7	809.5	531.7	392.9	309.7
0.08	12 482.4	6 232.3	4 148.9	2 482.3	1 232.3	607.3	399.1	294.9	232.5
0.10	9 986.1	4 986.1	3 319.3	1 986.0	986.0	486.1	319.4	236.1	186.2
0.20	4 993.6	2 493.5	1 660.2	993.5	493.5	243.5	160.2	118.6	93.6
0.30	3 329.4	1 662.7	1 107.1	662.7	329.3	162.7	107.1	79.4	62.7
0.40	2 497.3	1 247.3	830.6	497.3	247.3	122.3	80.6	59.8	47.3
0.50	1 998.0	998.0	664.7	398.0	198.0	98.0	64.7	48.0	38.0

Let ξ be the least positive zero of the right-hand side of equation (4.4.8) rewritten in terms of $X_t = N - Y_t$, i.e. ξ is the smallest positive root of

$$(1 - p\alpha)(N - \xi) = N(1 - \alpha)(1 - q^{N-\xi}); \qquad (4.4.10)$$

some values are shown in Table 4.4 when $N = 200$. Then $\xi < N$ if and only if $N > N_{p,\alpha}$, and the process $\{X_t\}$ has mean drift away from its absorbing state when $\xi < X_t \leq N$. Typically, we should have p small, in which case the right-hand side of (4.4.9) $\approx Np(1 - \alpha)$ and $N_{p,\alpha} \approx 1/[p(1 - \alpha)]$.

Table 4.4. *Least root ξ of (4.4.10) when $N = 200$*

$p =$	0.01	0.02	0.03	0.04	0.05
$1 - \alpha$					
0.10	200.0	200.0	200.0	200.0	197.2
0.20	200.0	200.0	184.9	171.7	165.4
0.30	200.0	178.8	153.6	144.7	140.8
0.40	200.0	146.5	127.5	121.3	118.8
0.50	198.0	118.4	103.9	99.7	98.0

Another approximation can be obtained by modifying (4.4.2) so as to study a process $\{\tilde{X}_t\}$ satisfying

$$\tilde{X}_{t+1} =_d \mathrm{Bin}(N - \mathrm{Bin}(N - \tilde{X}_t, p), \alpha); \qquad (4.4.11)$$

this is equivalent to changing the last row $(0\ 0\ \cdots\ 1)$ of R_2 below (4.4.5) to the terms of the binomial expansion $(\gamma + \alpha)^N$, so $\{\tilde{X}_t\}$ is a Markov chain on $\{0, \ldots, N\}$ with all states recurrent. Then

$$E\tilde{X}_t = [N - (N - E\tilde{X}_{t-1})p]\alpha = N\alpha(1-p)\frac{1 - (p\alpha)^t}{1 - p\alpha} + (p\alpha)^t E\tilde{X}_0. \quad (4.4.12)$$

Such a process has a stationary version with generic marginal r.v. $\tilde{X}$ for which

$$E\tilde{X} = \frac{N(1 - p)\alpha}{1 - p\alpha} \approx N\alpha, \qquad (4.4.13)$$

the approximation holding when p is small. See Exercises 4.1 and 4.2.

The process $\{\tilde{X}_t\}$ satisfies equation (4.4.7), so we might expect $E\tilde{X} \approx \xi$ because $\tilde{X}_t$ has mean drift always towards ξ, i.e. it has zero mean drift only when $\tilde{X}_t = \xi$. Comparison of (4.4.10) and (4.4.13) shows that, for p small, $\xi \approx N\alpha$ only if $q^{N-\xi} \approx 0$, which occurs only if α is not too large. See Exercise 4.3.

The duration time T until absorption in the state $X_t = N$ is considered separately for the two cases determined by the condition (4.4.9) and its complement. Crudely speaking, there is drift towards the state N when $N < N_{p,\alpha}$, whereas when $N > N_{p,\alpha}$, X_t will reach N only as a result of a rare excursion involving several large positive fluctuations away from $E\tilde{X}$.

For $N < N_{p,\alpha}$, the process $\{X_t\}$ has a drift to the absorbing state N with mean drift $E(X_{t+1} - X_t \mid X_t)$ lying between $N(1-p)\alpha - N(1-\alpha)q^N$ and 0. As a rough approximation then, we should have T of the order of $(N - X_0)/[N(1-p)\alpha] = Y_0/[N(1-p)\alpha]$; in fact a better approximation for T is given by $Y_0/[(1 - p\alpha)Y_0 - N(1 - \alpha)(1 - q^{Y_0})]$.

For $N > N_{p,\alpha}$, the process $\{X_t\}$ no longer has a mean drift towards the absorbing state so we must use some other approach. Recall that T is the first passage time into the state N for the process $\tilde{X}_t$ considered around (4.4.11), so we can approximate the order of T by the mean recurrence time of $\tilde{X}_t$ for the state N; this equals the reciprocal of $\Pr\{\tilde{X}_t = N\}$ when $\tilde{X}_t$ has its stationary distribution.

In both cases,

$$\Pr\{T = n\} \approx A\varpi^n \tag{4.4.14}$$

for sufficiently large n, where A is a positive constant and ϖ is the Perron–Frobenius eigenvalue (i.e. the eigenvalue of largest modulus) of the sub-stochastic matrix $\tilde{S}$ with elements defined at (4.4.6). There are graphs in Gani and Yakowitz (1993) illustrating (4.4.14) when $N = 7$. We have computed ET as

$$\Big(\sum_{j=1}^{n-1} + \sum_{j=n}^{\infty}\Big)j\Pr\{T = j\} \approx \sum_{j=1}^{n-1} j\Pr\{T = j\} + \frac{\Pr\{T = n\}}{1 - \varpi}\Big(n + \frac{\varpi}{1 - \varpi}\Big),\tag{4.4.15}$$

where ϖ is estimated by $\Pr\{T = n\}/\Pr\{T = n - 1\}$ provided these terms are not excessively small, and n is the number of transitions computed. If the terms are very small, then it is of no consequence, because the last term in (4.4.15) is negligible. Table 4.5 lists some values of ET starting from $X_0 = 1$ for $N = 200$ and the same p and α as in Table 4.4.

It is evident from the structure of the state space for the Markov chain X_t that the conditional distribution

$$q_i^t \equiv \Pr\{X_t = i \mid X_t \neq N\} \qquad (i = 0, \ldots, N - 1) \tag{4.4.16}$$

converges as $t \to \infty$ to a probability distribution $\{q_i\}$ say, known as the *quasi-stationary distribution* for X_t (Darroch and Seneta (1965)). Indeed,

Table 4.5. *Mean duration* ET *when* $N = 200$, $X_0 = 1$

$p =$ $1 - \alpha$	0.01	0.02	0.03	0.04	0.05
0.10	2.08	2.55	3.01	3.56	4.26
0.20	2.35	3.31	4.64	6.67	9.89
0.30	2.63	4.47	7.75	14.31	28.55
0.40	2.99	6.25	13.91	35.20	113.6
0.50	3.44	9.03	26.99	110.64	1538.0

general theory in Seneta (1981, Chapters 6 and 7) shows that $\Pr\{X_t \neq N\}$ $\approx A\varpi^{t+1}/(1 - \varpi)$ with A and ϖ as in (4.4.14), and the normalized left-eigenvector $\mathbf{q}$ for the eigenvalue ϖ has as its elements the terms of the limit distribution $\{q_i\}$, i.e. $\mathbf{q} = [q_0 \ \cdots \ q_{N-1}]'$. It is intuitively clear that when $N > N_{p,\alpha}$, $\mathbf{q}$ is approximately the same as the stationary distribution for the process $\tilde{X}$ considered earlier, and $\varpi \to 1$ as $N \to \infty$. See Exercise 4.5.

4.5 Final size of an epidemic with arbitrary infectious period

Comparison of the mathematical structure of the Reed–Frost chain binomial model with the Kermack–McKendrick model of the previous chapter, and the possibility of viewing of an epidemic as a 'branching process on a finite population', prompt a closer examination of the probabilistic features of both models. We show below that these models can be placed in a more general setting, and study their specific features as particular members of a broader class.

Suppose that we regard the population as a set of nodes in a graph, with each node either a susceptible, infective or removal; initially there are N susceptibles and 1 infective. Each node i is the hub of a (small) set of directed links which are 'activated' if i ever becomes infectious. The activation of a node's directed links transmits the infection to the nodes at the far ends of those links, turning any susceptible at the latter nodes into an infective but otherwise having no effect. Consequently, given the set of directed links for each node, we could in principle determine the total size of the epidemic: we would trace forwards the spread of infection along the links until eventually either the set of nodes that become infectious is exhausted, or there remain no susceptible nodes. In tracing the links from a given node, the change of that node to a removal is noted. Conversely, any node is ultimately infected if and only if there is a path backwards to the initial infective along some connected set of directed links.

We now impose on this structure some probabilistic assumptions that reflect the homogeneous mixing and independence properties underlying both the Kermack–McKendrick and Reed–Frost models. To do so, it is helpful to consider first the Kermack–McKendrick setting. Suppose that at some epoch in time a node I' is newly infected, there are X susceptibles, and we 'put on hold' the action of all infectives apart from I'. If I' spreads infection for a time S, then, according to the assumptions of the general stochastic epidemic in Section 3.3, each of the X susceptibles, independently of all others, becomes infected with probability $1 - e^{-\beta S}$. More widely, I' is linked to each node independently with the same probability $1 - e^{-\beta S}$, though a new infection results only when the target node is a susceptible. The number of directed links triggered by I''s infection, given S, is thus a binomial r.v. $\text{Bin}(N, 1 - e^{-\beta S})$. Now S, the period of infectiousness before I''s removal, is itself a random variable, distributed exponentially with mean $1/\gamma$. Thus, unconditionally, this r.v. is a mixture of these binomial distributions with mixing parameter S, while $\nu(X)$, the number of new infectives, is a mixture of the binomial r.v.s $\text{Bin}(X, 1 - e^{-\beta S})$, i.e. for $(k = 0, \ldots, X)$,

$$\Pr\{\nu(X) = k\} = \int_0^\infty \binom{X}{k} (1 - e^{-\beta s})^k e^{-\beta s(X-k)} \gamma e^{-\gamma s} \, ds. \qquad (4.5.1)$$

Let t be an index ('time' in the random walk we are about to describe) that counts the number of infectives whose immediate links have been traced up to the epoch $t - 0$, at which point there are X_t susceptibles, Y_t infectives and $Z_t = t$ removals. Thus, there are Z_t infectives whose links have been traced prior to $t - 0$. Provided that $Y_t \geq 1$, we then have

$$Y_{t+1} = Y_t - 1 + \nu(X_t), \qquad X_{t+1} = X_t - \nu(X_t), \qquad (4.5.2)$$

where the r.v.s $\{\nu(X_t) : t = 0, 1, \ldots\}$ are independent with the mixed binomial distribution (4.5.1), while if $Y_t = 0$, $Y_{t+1} = 0$ also.

We can easily evaluate the distribution of X_t. Set

$$p_i^t = \Pr\{X_t = i\}, \qquad p_k(i) = \Pr\{\nu(X_t) = k \mid X_t = i\}. \qquad (4.5.3)$$

Then when $Y_t \geq 1$, starting from $p_i^0 = \delta_{Ni}$,

$$p_j^{t+1} = \sum_{i=j}^{N-t} p_i^t p_{i-j}(i) \qquad (t = 0, \ldots, N). \qquad (4.5.4)$$

Modifications for the case where the initial number of infectives is larger than 1 are easily made (see Exercise 4.6).

Define
$$T = \inf\{t : X_t + t > N\}. \qquad (4.5.5)$$
Inspection of the construction underlying (4.5.2) shows that T is the total size of the epidemic (including the initial infectives), i.e. $T = N + 1 - X_T = Z_T$. It follows from (4.5.4–5) that the distribution of T is given by
$$\Pr\{T = k\} \equiv P_k = p_{N+1-k}^k = p_{N+1-k}^{k-1}p_0(N + 1 - k). \qquad (4.5.6)$$

In the argument above, we see that we can replace the exponential distribution of S by an arbitrary distribution for the infectious period, with d.f. $F(\cdot)$ say, leading to a different mixed binomial distribution on $k = 0, \ldots, X$, namely

$$\Pr\{\nu(X) = k\} = \int_0^\infty \binom{X}{k}(1 - \mathrm{e}^{-\beta s})^k \mathrm{e}^{-\beta s(X-k)}\, \mathrm{d}F(s). \qquad (4.5.7)$$

The special case in which $F(\cdot)$ is degenerate at $1/\gamma$, so that $\mathrm{E}S = 1/\gamma$ as for the exponential distribution, makes $\nu(X)$ a binomial r.v. $\mathrm{Bin}(X, 1 - \mathrm{e}^{-\beta/\gamma})$. Embedded in the resulting process $\{(X_t, Y_t)\}$ is a Reed–Frost epidemic, as we now indicate. Define $\{(\tilde{X}_n, \tilde{Y}_n)\}$ recursively, starting from $(\tilde{X}_0, \tilde{Y}_0, \tilde{Z}_0) = (N, I, 0)$, in such a way that in 'generation' time n those of the $\tilde{X}_n$ that become infectives by direct contact with one of the $\tilde{Y}_n$ infectives are identified, totalling $\tilde{Y}_{n+1} = \tilde{X}_n - \tilde{X}_{n+1}$ in all. At the same time, the $\tilde{Y}_n$ infectives become removals, i.e.

$$\tilde{Z}_{n+1} = \begin{cases} \tilde{Z}_n + \tilde{Y}_n & (\tilde{Y}_n > 0), \\ \tilde{Z}_n & (\text{otherwise}), \end{cases}$$
$$\tilde{X}_{n+1} = X_{\tilde{Z}_{n+1}}, \qquad \tilde{Y}_{n+1} = \tilde{X}_n - \tilde{X}_{n+1}.$$

This embedding is effectively the same as that used to define a Galton–Watson branching process in terms of a left-continuous random walk (Spitzer (1964) p. 234). We assert that $\{(\tilde{X}_n, \tilde{Y}_n)\}$ is a Reed–Frost epidemic process and leave the proof to the reader.

Daley (1990) exploited the representation at (4.5.2) to show that as the distribution for the infectious period S increases in the sense of stochastic, or decreasing convex, or a transform (Laplace–Stieltjes) ordering, the total size distribution increases in the sense of the same ordering (except that probability generating functions are the basis of the transform ordering). From a practical viewpoint, this implies that among infectious periods with the same mean for S, the total size is largest when S has the least variance, which is the case in the Reed–Frost model.

Exercise 4.6 indicates how to use the approach of this section to compute the total size distribution $\{P_k\}$. See e.g. Ball (1986) for another approach. Exercise 4.7 suggests a relation between the mean total size starting with $N + 1$ susceptibles to the distribution starting with N.

4.6 A pairs-at-parties model: exchangeable but not homogeneous mixing

The model described in this section is based on part of Daley and Gani (1999). It attempts to evaluate the importance of the usual homogeneous mixing assumption based on the Law of Mass Action. It also investigates the effect of pairwise interaction.

For the simplest construction, we assume a closed population of size $N = 2M$ individuals, of whom initially one is an infective and all others susceptibles. At discrete epochs in time $t = 1, 2, \ldots$, these individuals form M pairs, with each individual in contact with exactly one other individual at each time epoch. As a result of this pair formation, we assume that any susceptible in a susceptible–infective pair becomes an infective. Assuming that individuals, once infective, remain so, we can ask in the usual fashion how long it will take for all individuals to become infectives.

Assume that pair formation occurs at random. Denote the number of susceptibles after epoch t by X_t, with $X_0 = N - 1$. Then we can use indicator random variables and simple combinatorics to deduce that

$$\mathrm{E}(X_t - X_{t+1} \mid X_t) = \frac{X_t(N - X_t)}{N - 1}. \tag{4.6.1}$$

To find the distribution of the decrement $X_t - X_{t+1}$, we must count the number of ways of forming pairs, and in particular infective–susceptible pairs. i.e. *mixed* pairs. First, the possible number of distinct sets of M pairs which can be formed from the $2M$ distinct individuals equals

$$\frac{1}{M!} \binom{N}{2\ 2\ \cdots\ 2} = \frac{N!}{M!\,(2!)^M} = \frac{(2M)!}{M!\,2^M} = \frac{2^M \Gamma(M + \frac{1}{2})}{\Gamma(\frac{1}{2})}. \tag{4.6.2}$$

Next, the number of mixed pairs is odd or even according to whether the number of infectives $Y_t = N - X_t$ is odd or even, so irrespective of Y_0, Y_t is even for $t = 1, 2, \ldots$. Define $z_M(i) = \min(i, 2M - i)$ and set $Z_t = z_M(X_t)$. Then the number of ways of forming exactly j mixed pairs from the X_t

susceptibles and Y_t infectives is zero if $Z_t + j$ is odd, and

$$
\binom{Z_t}{j}\binom{2M - Z_t}{j} j! \times \left(\begin{array}{c} \text{the number of ways of forming} \\ \tfrac{1}{2}(Z_t - j) \text{ and } M - \tfrac{1}{2}(Z_t + j) \text{ non-mixed pairs} \end{array}\right)
$$

$$
= \frac{Z_t!\,(2M - Z_t)!}{j!\,(Z_t - j)!\,(2M - Z_t - j)!} \cdot \frac{(Z_t - j)!}{(\tfrac{1}{2}[Z_t - j])!\,2^{\frac{1}{2}(Z_t - j)}}
$$

$$
\times \frac{(2M - Z_t - j)!}{(M - \tfrac{1}{2}[Z_t + j])!\,2^{M - \frac{1}{2}(Z_t + j)}} \tag{4.6.3}
$$

otherwise. It now follows that the one-step transition matrix for the Markov chain $\{X_t : t = 1, 2, \ldots\}$ has elements $p_{i,i-j} = r_j(i, M)$ where, with $Z_t = z_M(X_t)$ as above,

$$
r_j(i, M) \equiv \Pr\{X_{t+1} = X_t - j \mid X_t = i, M\}
$$

$$
= \frac{\binom{Z_t}{j}\binom{2M - Z_t}{j} \dfrac{j!\,(Z_t - j)!}{(\tfrac{1}{2}[Z_t - j])!\,2^{\frac{1}{2}(Z_t - j)}} \cdot \dfrac{(2M - Z_t - j)!}{(M - \tfrac{1}{2}[Z_t + j])!\,2^{M - \frac{1}{2}(Z_t + j)}}}{\dfrac{(2M)!}{M!\,2^M}}
$$

$$
= \begin{cases} \dfrac{2^j\,Z_t!\,(2M - Z_t)!\,M!}{j!\,(\tfrac{1}{2}[Z_t - j])!\,(M - \tfrac{1}{2}[Z_t + j])!\,(2M)!} = \dfrac{2^j \binom{M}{j\ \ \tfrac{1}{2}(Z_t - j)\ \ M - \frac{1}{2}(Z_t + j)}}{\binom{2M}{Z_t}} \\ \qquad\qquad\qquad\qquad\qquad\qquad (j = Z_t, Z_t - 2, \ldots, 1 \text{ or } 0), \\[2mm] 0 \qquad\qquad\qquad\qquad\qquad\qquad\qquad \text{otherwise.} \end{cases}
$$

$$\tag{4.6.4}$$

We can now use this Markov chain to find numerically the distribution of the time T until all $2M$ individuals are infective.

The assumption that transmission of infection occurs in every infective–susceptible pair is unrealistic. If infection occurs with probability β' say, then by using indicator variables we should have in place of (4.6.1) the relation

$$
\mathrm{E}(X_t - X_{t+1} \mid X_t) = \frac{\beta' X_t (N - X_t)}{N - 1}. \tag{4.6.5}
$$

The transition probabilities $p_{i,i-j}^{\beta'}$ say, are now binomial mixtures of the terms $r_j(i, M)$, because from the random number K_t of mixed pairs formed by the X_t susceptibles and $N - X_t$ infectives, the number of new infectives is a binomially distributed r.v. $\mathrm{Bin}(K_t, \beta')$. We have

$$
p_{i,i-j}^{\beta'} = \sum_{k=j}^{\min(i, N-i)} \binom{k}{j} \beta'^j (1 - \beta')^{k-j} r_k(\min(i, N - i), M). \tag{4.6.6}
$$

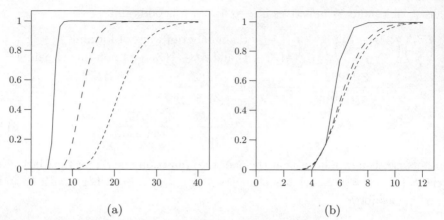

(a)   (b)

Figure 4.3. Duration time distributions for the pairs-at-parties model with $\beta' = 1$ (——), $\beta' = 0.5$ (– – –), and $\beta' = 0.3$ (- - - -), for $N = 20$. (a) Actual time $\Pr\{X_t = 0\}$, (b) rescaled time $\Pr\{X_{t/\beta'} = 0\}$.

Figure 4.3 plots the distrubution of the duration time of an epidemic in this model for three values of β', with values rescaled in part (b) of the figure indicating convergence as $\beta' \downarrow 0$ to a limit in which the effect of exactly M pairs being formed in each time unit largely disappears. These distributions can also be illustrated by plotting the mean numbers of new infectives in a time unit (see Figure 4.4). Rescaling again emphasizes similarities and suggests convergence (see Exercise 4.8).

We now attempt to understand better the effect of the pair-formation aspect of the model relative to 'classical' homogeneously mixing models, subject of course to appropriate choice of such a classical-style model. For a start, we observe that in the pairs-at-parties model every individual in the closed population is either susceptible or infective, and that once infected, an individual remains so forever. In this respect the model resembles the simple stochastic epidemic $X(t)$ of Section 3.1 starting from $N-1$ susceptibles and 1 infective, with transmission rate β which we must determine appropriately. We deduce from Section 3.1 that

$$\frac{d}{dt}(EX(t) \mid X(t-) = i) = \beta i(N - i) ; \qquad (4.6.7)$$

we can immediately see the similarity of functional form with the right-hand side of (4.6.5). This derivative best approximates the discrete-time mean decrement at (4.6.5) (which includes the case $\beta' = 1$ in (4.6.1)) by setting $\beta = \beta'/(N - 1)$. The deterministic analogue of this stochastic model gives the logistic growth curve as in Section 2.1.

However, since the pairs-at-parties model is a discrete-time model, with exactly $M = \frac{1}{2}N$ pairs formed in each unit of time, we should use a discrete time analogue of this simple epidemic model. We consider two possibilities. For the first we start with the discrete time approximating process $\{X_t^A\}$ defined by $X_0^A = N - 1$ and the one step transition probabilities

$$
p_{ij} = \begin{cases} \dfrac{\beta' i(N - i)}{\frac{1}{2}N(N - 1)} & \text{if } j = i - 1, \\[2mm] 1 - p_{i,i-1} & \text{if } j = i, \\[1mm] 0 & \text{otherwise.} \end{cases} \tag{4.6.8}
$$

We recognize that the term $p_{i,i-1}$ equals the product of the probabilities that a randomly chosen pair is a mixed pair and that there is infection transmission. Since M pairs are formed in each time unit of the pairs-at-parties process $\{X_t\}$ it is appropriate that it be compared with the process $\{\tilde{X}_t\} \equiv \{X_{Mt}^A\}$.

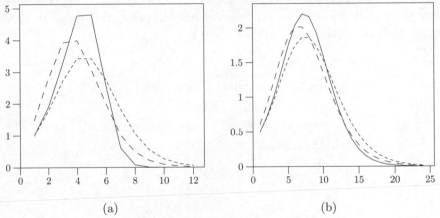

(a)   (b)

Figure 4.4. Mean numbers of new infectives in pairs-at-parties model (———), approximating discrete simple epidemic model ($---$), and approximating Reed–Frost-style simple epidemic ($----$), for $N = 20$ and (a) $\beta' = 1$, (b) $\beta' = 0.5$.

Figure 4.4 compares the two processes $\{X_t\}$ and $\{\tilde{X}_t\}$ for $N = 20$ and the two cases $\beta' = 1$ and $\beta = 0.5$, plotting for each time unit the mean decrements $\mathrm{E}(X_t - X_{t-1})$, i.e. the mean numbers of new infectives. The figure also shows the corresponding data for the other discrete-time process $\{\bar{X}_t\}$ that is a simple epidemic analogue of the Reed–Frost model of Sections 4.1–2. Conditional on $\bar{X}_t$, $\bar{X}_{t+1}$ is a binomially distributed r.v.

$\text{Bin}(\bar{X}_t, \bar{q}^{N-\bar{X}_t})$, where $\bar{q}$ denotes the probability that a given susceptible is not infected by a given infective in the time interval $(t, t+1)$. This process $\bar{X}_t$ has mean decrement

$$\mathrm{E}(\bar{X}_t - \bar{X}_{t+1} \mid \bar{X}_t) = \bar{X}_t[1 - \bar{q}^{N-\bar{X}_t}] = \bar{X}_t \bar{p}(1 + \bar{q} + \cdots + \bar{q}^{N-\bar{X}_t-1})$$
$$\approx \bar{X}_t(N - \bar{X}_t)\bar{p}. \tag{4.6.9}$$

By choosing $\bar{p} = \beta'/(N-1)$ we approximate the decrement (4.6.5), exactly for $\bar{X}_t = N - 1 = \bar{X}_0$; otherwise (4.6.9) is a lower bound. Thus, we could expect this simple epidemic analogue of a Reed–Frost epidemic to evolve more slowly than the pairs-at-parties model.

Figure 4.5 provides another comparison of the processes $\{X_t\}$, $\{\tilde{X}_t\}$ and $\{\bar{X}_t\}$, by plotting the increments $\Pr\{X_t = 0\} - \Pr\{X_{t-1} = 0\}$ of the d.f. shown in Figure 4.3, in the two cases $\beta' = 1$ and 0.5 as for Figure 4.4. Figure 4.4 indicates that the spread of infection in the pairs-at-parties model is more rapid than the Reed–Frost simple epidemic analogue, as noted below (4.6.9). Compared with the simple epidemic analogue, its initial spread is slower; in the middle and later stages, however, its spread is faster so that the population becomes totally infected more rapidly (this latter point is underlined in Figure 4.5).

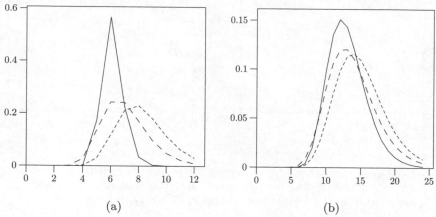

(a)   (b)

Figure 4.5. Increments $\Pr\{X_t = 0\} - \Pr\{X_{t-1} = 0\}$ in the duration time distribution of pairs-at-parties model (———), approximating discrete simple epidemic model ($- - -$), and approximating Reed–Frost-style simple epidemic ($----$), for $N = 20$ and (a) $\beta' = 1$, (b) $\beta' = 0.5$.

Decreasing β' has the effect of increasing the uncertainty of transmission of infection. All three Figures 4.3–5 indicate that as β' decreases, the pairs-at-parties model resembles a classical model more closely.

By way of summary, these properties indicate that, compared with standard homogeneous mixing models, an epidemic spread via the 'regularization' of pair-formation for all individuals in each discrete time unit, leads to a more predictable and ultimately faster spread of infection. However, the effect of pair-formation in each time unit is not great.

4.7 Exercises and Complements to Chapter 4

4.1 (a) Use a sketch graph to check that when (4.4.9) holds, the root ξ of equation (4.4.10) lies between N and $\xi_0 \equiv N\alpha(1-p)/(1-p\alpha)$.

(b) Expand the term $q^{N-\xi}$ when $(N-\xi_0)|\ln(1-p)|$ is small (i.e. $(N-\xi_0)p$ is small) and deduce that

$$N - \xi \approx 1 + \frac{2}{p}\left[1 - \frac{1-p\alpha}{Np(1-\alpha)}\right].$$

Compare with the numerical values in Table 4.4.

4.2 Show that for a stationary process $\{X_t\}$ satisfying (4.4.11),

$$[1 - (p\alpha)^2]\operatorname{var}\tilde{X} = \alpha(1-\alpha)(N - p\mathrm{E}\tilde{Y}) + \alpha^2 pq\mathrm{E}\tilde{Y},$$

where $\tilde{Y} = N - \tilde{X}$. What is the asymptotic behaviour of $1 - \varpi$ for large N? Investigate conditions for a 'quasi-stable' $\tilde{Y}$ that is $O(1)$.

4.3 Compare the stationary mean $\mathrm{E}\tilde{X}$ at (4.4.13) with the least root ξ of (4.4.10) given in Table 4.4.

4.4 Investigate whether martingale and/or transform methods may assist in studying the process $\{X_t\}$ of Section 4.4, in particular first passage time variables and the value of ξ (or other quantity) as an approximation.

4.5 Show that the total size distribution $\{P_k\}$ of an epidemic starting from I infectives and otherwise as in Section 4.5 can be computed from

$$p_i^0 = \delta_{Ni}, \qquad p_j^{t+1} = \sum_{i=j}^{\min(N,N+I-t-1)} p_i^t p_{i-j}(i) \quad (j+t+1 < N+I),$$

$$P_k = p_{N+I-k}^{k-I} \quad (k = I, \ldots, N+I).$$

4.6 (a) Show that the total size distribution $\{P_k\}$ of the stochastic carrier epidemic model of Section 3.6 can be computed from $P_k = P_{n-k,0}$ where, starting from $P_{nb} = 1$, the quantities $P_{ij} = \Pr\{\text{for some } t \text{ there are } i \text{ susceptibles and } j \text{ carriers}\}$ are defined recursively by

$$
\begin{aligned}
P_{ib} &= p_{i+1}P_{i+1,b} & (i &= n-1,\dots,0), \\
P_{nj} &= q_n P_{n,j+1} & (j &= b-1,\dots,0), \\
P_{ij} &= p_{i+1}P_{i+1,j} + q_i P_{i,j+1} & (i &= n-1,\dots,1; j = b-1,\dots,1), \\
P_{i0} &= q_i P_{i1} & (i &= n,\dots,1),
\end{aligned}
$$

in which $p_i = i/(i+\rho) = 1 - q_i$.

(b) Justify the alternative computational scheme based on $P_k = p_{n-k}^{(0)}$ where $p_i^{(b)} = \delta_{ni}$ and for $j = b,\dots,1$ and $i = n,\dots,0$,

$$
\begin{aligned}
p_i^{(j-1)} &= \sum_{r=0}^{n-i} (p_{i+r} \cdots p_{i+1} q_i) p_{i+r}^{(j)} \\
&= q_i(p_i^{(j)} + p_{i+1}(p_{i+1}^{(j)} + p_{i+2}(p_{i+2}^{(j)} + \cdots (p_{n-1}^{(j)} + p_n p_n^{(j)}) \cdots))), \\
&= q_i\left(p_i^{(j)} + \frac{p_{i+1}}{q_{i+1}} p_{i+1}^{(j-1)}\right) \qquad (i \le n-1).
\end{aligned}
$$

[*Remark:* Either of these computational schemes is numerically more stable than the explicit formula at (3.6.12).]

4.7 In the Markovian model for a general stochastic epidemic process $\{(X,Y)_t : 0 \le t < \infty\}$ discussed in Section 3.3, starting from $(X,Y)_0 = (N,1)$, let $\mathcal{H}_t$ denote the increasing σ-fields determined by the sample paths $\{(X,Y)_u : 0 \le u < t\}$. Regard a similar model $(\tilde{X},\tilde{Y})_t$ with $(\tilde{X},\tilde{Y})_0 = (N+1,1)$ as starting with the same $(N,1)$ individuals as determine $\mathcal{H}_t$ augmented by a distinguished individual that is initially susceptible and that has no impact on the sample paths $(X,Y)_t$ for precisely as long as it remains susceptible. Show that

$$
\begin{aligned}
p_{N+1}(t) &\equiv \Pr\{\text{distinguished individual is susceptible at } t\} \\
&= \mathrm{E}[\exp(-\beta \textstyle\int_0^t Y(u)\,\mathrm{d}u)\,|\,\mathcal{H}_t].
\end{aligned}
$$

From this it is plausible that

$$
p_{N+1}(\infty) = \frac{\mathrm{E}\tilde{X}_\infty}{N+1} = \mathrm{E}\left[\left(\frac{\gamma}{\gamma+\beta}\right)^{N+1-X_\infty}\right];
$$

compare with the argument in Ball (1986). Cf. also (2.3.7) and Exercise 5.6.

4.8 Investigate appropriately rescaled limits of the pairs-at-parties model and of the two simple epidemic analogues of Section 4.6, for (a) $N \to \infty$, and (b) $\beta' \to 0$.

5

Rumours: Modelling Spread and its Cessation

This chapter is devoted to further models of spread in a population, most of them appealing to the Law of Mass Action. Our aim is to exemplify the modelling principles found useful in other problems involving the spread of an attribute through a population. It is important to note that except for models in which the only 'mechanism' is that of spreading, as for example in the case of a simple epidemic, the range of behaviour exhibited by processes with a removal mechanism is quite varied.

The two key features of previous models involve the spread of a disease and the removal of infectious individuals. We have given some emphasis in Chapters 2, 3 and 4 to the spread of disease by other than homogeneous mechanisms. In this chapter we look also at a variety of removal mechanisms, such as may apply to the spread of a rumour (an 'infection of the mind'). We show that different removal mechanisms can lead to somewhat different conclusions from those of earlier chapters, where threshold phenomena were of particular interest.

5.1 Rumour models

The earliest references in the probability literature to a rumour model appear in the work of Rapoport and co-workers from 1948 onwards (see Bartholomew (1967) for references), in Feller (1957, Exercises 11.10.21–22) though not in his first (1950) edition, and in Kendall (1957). Here we take as our basic model that described in Daley and Kendall (1965) (called [DK] below), where the original motivation for its formulation was the possible similarity in the spread of physiological and psychological infections (cf. Daley and Kendall, 1964). The analysis that ensued highlighted a major difference in modelling the way that spreading ceases for the two types of 'infection'.

As in the simpler models of Chapters 2 and 3, we consider a closed homogeneously mixing population of $N+1$ individuals. At any time they can be classified as belonging to one of three mutually exclusive and exhaustive categories consisting at time $t > 0$ of

(a) $X(t)$ individuals who are ignorant of the rumour;

(b) $Y(t)$ individuals who are actively spreading the rumour; and

(c) $Z(t)$ individuals who know the rumour but have ceased spreading it.

Initially, $X(0) = N$, $Y(0) = 1$ and $Z(0) = 0$, while for all t, $X(t) + Y(t) + Z(t) = N + 1$. We refer to these three types of individuals as ignorants, spreaders and stiflers respectively; they are the equivalents of susceptibles, infectives and removals of the general epidemic model of Chapter 3, but we model their behaviour somewhat differently.

The rumour is propagated through the population by contact between ignorants and spreaders, following the law of mass action just as in Chapter 3. Specifically, assume that any spreader involved in any pairwise meeting attempts to 'infect' the other individual involved in the meeting; this 'other individual' is either an ignorant, a spreader or a stifler. In the first case, the ignorant becomes a spreader; in the other two cases, either or both of those involved in the meeting learn that the rumour is 'known' and so decide not to tell the rumour any more, thereby joining the stiflers as a result of this 'stifling experience'. When the pairwise meeting rate is β, ignorant–spreader, spreader–spreader and stifler–spreader meetings occur at time t at relative rates $\beta X(t) Y(t)$, $\frac{1}{2}\beta Y(t)[Y(t) - 1]$, and $\beta Y(t) Z(t)$ respectively. It is convenient to write such changes as may occur in a (small) time interval $(t, t + h)$ in the form

$$\Delta_h(X, Y)(t) \equiv (X, Y)(t + h) - (X, Y)(t), \qquad (5.1.1)$$

so for example an ignorant–spreader meeting yields $\Delta_h(X, Y)(t) = (-1, 1)$. We use the meeting rates to set the transition rates for changes in the state of the population, and so deduce the relations, with the approximations neglecting terms that are $o(h)$,

$$\Pr\{\Delta_h(X, Y)(t) = (-1, 1) \mid (X, Y)(t) = (x, y)\} = \beta xyh,$$
$$\Pr\{\Delta_h(X, Y)(t) = (0, -2) \mid (X, Y)(t) = (x, y)\} = \tfrac{1}{2}\beta y(y - 1)h,$$
$$\Pr\{\Delta_h(X, Y)(t) = (0, -1) \mid (X, Y)(t) = (x, y)\} = \beta yzh, \qquad (5.1.2)$$
$$\Pr\{\Delta_h(X, Y)(t) = (0, 0) \mid (X, Y)(t) = (x, y)\} = 1 - \beta y(N - \tfrac{1}{2}[y - 1])h,$$

while all other transitions have probability $o(h)$. It is clear here that β plays the role of a time constant, so by suitable choice of time unit we may assume that $\beta = 1$.

We shall be interested in the proportion f of the ignorant population $X(0) = N$ which eventually learns the rumour, so that

$$\lim_{t \to \infty} X(t) = N - Nf, \quad \lim_{t \to \infty} Y(t) = 0, \quad \lim_{t \to \infty} Z(t) = 1 + Nf. \quad (5.1.3)$$

We can study the properties of f both in a deterministic version of the model described by equations (5.1.2) (cf. Chapter 2 and Section 5.2 below), and an embedded jump chain argument (cf. Sections 3.4.2–3 and 5.3). It is also convenient to use the present context to describe an argument due to D.G. Kendall leading to a quicker computation of asymptotic properties of the model for larger population sizes (see Section 5.4).

We now describe two simple variants of the basic [DK] model. For the first, which we call the k-fold stifling model, assume that a spreader does not decide to stop propagating the rumour until being involved in k stifling experiences as described earlier. Then by identifying the $Y(t)$ spreaders as belonging to one of the k mutually exclusive categories of spreaders who have had j stifling experiences ($j = 0, \ldots, k-1$), we can still give a Markovian description of the process, using the larger, $(k+1)$-dimensional vector $(X, Y_1, \ldots, Y_k)(t)$ where $(Y_1 + \cdots + Y_k)(t) = Y(t) = N + 1 - X(t) - Z(t)$ as earlier. See Exercise 5.3 for a deterministic version of this model.

For the second variant, which we call the (α, p)-probability variant, observe that the [DK] model is certainly simplistic in supposing that (a) every pairwise meeting involving a spreader results in the spreader attempting to spread the rumour, and (b) a spreader becomes a stifler as a result of exactly one stifling experience. Suppose instead that a spreader involved in a pairwise meeting attempts to spread the rumour with probability p, and that when such an attempt is made any spreader so involved decides with probability α to become a stifler, independently for each spreader and each meeting. The basic model has $p = \alpha = 1$; we now suppose that $0 < p \leq 1$ and $0 < \alpha \leq 1$. Then when $(X, Y)(t) = (x, y)$, there occurs in $(t, t + h)$ either an (X, Y) meeting resulting in $\Delta_h(X, Y) = (-1, 1)$ with probability $pxyh$ (neglecting $o(h)$ terms), or a (Y, Y) meeting resulting in $\Delta_h(X, Y) = (0, -1)$ or $(0, -2)$ with respective probabilities $p(2-p)\alpha(1-\alpha)y(y-1)h$ and $p(2-p)\alpha^2 \frac{1}{2}y(y-1)h$, or a (Y, Z) meeting resulting in $\Delta_h(X, Y) = (0, -1)$ with probability $p\alpha yzh$, or no change with probability $1 - p[(1+\alpha)x + (1 - \frac{1}{2}p)\alpha(2-\alpha)(y-1)]yh$.

Another model which has gained some currency, if only because of its simplicity and appearance in an undergraduate text, is due to Maki and Thompson (1973). As before, the population is classified and counted as (X, Y, Z); a continuous time Markov process version of the model is then

as follows (Watson, 1988). The rumour is spread by directed contact of the
$Y(t)$ spreaders at time t with others in the population. The outcome of
contact of a specified spreader with (a) an ignorant is that the ignorant becomes a spreader, and (b) another spreader or a stifler, is that the initiating
spreader becomes a stifler. No other micro-level transitions occur. Then
the model has just two elementary transitions, with $\Delta_h(X,Y) = (-1,1)$
or $(0,-1)$ at infinitesimal rates $XYh + o(h)$ and $Y(Y - 1 + Z)h + o(h)$
respectively, i.e. omitting terms $o(h)$,

$$\Pr\{\Delta_h(X,Y)(t) = (-1,1) \mid (X,Y)(t) = (x,y)\} = xyh,$$
$$\Pr\{\Delta_h(X,Y)(t) = (0,-1) \mid (X,Y)(t) = (x,y)\} = y(y+z-1)h, \quad (5.1.4)$$
$$\Pr\{\Delta_h(X,Y)(t) = (0,0) \mid (X,Y)(t) = (x,y)\} = 1 - Nyh.$$

Notice that because there is now *directed* contact of the initiating spreader,
the term $\frac{1}{2}y(y-1)$ of equations (5.1.2) is replaced by $y(y-1)$ in (5.1.4). The
model is otherwise like the [DK] model in assuming that it is only through
interaction between the initiating spreader and others of the population that
a spreader becomes a stifler. The resulting deterministic analysis is similar
(see the next section and Exercise 5.4), but not so the stochastic analysis
(see Section 5.3 and Exercise 5.7).

Both the simple epidemic model and the general epidemic model discussed
in Chapter 3 have been suggested as models to describe the spread of a rumour (e.g. Goffman (1965), Goffman and Newill (1964, 1967), Bartholomew
(1973, Chapters 9 and 10)). Recall that the general epidemic model has
two basic transitions possible in a small interval of time of length h, namely
$\Delta_h(X,Y) = (-1,1)$ or $(0,-1)$ at rates βxy and γy respectively. Clearly the
first transition can result from an (X,Y) contact, but the second requires
no interaction between individuals in the population at all. It is enough for
the cessation of rumour-spreading to occur purely as a result of a spreader's
'forgetting', irrevocably, to tell the rumour to those of the population with
whom (s)he comes into contact. Now forgetfulness, or disinclination ever
to tell the rumour, are certainly features we may wish to model as factors
contributing to the decline in the spread of the rumour. But it seems an
unrealistic description of human behaviour to make it the sole mechanism
causing the cessation of a rumour's spreading, in the same way as total
reliance on the stifling mechanism may be unrealistic. Just as diseases may
vary in their potency, so rumours may vary in the urgency with which individuals communicate them. On balance we may wish to use both stifling
and forgetfulness mechanisms (for surely, some items of news are eminently
forgettable!); one possible way of doing so is indicated in Exercise 5.5. It

would then be reasonable to expect the relative rates of pariwise contact (for both spreading and stifling) and of individual forgetfulness to affect the extent of the spread of the rumour.

Threshold phenomena such as occur in branching processes or the spread of epidemics (see e.g. Chapters 2 and 3) depend on a balance between spreading on the one hand and cessation of spread on the other. If, as in the basic [DK] models, the cessation depends on interaction of the spreaders with themselves or stiflers in the population, then the effect of the cessation mechanism is negligible relative to that of the spreading mechanism when the numbers of spreaders and stiflers are small. On the other hand, when cessation of contagious spread occurs as a result of the evolution of a spreader independently of the rest of the population, with spreading dependent on the state of the population, then it is the state of the rest of the population, relative to the dynamics of spread and its cessation amongst the spreaders themselves, that determines the fate of the spread. In this case, conditions for threshold criteria exist, whether for the spread of a disease or a rumour, as in the general epidemic model.

We now describe a distinctly different family of models for the spread of news or a rumour in a population. For convenience we assume that the population is of constant size $N + 1$, its members being classified as ignorants, spreaders and former spreaders (e.g. stiflers or removed cases), much as before; initially there are N ignorants and 1 spreader. Let each individual becoming a spreader, including the initial spreader, be identified by a distinct integer-valued index r. Spreader r spreads the rumour to K_r individuals chosen at random (without replacement, for definiteness) from the rest of the population; $\{K_r : r = 1, 2, \ldots\}$ is a family of independent identically distributed integer-valued random variables with distribution $\{f_k = \Pr\{K_r = k\}, \ k = 0, 1, \ldots\}$ and mean $m = \mathrm{E}K_r$. Those of the K_r individuals who are ignorants become spreaders, while the others are not affected by the contact. After making these K_r contacts, spreader r plays no further part in spreading the rumour. A convenient identification of the indices is that matching the order in which the r.v.s $\{K_r\}$ are taken into the analysis. Then, writing (X_r, Y_r) for the numbers of ignorants and spreaders just before the K_r contacts occur, we have for $Y_r \geq 1$,

$$X_{r+1} = X_r - J_r(K_r), \qquad Y_{r+1} = Y_r - 1 + J_r(K_r), \qquad (5.1.5)$$

where $J_r(K_r)$ denotes the number of contacts with ignorants amongst the

K_r contacts of spreader r. These assumptions give

$$\Pr\{J_r(K_r) = j \mid X_r = i\} = \sum_{k=j}^{N} f_k \binom{i}{j}\binom{N-i}{k-j} / \binom{N}{k}, \qquad (5.1.6)$$

for r such that $Y_r \geq 1$. Recognizing the hypergeometric distribution probabilities as the coefficients of f_k, we have $E(J_r(K_r) \mid X_r = i, Y_r \geq 1) = \sum_k f_k k(i/N) = mX_r/N$. The relations (5.1.5) are similar to those at equation (4.5.2) where we considered the analysis of a variant of the general epidemic model by means of an embedded random walk. The same approach is applicable here.

Such a model is most aptly described as a branching process *on* a finite population. It can certainly be used to describe the so-called chain letter process. It also includes the general epidemic model when $\{f_k\}$ is the geometric distribution $\{\rho N^{k-1}/(N+\rho)^k : k = 0, 1, \ldots\}$) as far as the ultimate extent of the spread of the news or rumour is concerned. There exist both deterministic and stochastic threshold theorems for which a major outbreak can occur only if $m > 1$. Chapter 10.3 of Bartholomew (1973) includes discussion that refers to related work of Rapoport and co-workers.

5.2 Deterministic analysis of rumour models

Except for the branching process model described at the end of the last section, the models we have sketched for the spread of news or a rumour can be formulated as Markov processes in continuous time. Their analysis by explicit algebra does not proceed easily; in particular their transition probabilities are not readily accessible for the range of parameter values of interest, most notably the initial number of ignorants N. We resort in the first instance to deterministic versions of the models.

For the deterministic version of (5.1.1) we consider the continuous functions $x(t)$, $y(t)$ and $z(t)$, differentiable in t, that have the same initial values $x(0) = X(0) = N$, $y(0) = Y(0) = 1$, $z(0) = Z(0) = 0$ and satisfy $x(t) + y(t) + z(t) = N + 1$ for a closed population. The rates of change of x and y are assumed to coincide with the rates of change of the conditional mean functions such as $\lim_{h \to 0} E(X(t+h) \mid (X, Y)(t) = (i, j))$ at the lattice points (i, j), 'smoothly' interpolated between. These limits are assumed to be given as below:

$$\dot{x} = \sum_{\text{simple transitions}} (\text{change in } x) \times (\text{rate of change}) = (-1)xy, \qquad (5.2.1a)$$

and similarly,

$$\dot{y} = (+1)xy + (-2)\tfrac{1}{2}y(y-1) + (-1)yz = y(x-y+1-z) = y(2x-N). \quad (5.2.1\text{b})$$

These two equations yield

$$\frac{dy}{dx} = -2 + \frac{N}{x}, \qquad (5.2.2)$$

whose solution consistent with the initial conditions is

$$2x(t) + y(t) + N \ln \frac{N}{x(t)} \equiv \lambda\big(x(t), y(t)\big) = 2N + 1 \qquad \text{(all } t > 0\text{)}. \quad (5.2.3)$$

It follows from (5.2.3) that the limit $\lim_{t\to\infty} x(t)/N = \theta_N$ say, analogous to the proportion f at (5.1.3) of ignorants who never hear the rumour, satisfies

$$-1 = 2N(1 - \theta_N) + N \ln \theta_N, \qquad (5.2.4)$$

and that $\lim_{N\to\infty} \theta_N = \theta$ satisfies

$$2(1 - \theta) + \ln \theta = 0. \qquad (5.2.5)$$

This is the same as the equation for the deterministic model of a general epidemic considered in Chapter 2.3, having relative removal rate $\tfrac{1}{2}N$ (cf. equations (2.3.6) and (2.3.7)). Unlike the epidemic model, the rumour model no longer has a family of processes with a parameter determining threshold behaviour. Instead, the analogy is with a single process; it is not difficult to check that the dependence on N of the root θ_N of (5.2.4) is $O(N^{-1})$ (see Exercise 5.1).

In a similar fashion, the general (α, p)-probability variant of the basic [DK] model leads to the pair of differential equations

$$\dot{x} = (-1)pxy,$$
$$\dot{y} - (+1)pxy + (-1)[p(2-p)2\alpha(1-\alpha)\tfrac{1}{2}y(y-1) + p\alpha yz]$$
$$+ (-2)p(2-p)\alpha^2 \tfrac{1}{2}y(y-1)$$
$$= py[x - \alpha(z + (2-p)(y-1))].$$

In this case, the analogue of equation (5.2.2) is

$$\frac{dy}{dx} = -(1+\alpha) + \frac{\alpha(N-1+p)}{x} + \frac{\alpha(1-p)y}{x}. \qquad (5.2.6)$$

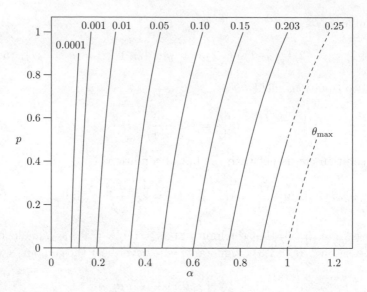

Figure 5.1. Contours of $\theta(\alpha, p)$, the proportion of a large population not hearing a rumour with uncertain spreading $(p < 1)$ and stifling $(\alpha < 1)$. The values at the top of each curve are of $\theta(\alpha, p)$, the smaller positive root in θ of equation (5.2.8) (see Exercise 5.2 for $\theta_{\max}$).

This is still a first order linear differential equation, with the general solution

$$y = 1 - \frac{(1 + \alpha)x}{1 - \alpha(1 - p)} - \frac{N}{1 - p} + \lambda_{N,\alpha,p} x^{\alpha(1-p)}$$

for some constant $\lambda_{N,\alpha,p}$ of integration which is determined by the initial conditions, yielding

$$y = 1 - \frac{(1 + \alpha)x}{1 - \alpha(1 - p)} + \frac{N}{1 - p}\left[\frac{2 - p}{1 - \alpha(1 - p)}\left(\frac{x}{N}\right)^{\alpha(1-p)} - 1\right]. \quad (5.2.7)$$

The proportion θ_N of ignorants who never hear the rumour behaves much as the root of equation (5.2.4), but with limit $\theta \equiv \theta(\alpha, p) = \lim_{N \to \infty} \theta_N$ now satisfying

$$(2 - p)\theta^{\alpha(1-p)} - (1 + \alpha)(1 - p)\theta = 1 - \alpha(1 - p). \quad (5.2.8)$$

The contour curves in Figure 5.1 depict the non-unit root $\theta(\alpha, p)$ as a function of α and p; always, $0 < \theta(\alpha, p) \le \theta_{\max}$, where $\theta_{\max} \approx 0.284\,668$ is the smaller positive root of $\theta(1 - 2\ln\theta) = 1$ arising from the limit $\alpha \to 1$ and $p \to 0$ (see also Exercise 5.2).

The deterministic analysis of Maki and Thompson's model is sketched in Exercise 5.4.

5.3 Embedded random walks for rumour models

We now return to [DK]'s stochastic model described by the Markov chain with infinitesimal transition rates as at (5.1.2). The main vehicle for studying the final state of this process (e.g. [DK] and Pittel (1990)) has been the Markov chain embedded at the jump points occurring at times $t_1, \ldots, t_n$, $\ldots, t_M$ (cf. Section 3.4.2 above), where M is the total number of jumps. We note that because the state space is finite and the process is 'strictly evolutionary' in the sense of having well-ordered sample paths, M must be finite.

Denote the states immediately after these jump epochs by $\{(X, Y)_n : n = 0, 1, \ldots\}$, with $(X, Y)_0 = (N, 1)$, so that when for some particular n we have $(X, Y)_n = (X, Y)(t_n+) = (i, j)$,

$$(X, Y)_{n+1} = (X, Y)_n + \begin{cases} (-1, +1) & \text{with probability } i/f_{ij}, \\ (0, -1) & \text{with probability } (N+1-i-j)/f_{ij}, \\ (0, -2) & \text{with probability } \frac{1}{2}(j-1)/f_{ij}, \end{cases}$$
(5.3.1)

where $f_{ij} = N - \frac{1}{2}(j-1)$. Note that the first case is excluded if $i = 0$, when the probability equals zero, or $j = 0$, while the last case is excluded if $j \leq 1$. This embedded jump process is a random walk on that part of the two-dimensional integer lattice for which $0 \leq i \leq N$, $0 \leq j \leq N+1-i$, and the states $\{(i, 0) : i = 0, \ldots, N-1\}$ are absorbing. From equations (5.3.1) we can derive equations for the probabilities P_{ij} on the path of a rumour, defined by

$$\begin{aligned} P_{ij} &= \Pr\{(X, Y)(t) = (i, j) \text{ for some } t\} \\ &= \Pr\{(X, Y)_n = (i, j) \text{ for some } n\}. \end{aligned}$$
(5.3.2)

The Markov process $\{(X, Y)(t)\}$ is strictly evolutionary in the sense that, once a state (i, j) is visited and left, it is never visited again. Hence the probabilities P_{ij} satisfy a set of equations, derived by a forward decomposition argument, of the general form

$$P_{ij} = \sum P_{(i,j)-\Delta} \Pr\{\text{next jump is } \Delta \mid \text{present state is } (i, j) - \Delta\}, \quad (5.3.3)$$

where Δ denotes one of the three jumps $(-1, 1)$, $(0, -1)$ and $(0, -2)$ at equation (5.3.1). Specifically, starting from $P_{N1} = P_{N-1,2} = 1$, we have for

$i = 0, \ldots, N - 1,$

$$
P_{ij} = \begin{cases}
\dfrac{i+1}{N - \frac{1}{2}(N - i - 1)} P_{i+1,N-i} & (j = N - i + 1), & (5.3.4a) \\[2ex]
0 & (j = N - i), & (5.3.4b) \\[2ex]
\dfrac{i+1}{N - \frac{1}{2}(j-2)} P_{i+1,j-1} + \dfrac{N - i - j}{N - \frac{1}{2}j} P_{i,j+1} + \dfrac{\frac{1}{2}(j+1)}{N - \frac{1}{2}(j+1)} P_{i,j+2} & & \\[1ex]
& (2 \le j \le N - 1 - i), & (5.3.4c) \\[2ex]
\dfrac{N - i - j}{N - \frac{1}{2}j} P_{i,j+1} + \dfrac{\frac{1}{2}(j+1)}{N - \frac{1}{2}(j+1)} P_{i,j+2} & (j = 0, 1). & (5.3.4d)
\end{cases}
$$

From these relations, in the same way as the distribution of the size of the general epidemic process was derived in Section 3.4.3, we can find the distribution

$$
\{P_{i0}\} = \{\Pr\{\text{rumour ends with } i \text{ ignorants}\} : i = 0, 1, \ldots, N - 1\}. \quad (5.3.5)
$$

Figure 5.2(a) illustrates the complementary distribution $\{P_{N-i,0}\}$ of the number of ignorants hearing the rumour in this model, for two initial sizes $N = 50$ and 100. The scales have been changed as indicated in the figure for $N = 100$, to facilitate comparison of the two distributions.

In [DK] it was concluded that the proportion $\xi_N = X(\infty)/N$ of ignorants left when the rumour stops spreading has

$$
\begin{aligned}
\mathrm{E}\,\xi_N &\approx 0.203\,188 + 0.273\,843/N = \theta + 0.273\,843/N, \\
N \operatorname{var} \xi_N &\approx 0.310\,681 + 1.232\,700/N.
\end{aligned} \quad (5.3.6)
$$

Observe that the correction term added to $\theta = 0.203\,188$, the solution of equation (5.2.5), shows that θ_N, the solution of (5.2.4) (see Exercise 5.1), is such that $\theta_N \ne \mathrm{E}\,\xi_N$, nor is there any good reason that equality should hold. In Section 5.4 we note that

$$
\frac{\theta(1-\theta)[(1-\theta)^2 + \theta^2]}{(1-2\theta)^2} = 0.310681 \approx N \operatorname{var} \xi_N. \quad (5.3.7)
$$

For the [DK] model the general form of equation (5.3.4) involves three terms on the right-hand side. For the Maki–Thompson model, however, while the same deterministic equation (5.2.2) applies, the analogous equation has only two terms, corresponding to the simpler possible transitions

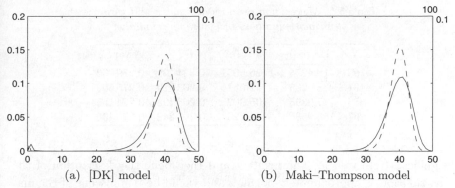

(a) [DK] model   (b) Maki–Thompson model

Figure 5.2. Frequency polygons of the distribution of the numbers of ignorants ultimately hearing a rumour in two rumour models, for $N = 50$ (——, scales as shown) and $N = 100$ (– – –, double the abscissa scale, halve the ordinate scale, as indicated at top right-hand corners).

as at (5.1.4). Specifically, starting from $P_{N1} = P_{N-1,2} = 1$ as before, we now have for $i = 0, \ldots, N - 1$,

$$
P_{ij} = \begin{cases}
\dfrac{i+1}{N} P_{i+1,N-i} & (j = N - i + 1), & (5.3.8\text{a}) \\[2mm]
\dfrac{i+1}{N} P_{i+1,j-1} + \left(1 - \dfrac{i}{N}\right) P_{i,j+1} & (2 \leq j \leq N - i), & (5.3.8\text{b}) \\[2mm]
\left(1 - \dfrac{i}{N}\right) P_{i,j+1} & (j = 0, 1). & (5.3.8\text{c})
\end{cases}
$$

In principle, generating function methods could now be used to study these equations and develop a routine for evaluating P_{i0}. But it is unquestionably more practical to proceed directly to their numerical evaluation (see Table 5.1 for some values of moments), and to contrast their stochastic behaviour for larger N using the diffusion arguments presented in Section 5.4 (cf. Exercise 5.7). By fitting quadratics in $1/N$ to the last two columns of Table 5.1 for $N = 191, 383$ and 767, we obtain in place of (5.3.6)

$$
\begin{aligned}
\mathrm{E}\,\xi_N &\approx 0.203\,188 + 0.117\,20/N + 0.6606/N^2, \\
N\,\mathrm{var}\,\xi_N &\approx 0.272\,735 + 0.529\,86/N + 5.5823/N^2.
\end{aligned}
\tag{5.3.9}
$$

These results differ from the relations at (5.3.6) for the [DK] model except for the commonality of $\theta = 0.203\,188$ in $\mathrm{E}\,\xi_N$. The values for N in the table are used to facilitate direct comparison with [DK]'s Table 1. Note that the moments given are of $X(\infty)$ conditioned to be less than $N - \sqrt{N}$: conditioning is necessary because otherwise the term $P_{N-1,0} = 1/N^2$ contributes

Table 5.1. *Maki–Thompson model: mean and variance of ultimate numbers of ignorants remaining*

N	$EX(\infty)$	$\operatorname{var} X(\infty)$	$E\xi_N$	$N\operatorname{var}\xi_N$
95	19.4274	26.5051	0.204 499	0.279 002
191	38.9295	52.6515	0.203 819	0.275 662
383	77.9398	105.002	0.203 498	0.274 155
767	155.963	209.725	0.203 342	0.273 435

significantly to $\operatorname{var}\xi_N$. The result would then belie the description of the distribution as approximately normal, and would be reminiscent of the major/minor humps of the final size distribution of the general epidemic (cf. Figure 3.2). Pittel (1990) illustrates ways around the complications that result from this fact when attempting to use a moment method for proving asymptotics of the final size distribution. Watson (1988) remarks that the fact that the asymptotic value of $N\operatorname{var}\xi_N$ for the Maki–Thompson model is smaller than for the [DK] model 'accords with the change to smaller more frequent jumps in the removal process'.

Figure 5.2(b) complements part (a) by presenting the distribution for the Maki–Thompson model. The probability of very few ignorants ever hearing the rumour, which is approximately $\frac{1}{2}N^{-1}$ for the [DK] model and N^{-2} for the Maki–Thompson model, shows as a small peak in (a) and not at all in (b), at the scale of the diagram and for the values of N used.

Both the general epidemic and Maki–Thompson models have embedded random walks that are of a simpler structure than that in the [DK] model. Specifically, because the process is strictly evolutionary and the jumps are to 'adjacent' states, much as in a birth-and-death process, the 'time' argument n of the embedded jump process can be used to reduce the dimension of the state space, from a two-dimensional to a one-dimensional lattice. To study such processes we replace the embedded jump process $\{(X,Y)_n\}$ by $\{(X',Y')_n\}$ which is defined as starting from the same initial state and as having one-step transitions to $(-1,1)$ and $(0,-1)$ with the same probabilities as for $\{(X,Y)_n\}$. But now $\{(X',Y')_n\}$ is no longer confined to a first passage into the states $(0,j)$ $(j=0,\ldots,N)$; rather,

$$(X',Y')_n \mapsto (X',Y')_{n+1} + \begin{cases} (-1,1) & \text{with probability } X'_n/N, \\ (0,-1) & \text{with probability } 1 - X'_n/N. \end{cases} \tag{5.3.10}$$

Clearly, $(X,Y)_n = (X',Y')_n$ for $n = 0,\ldots,M$.

Now, after n jumps starting from $(X',Y')_0 = (N,1)$, it must be the case, since these n jumps have increments that are either $(-1,1)$ or $(0,-1)$, that

$n = N - X'_n + (1 + N - X'_n - Y'_n)$, or $2X'_n + Y'_n + n = 2N + 1$. From this relation we deduce that $M = \inf\{n : n = 2N + 1 - 2X'_n\}$.

Also, conditional on the σ-field $\mathcal{F}_n \equiv \sigma(X'_0, \ldots, X'_n)$, the expected decrement in $\{X'_n\}$ equals X'_n/N, or equivalently, $\mathrm{E}(X'_{n+1} \mid \mathcal{F}_n) = X'_n(1 - N^{-1})$. This means that the functional $V_n = [N/(N-1)]^n X'_n$ satisfies

$$
\begin{aligned}
\mathrm{E}(V_{n+1} \mid \mathcal{F}_n) = \mathrm{E}(V_{n+1} \mid X'_n) &= \mathrm{E}\left[\left(\frac{N}{N-1}\right)^{n+1} X'_{n+1} \,\Big|\, X'_n\right] \\
&= \left(\frac{N}{N-1}\right)^n X'_n = V_n,
\end{aligned}
\tag{5.3.11}
$$

implying that $\{V_n\}$ is a martingale with respect to the σ-fields $\{\mathcal{F}_n\}$ on which M is a stopping time.

Similarly, $\mathrm{E}([X'_{n+1} - X'_n]^2 \mid \mathcal{F}_n) = X'_n/N$ so that

$$
\begin{aligned}
\mathrm{E}(X'^2_{n+1} \mid \mathcal{F}_n) &= 2X'_n \mathrm{E}(X'_{n+1} \mid \mathcal{F}_n) - X'^2_n + \frac{X'_n}{N} \\
&= X'^2_n\left(1 - \frac{2}{N}\right) + \mathrm{E}(X'_n - X'_{n+1} \mid \mathcal{F}_n)
\end{aligned}
$$

and

$$
\mathrm{E}(X'^2_{n+1} - X'_{n+1} \mid \mathcal{F}_n) = (X'^2_n - X'_n)\left(1 - \frac{2}{N}\right),
$$

and therefore $\{[N/(N-2)]^n(X'^2_n - X'_n)\}$ is also a martingale.

Sudbury (1985) uses this pair of martingales in conjunction with the stopping time M to prove that as $N \to \infty$, $\xi_N \to \theta$ in probability. This is a weaker statement than the convergence in distribution of $\sqrt{N}(\xi_N - \theta)$. Exercise 5.6 sketches a pair of martingales for the analogous embedded jump process $\{(X', Y')_n\}$ defined on a general epidemic.

5.4 A diffusion approximation

Daley and Kendall (1965) outlined an heuristic method for evaluating var $X(\infty)$, the variance of the number of ignorants remaining when spreading stops. The major step in the procedure is to find the variation in Λ, the stochastic analogue of the deterministic 'constant of integration' λ in (5.2.3). We describe the mechanics of the procedure; mathematical details of the martingale and limit arguments involved can be found in Barbour (1972, 1974) and e.g. Watson (1988). Martingale arguments have also been noted by Pittel (1990) and Lefèvre and Picard (1994).

The essence of Kendall's Principle of Diffusion of Arbitrary Constants, as it applies to pure jump Markov population processes such as epidemics or predator–prey models, embodies two features, one reflecting the mean behaviour of the process and the other the variability about that mean behaviour. The mean behaviour is represented by the so-called deterministic path or deterministic version of the model; ideally, this is represented by an 'invariant of the motion', to borrow a phrase from classical applied mathematics. Its probabilistic analogue is a martingale. The variability can be regarded as a diffusion on adjacent paths, each path characterized by a different starting point. The local probabilistic analogue is the quadratic variation of the martingale. The total variation is then the result of accumulating this local variability as the process evolves along its deterministic path.

In the rest of this section we illustrate this approach as it applies to the [DK] rumour model and the general epidemic. Three more applications are stated as exercises.

By analogy with (5.2.3), but recalling that the rumour process $(X, Y)(t)$ is lattice-valued, we start by writing

$$\Lambda(t) = 2X(t) + Y(t) + N\left[\frac{1}{N} + \cdots + \frac{1}{X(t) + 1}\right]$$

$$\approx \lambda(X(t), Y(t)) = 2X(t) + Y(t) + N\ln\frac{N}{X(t)},$$

(5.4.1)

where $\Lambda(\cdot)$ is clearly a random variable. Recall from (5.2.3) that $\lambda(t) = \lambda(x(t), y(t)) \equiv 2x(t) + y(t) - N\ln[x(t)/N] = 2N + 1$ (all $t \geq 0$) for $(x(t), y(t))$ denoting the deterministic path. We use this relation later in the form

$$y(t) - 1 = 2[N - x(t)] + N\ln\frac{x(t)}{N}.$$

(5.4.2)

Now the process $\Lambda(t)$ is a martingale with respect to the σ-fields $\{\mathcal{F}_{t-}\} \equiv \{\sigma(\{(X, Y)(s) : s < t\})\}$, as is verified by evaluating

$\mathrm{E}(d\Lambda(t) \mid \mathcal{F}_{t-})$

$$= \left[\left(-1 + \frac{N}{X(t)}\right)X(t)Y(t) + (-1)Y(t)Z(t) + (-2)\tfrac{1}{2}Y(t)[Y(t) - 1]\right]dt$$

$$= Y(t)(N - X(t) - Z(t) - Y(t) + 1)\,dt = 0.$$

(5.4.3)

To find its quadratic variation we find $\mathrm{E}([d\Lambda(t)]^2 \mid \mathcal{F}_{t-})$, namely

$$\left[\left(-1 + \frac{N}{X(t)}\right)^2 X(t)Y(t) + Y(t)Z(t) + 2Y(t)[Y(t) - 1]\right]dt$$

$$= Y(t)\left[N - 2N + \frac{N^2}{X(t)} + Y(t) - 1\right]dt.$$

(5.4.4)

In order to compute the total quadratic variation over the evolution of the spread of the rumour, we replace the stochastic process $(X, Y)(t)$ on the right-hand side by its deterministic version $\big(x(t), y(t)\big)$ given by equation (5.4.2) with $N \geq x(t) \geq N\theta$ and $\dot{x}(t) = -x(t)y(t)$. These substitutions give

$$
\begin{aligned}
\operatorname{var} \Lambda(\infty) &\approx \int_{x=N\theta}^{N} \frac{\mathrm{E}\big([\mathrm{d}\Lambda(t)]^2 \mid \mathcal{F}_{t-}\big)\big|_{(X,Y)(t)=(x,y)(t)}}{\dot{x}(t)} \\
&= \int_{N\theta}^{N} \frac{1}{x}\left[-N + \frac{N^2}{x} + 2(N - x) + N \ln \frac{x}{N}\right] \mathrm{d}x \\
&= N \int_{\theta}^{1} \frac{1 - 2u + 1/u + \ln u}{u} \, \mathrm{d}u \\
&= N\left[-\ln\theta - 2(1 - \theta) + \frac{1 - \theta}{\theta} - \tfrac{1}{2}(\ln\theta)^2\right] \\
&= \frac{N(1 - \theta)(1 - 2\theta + 2\theta^2)}{\theta},
\end{aligned}
\tag{5.4.5}
$$

using (5.2.5) at the last step. Since $|\mathrm{d}\lambda/\mathrm{d}x|_{x=N\theta} = (1 - 2\theta)/\theta$, we arrive finally at

$$
\operatorname{var} X(\infty) \approx \left(\frac{\mathrm{d}x}{\mathrm{d}\lambda}\bigg|_{x=N\theta}\right)^2 \operatorname{var} \Lambda(\infty) \approx \frac{N\theta(1 - \theta)[(1 - \theta)^2 + \theta^2]}{(1 - 2\theta)^2}, \tag{5.4.6}
$$

which is the source of the approximation at (5.3.7).

Another way of linking (5.4.5) and (5.4.6) is as follows. Recall that in the evolution of $\{(X, Y)(t) : t \geq 0\}$, the rumour stops spreading at time $t = T \equiv \inf\{t > 0 : Y(t) = 0\}$, when $X(T-) = X(T+) = X(\infty)$. Since $\{\Lambda(t), \mathcal{F}_{t-}\}$ is a bounded martingale, the optional stopping theorem gives $\mathrm{E}\Lambda(T+) = \mathrm{E}\Lambda(0) = 2N + 1$. From the definition of Λ at (5.4.1) it therefore follows that

$$
\mathrm{E}[\Lambda(T+) - \Lambda(0)] = 0 = 2\mathrm{E}X(\infty) + N\mathrm{E}\left[\frac{1}{N} + \cdots + \frac{1}{X(\infty) + 1}\right] - 2N - 1,
$$

so defining θ_N by $N\theta_N = \mathrm{E}X(\infty)$,

$$
2(1 - \theta_N) = 1 + \mathrm{E}\left[\sum_{i=X(\infty)+1}^{N} \frac{1}{i}\right] \approx 1 + \mathrm{E}\ln\frac{N}{X(\infty)} \approx 1 + \ln\frac{1}{\theta_N} + O(N^{-1}).
$$

Let $X(\infty) = \mathrm{E}X(\infty) + W \approx N\theta_N + W$ for some random deviation W. Then

$$
\Lambda(\infty) - \Lambda(0) = 2[\mathrm{E}X(\infty) + W - N] - 1 - N\sum_{i=\mathrm{E}X(\infty)+W}^{N} \frac{1}{i} \approx W f'\big(\mathrm{E}X(\infty)\big),
$$

where $f(x) = 2x + N\ln(N/x)$, so $f'(x) = 2 - N/x$. Hence,

$$\text{var}\,\Lambda(\infty) \approx \text{var}\,W[f'(\mathrm{E}X(\infty))]^2 = \left(\frac{1-2\theta}{\theta}\right)^2 \text{var}\,X(\infty),$$

from which (5.4.6) follows.

The same relation (5.4.6) follows in a discrete time setting for the jump process $\{(X,Y)_n\}$ considered in Section 5.3, where we now use

$$\Lambda_n = 2X_n + Y_n + N\left[\frac{1}{N} + \cdots + \frac{1}{X_n+1}\right] \tag{5.4.7}$$

and the σ-fields $\{\mathcal{F}_n\} \equiv \{\sigma(\{(X,Y)_r, r = 0,\ldots,n\})\}$. It is easy to check that $\mathrm{E}(\Lambda_{n+1} - \Lambda_n \mid \mathcal{F}_n) = 0$, i.e. $\{\Lambda_n, \mathcal{F}_n\}$ is a martingale.

We now apply the same argument as from (5.4.1) to the general epidemic model, with

$$\begin{aligned}
\Lambda(t) &= X(t) + Y(t) + \rho\left[\frac{1}{N} + \cdots + \frac{1}{X(t)+1}\right] \\
&\approx X(t) + Y(t) + \rho\ln\frac{N}{X(t)},
\end{aligned} \tag{5.4.8}$$

for this model (cf. equation (2.3.6)). The jumps of $(X,Y)(\cdot)$ give

$$\mathrm{d}\Lambda(t) \mid \mathcal{F}_{t-} = \begin{cases} \dfrac{\rho}{X(t)} & \text{at rate } \beta X(t)Y(t)\,\mathrm{d}t, \\ -1 & \text{at rate } \gamma Y(t)\,\mathrm{d}t. \end{cases} \tag{5.4.9}$$

From this the martingale condition $\mathrm{E}(\mathrm{d}\Lambda(t) \mid \mathcal{F}_{t-}) = 0$ is readily verified, and its quadratic variation is computed, formally, as

$$\frac{\mathrm{d}\,\text{var}\,\Lambda}{\mathrm{d}t} = \left(\frac{\rho}{X(t)}\right)^2 \beta X(t)Y(t) + \gamma Y(t) = \beta Y(t)\left[\rho + \frac{\rho^2}{X(t)}\right]. \tag{5.4.10}$$

Then, using $\dot{x} = -\beta xy$ from (2.3.1), and assuming that $\kappa \equiv \rho/N < 1$,

$$\begin{aligned}
\text{var}\,\Lambda(\infty) &\approx \int_{N\theta}^{N} \frac{\rho + \rho^2/x}{x}\,\mathrm{d}x = -\rho\ln\theta + \frac{\rho^2(1-\theta)}{N\theta} \\
&= N(1-\theta)\left[1 + \frac{(\rho/N)^2}{\theta}\right] = \frac{N(1-\theta)(\theta+\kappa^2)}{\theta},
\end{aligned} \tag{5.4.11}$$

where we have used $\rho\ln\theta + N(1-\theta) = 0$ to deduce the last equation (cf. e.g. equation (2.3.7)). Finally, as an analogue of (5.4.6),

$$\text{var}\,X(\infty) \approx \frac{N\theta(1-\theta)(\theta+\kappa^2)}{(\kappa-\theta)^2}, \tag{5.4.12}$$

where $\kappa = \rho/N$ with $\theta < \kappa < 1$.

The epidemic model with $\kappa = \frac{1}{2}$ has the same deterministic path as the basic [DK] rumour model. Then the right-hand side of (5.4.12) equals $N\theta(1-\theta)(1+4\theta)/(1-2\theta)^2$, with the same value of $\theta \approx 0.203$ as in Sections 5.2–3. This asymptotic variance is clearly larger than (5.4.6), as is consistent with the somewhat different behaviour in the initial stages of a general epidemic process conditional on a major outbreak and of the [DK] rumour model process. In the latter, almost all transitions in the early stage of the process are of ignorants becoming spreaders, while in the former the ratio of transitions that increase the number of spreaders to those that decrease their number, is about $1 : \kappa$.

The Maki–Thompson model is a third model with the same deterministic version but, as its stochastic origins are again different, so too is its asymptotic variance (see Exercise 5.9).

The deterministic versions of the k-fold stifling and (α, p)-probability variants of the [DK] model described in Section 5.1 lead to the same proportion of surviving ignorants when the rumour stops spreading for the values $(\alpha, p) = (k^{-1}, 1)$. The asymptotic variance $N \operatorname{var} \xi_N$ is accessible algebraically in the $(\alpha, 1)$-variant (see Exercise 5.7), but only numerically for the k-fold variant (see Exercise 5.8).

5.5   P.g.f. solutions of rumour models

In view of our earlier exposition of probability generating function methods for studying stochastic models for epidemics, it is proper to note the extent of their applicability to the models described in Section 5.1.

Because all the models are strictly evolutionary and the state space is finite, it is in principle possible to find $\Pr\{(X,Y)(t) = (i,j) \mid (X,Y)(0) = (N,1)\}$ by enumerating the finite set of paths that connect $(N,1)$ to (i,j) and have non-zero probability of passage. The extent to which such computations can be organized and presented conveniently depends on whether the algebraic form of the probabilities and rates involved can be simplified sufficiently. These remarks apply equally to the results derived earlier using p.g.f. methods.

P.g.f. solutions are worthwhile when they afford a simplification of information found by other means (cf. remarks above), or if they provide a solution not available by another route. This, of course, is on condition that the solution provides some further understanding of the problem at hand. Certainly (cf. equation (3.3.6)) equations for the p.g.f. provide a useful summary of the information needed to derive equations for the moments of the process concerned.

Consider the [DK] model by way of example. As a continuous time Markov chain model it has the infinitesimal transition rates at (5.1.2). Defining $p_{ij}(t) \equiv \Pr\{(X,Y)(t) = (i,j) \mid (X,Y)(0) = (N,1)\}$ we readily deduce from the forward Kolmogorov equations that

$$\frac{\mathrm{d}\,p_{ij}(t)}{\mathrm{d}t} = (i+1)(j-1)p_{i+1,j-1}(t) + (N-i-j)(j+1)p_{i,j+1}(t)$$
$$+ \tfrac{1}{2}(j+1)(j+2)p_{i,j+2}(t) - j[N - \tfrac{1}{2}(j-1)]p_{ij}(t), \quad (5.5.1)$$

where the first term on the right-hand side vanishes for $j = 1$. From these equations it is easy to find a differential equation for the moments (see Exercise 5.10). If we introduce the generating function $F(v,w,t) = \mathrm{E}(v^{X(t)}w^{Y(t)})$ ($|v| \le 1$, $|w| \le 1$), standard manipulation leads to a partial differential equation of first order in t and second order in v and w. Pearce (1998) has shown how this can be solved, by a procedure somewhat more involved than the analogous one for the general epidemic (cf. Section 3.3.1). His method has overtones that recall the recurrence relations of Section 5.3, and for the same reason, namely, the strictly evolutionary nature of the process. His setting is more general and includes both the Maki–Thompson model and the (α, p)-variant of the [DK] model.

Introduce

$$f_i(w,t) = \sum_{j=0}^{\infty} p_{ij}(t)w^j \qquad (|w| \le 1).$$

Then from (5.5.1) we have

$$\frac{\partial f_i(w,t)}{\partial t} = (i+1)w^2\frac{\partial f_{i+1}}{\partial w} + \left(N(1-w)-i\right)\frac{\partial f_i}{\partial w} + \tfrac{1}{2}(1-w)^2\frac{\partial^2 f_i}{\partial w^2}.$$

Forming the Laplace transforms $\Phi_i(w,\theta) = \int_0^{\infty} \mathrm{e}^{-\theta t} f_i(w,t)\,\mathrm{d}t$ and using the initial conditions $\Phi_i(w,0) = \delta_{Ni}w$ gives

$$\theta\Phi_i(w,\theta) - \delta_{Ni}w = (i+1)w^2\frac{\partial\Phi_{i+1}}{\partial w} + \left(N(1-w)-i\right)\frac{\partial\Phi_i}{\partial w} + \tfrac{1}{2}(1-w)^2\frac{\partial^2\Phi_i}{\partial w^2}.$$

The function $\Phi_i(w,\theta)$ is a polynomial in w of degree $N+1-i$, in which the coefficients are functions of θ and can be determined by a set of recurrence relations. The analysis is an algebraic *tour de force*, describing the manipulations that are possible for strictly evolutionary Markov chains, using square matrices of order up to $3(N+1)$. A formal solution for the $\Phi_i(w,\theta)$ is obtained. See Pearce (2000) for details.

5.6   Exercises and Complements to Chapter 5

5.1 Show that the root θ_N of equation (5.2.4) satisfies $\theta_N = \theta + C/N + O(N^{-2})$, where $\theta = 0.203\,188...$ and $C = \theta/(1 - 2\theta) \approx 0.34$.

5.2 Consider the non-unit root $\theta(\alpha, p)$ of equation (5.2.8). Rearrange the equation and take limits so as to deduce that $\theta(\alpha) \equiv \lim_{p \to 1} \theta(\alpha, p)$ satisfies the equation $(1 + \alpha^{-1})(1 - \theta) = -\ln\theta$ (this equation coincides with (5.2.5) when $\alpha = 1$). Conclude also that $\theta(\alpha, p) < \theta_{\max}$ on $0 < p \le 1$, $0 < \alpha \le 0$, where $\theta_{\max}$ is the smaller positive root of $\theta(1 - 2\ln\theta) = 1$, attained when $\alpha \to 1$ and $p \to 0$.

5.3 Formulate a deterministic version of the k-fold stifling model for which the function $y_i(t)$ $(i = 1, \ldots, k)$ denotes the number of spreaders that have had contact with a spreader or stifler on $i - 1$ occasions. Setting $y = y_1 + \cdots + y_k$, the differential equations are

$$\dot{x} = -xy,$$
$$\dot{y}_1 = xy - y_1(y - 1 + z),$$
$$\dot{y}_i = (y_{i-1} - y_i)(y - 1 + z) \qquad (i = 2, \ldots, k),$$
$$\dot{z} = y_k(y - 1 + z).$$

Deduce that the quantities $x(t)$, $y_i(t)$ $(i = 1, \ldots, k)$ satisfy

$$(k+1)x(t) + ky_1(t) + \cdots + y_k(t) + N\ln\left(N/x(t)\right) = (k+1)N + k \quad \text{(all } t \ge 0),$$

and that the analogue θ_k of θ at (5.2.5) is the root in $(0, 1)$ of

$$(k+1)(1 - \theta) + \ln\theta = 0.$$

Interpret the equality of θ_k and $\theta(k^{-1})$ as in Exercise 5.2 in terms of the respective models defining them. [DK] illustrates the solution curves y and y_i $(i = 1, 2, 3)$ in the case $k = 3$.

5.4 (*Maki–Thompson model*). Show that the analogues of equations (5.2.1) that follow from the transition probabilities at (5.1.4) are

$$\dot{x} = (-1)xy = -xy,$$
$$\dot{y} = (+1)xy + (-1)y(N - x) = y(2x - N).$$

Conclude that dy/dx satisfies equation (5.2.2) so the same solution (5.2.3) and other consequences follow. Investigate the time $t_N = \inf_t\{y(t) < 1\}$. [Maki and Thompson's original formulation is as a discrete time model in which exactly one pairwise contact occurs at each discrete epoch in time. This corresponds to scaling time in our formulation by $N(N + 1)$.]

5.5 *([DK] model with forgetfulness).* Modify the [DK] model as follows. Assume that pairwise meetings occur at rate β per unit time, and that each spreader may also become a stifler by means of 'forgetfulness' or 'loss of interest' at a rate γ per unit time, independently for each individual and of any interaction with others in the population. To reflect this assumption, replace the last two equations at (5.1.2) by

$$\Pr\{\Delta_h(X, Y)(t) = (0, -1) \mid (X, Y)(t) = (x, y)\} = (\beta yz + \gamma y)h,$$
$$\Pr\{\Delta_h(X, Y)(t) = (0, 0) \mid (X, Y)(t) = (x, y)\} = 1 - \beta y(N + \rho - \tfrac{1}{2}[y - 1])h,$$

where $\rho = \gamma/\beta$. Deduce that for a deterministic version of the model, in place of equation (5.2.2) we should have

$$\frac{dy}{dx} = -2 + \frac{N + \rho}{x}.$$

Hence conclude that, unless the individual rate of forgetfulness $\gamma < \beta N$, the rumour spreads to only a small fraction of the population, and that no matter how small γ is, about 80% at most of the population would hear the rumour.

5.6 (cf. end of Section 5.3, around equation (5.3.10)). Extend the state space $\mathcal{X}_{NI}$ to $\{(i, j) : i = 0, \dots, N, \ j = I + N - i, I + n - i - 1, \dots, 0, -1, \dots\}$ on which a random walk $\{(X', Y')_n\}$ is defined so as to coincide on $\mathcal{X}_{NI}$ with the embedded random walk jump process defined on the general epidemic model of Chapter 3 (see the start of Section 3.4.3). Show that the processes $\{V_n\}$ and $\{W_n\}$ defined by

$$V_n = \prod_{r=0}^{n-1} \frac{X'_{r+1}}{X'_r} \left(1 + \frac{1}{X'_r + \rho - 1}\right)$$

and

$$W_n = \prod_{r=0}^{n-1} \frac{X'_{r+1}(X'_{r+1} - 1)}{X'_r(X'_r - 1)} \left(1 + \frac{2}{X'_r + \rho - 2}\right)$$

are martingales with respect to the σ-fields $\{\mathcal{F}_n\} \equiv \{\sigma(X'_0, \dots, X'_n)\}$. Find a stopping time M such that $N - X'_M$ is the final size of the general epidemic.

5.7 *(Variance of final number with uncertain stifling).* For the $(\alpha, 1)$-probability variant of the [DK] model with deterministic version following the differential equation (5.2.6), the function $\lambda(x, y) = (1 + \alpha)x + y - \alpha N \ln x$ is invariant along the path. Use the method of Section 5.4 to find

$$\text{var}\, X(\infty) \approx \frac{N\theta(1 - \theta)(2\alpha^2 + [2(1 - \alpha) - \alpha(1 + \alpha)^2]\theta + \alpha(1 + \alpha)^2\theta^2)}{2[\alpha - (1 + \alpha)\theta]^2},$$

where θ is the non-unit real root of $(1 + \alpha)(1 - \theta) + \alpha \ln \theta = 0$ (so, $\theta = \theta(\alpha)$ in the context of Exercise 5.2).

5.8 *(Variance of final number with k-fold stifling).* Consider the k-fold stifling variant of the [DK] model and use standardized variables $x(t) = X(t)/N$, $y_i(t) = Y_i(t)/N$. Construct differential equations analogous to those of Exercise 5.3 in conjunction with the procedure of Section 5.4 to conclude that $X(\infty)$, the number of ignorants never hearing the rumour, has approximate variance

$$\operatorname{var} X(\infty) \approx N \left(\frac{\theta_k}{1 - (k+1)\theta_k} \right)^2 \int_0^\infty y(x^{-1} - 1 + y) \, \mathrm{d}t.$$

Here, θ_k is as in Exercise 5.3, $x(0) = 1$, $y \equiv y(t) = y_1 + \cdots + y_k$, $y_1(0) \approx 0$ (e.g. $y_1 = 10^{-6}$), $y_i(0) = 0$ $(i = 2, \ldots, k)$, and for $0 < t < \infty$, $\dot{x} = -xy$, $\dot{y}_1 = xy - y_1(1 - x)$, and $\dot{y}_i = (y_{i-1} - y_i)(1 - x)$ $(i = 2, \ldots, k)$. [Computation gives $\operatorname{var} X(\infty) \approx 0.073\,80N$ $(k = 2)$, $0.021\,99N$ $(k = 3)$.]

5.9 *(Variance of final number in Maki–Thompson model).* Apply the calculus of Section 5.4 to the model with transition rates at (5.1.4) to deduce that

$$N \operatorname{var} \xi_N \to \frac{\theta(1 - \theta)}{1 - 2\theta} = 0.272\,736.$$

5.10 *(Differential equations for first moments).* Show that the first moments for both the [DK] and Maki–Thompson models satisfy the same pair of equations (cf. equations (3.3.6) for the general epidemic model), namely

$$\frac{\mathrm{d}\,EX(t)}{\mathrm{d}t} = -EX(t)\,EY(t) - \operatorname{cov}(X(t), Y(t)),$$

$$\frac{\mathrm{d}\,EY(t)}{\mathrm{d}t} = 2EX(t)\,EY(t) - EY(t) + 2\operatorname{cov}(X(t), Y(t)).$$

6

Fitting Epidemic Data

When epidemic models are used in practice, it is essential to know how well they fit the available data. This is particularly important if reliable predictions are to be made, for example, of the number of AIDS cases to be expected during the next year. Comprehensive accounts of the fitting of various models to sets of epidemic data are given in Bailey (1975), Becker (1989) and Anderson and May (1991), among others. We have already illustrated how certain models were developed to explain observed data. In Chapter 1 we modelled Bernoulli's data in Table 1.3, reviewed Abbey's work on Aycock's data in Table 1.5, and gave Enko's data in Table 1.6 (see Exercise 1.3) and Wilson and Burke's Providence RI data in Table 1.7 (see Exercise 1.4). Further examples were given in Section 2.8 (Saunders's data on rabbit populations affected by myxomatosis) and Section 4.2 (Enko's measles data again). This chapter provides a more extensive discussion of epidemic data fitting: we illustrate its principles with five simple examples, two in which the models are deterministic, and three in which they are stochastic. Readers seeking further details are referred to the previously mentioned books.

In a sense, this chapter serves to introduce the succeeding, final chapter which considers the control of epidemics: how can we use an epidemic model to evaluate possible strategies for countering a particular epidemic phenomenon? Simple models typically start with an elementary scenario; this may be modified subsequently to bring the model closer to the real-world context in which the phenomenon is occurring. For example, in most epidemics, those gathering the data may assume a given initial scenario, which is later changed. This implies that subsequent data are no longer directly comparable with the initial data. Also, in a very real sense, epidemic models vary with the historical period which furnishes their setting: one must recognize that many epidemics today typically occur in communities where living conditions have changed much over the past few centuries.

Such change has been particularly rapid during the twentieth century, with faster transportation methods and different life styles that affect both infection and removal rates.

6.1 Influenza epidemics: a discrete time deterministic model

The use of deterministic models of the Kermack–McKendrick type (see Section 2.3) for influenza epidemics, with modifications for the transfer of infectives between major population centres, dates back to the work of Baroyan *et al.* (1967, 1971, 1977) in the former USSR. Bailey (1975, Chapter 19) describes their methods. In Britain, Spicer (1979) modified this approach to obtain a discrete time model applicable to influenza epidemics, and to deaths due to influenza and influenzal pneumonia in England and Wales, and Greater London. We referred to this work briefly in Section 2.8; here we outline his results in greater detail, including some numerical work. The model is a discrete time version of the general epidemic model in Section 2.3, but with a more general removal rate.

Using the same notation as in Section 2.8, let us consider the discrete time model where $t = 0, 1, \ldots$, refers to time in days. If in the population there are, on day t, a total of Y_t infectives with influenza and x_t susceptibles, then the number y_{t+1} of new infectives produced at time $t + 1$ will be

$$y_{t+1} = \beta x_t Y_t, \tag{6.1.1}$$

where β is the infection parameter. Let ψ_j be the proportion of infectives who are still infectious and mixing in the population j days after initially contracting the disease. Baroyan and co-workers found empirical estimates of these ψ_j as below (with $\psi_j = 0$ for $j \geq 6$, i.e. no individual is infectious for longer than 6 days):

j	0	1	2	3	4	5	6
ψ_j	1.0	0.9	0.55	0.3	0.15	0.05	0.0

We follow Spicer in assuming that these estimates hold universally.

The deterministic model starting with x_0 susceptibles and $Y_0 = y_0$ infectives thus leads to the calculations in Table 6.1, where it is clear that

$$y_{t+1} = \beta x_t Y_t = \beta x_t \sum_{u=0}^{\min(5,t)} y_{t-u}\psi_u, \tag{6.1.2}$$

$$x_{t+1} = x_t - y_{t+1}.$$

Table 6.1. *Progress of an influenza epidemic*

t	Total number of infectives Y_t	Susceptibles x_t	New cases y_t
0	$\psi_0 y_0 = Y_0$	x_0	0
1	$\psi_0 y_1 + \psi_1 y_0 = Y_1$	$x_1 = x_0 - y_1$	$y_1 = \beta x_0 Y_0$
2	$\psi_0 y_2 + \psi_1 y_1 + \psi_2 y_0 = Y_2$	$x_2 = x_1 - y_2$	$y_2 = \beta x_1 Y_1$
3	$\psi_0 y_3 + \psi_1 y_2 + \psi_2 y_1 + \psi_3 y_0 = Y_3$	$x_3 = x_2 - y_3$	$y_3 = \beta x_2 Y_2$
$\vdots$	$\vdots$	$\vdots$	$\vdots$
t	$\psi_0 y_t + \psi_1 y_{t-1} + \cdots + \psi_5 y_{t-5} = Y_t$	$x_t = x_{t-1} - y_t$	$y_t = \beta x_{t-1} Y_{t-1}$

Suppose that the proportion of individuals dying j days after infection is $\kappa \varphi_j$, where $\sum_{j=0}^{\infty} \varphi_j = 1$, so that $\kappa = \Pr\{\text{death from influenza} \mid \text{individual is infected by influenza}\}$. Then the number ζ_t of deaths between times $t-1$ and t is given by

$$\zeta_t = \kappa \sum_{u=0}^{t} y_{t-u} \varphi_u, \qquad (6.1.3)$$

where the φ_u are based on empirical observations, and κ is taken as 2×10^{-4}, a rough estimate of the influenza death rate. Note that ζ_t here refers to a subset of all removals whereas $z(t)$ as in (2.3.3) refers to all removals up to time t.

Spicer (1979) reports that, for his analysis, given that notification of deaths occurs weekly in England and Wales, the time unit was changed from one day to one week. He states that this 'does not seriously affect the model owing to the short infectious period of influenza, and it introduces a useful smoothing effect'. In order to use the data on the ψ_j we must calculate the evolution of the epidemic via (6.1.2) and (6.1.3) on a daily basis, and then accumulate them over a week to obtain

$$y'_T = \sum_{t=7T}^{7T+6} y_t \quad \text{and} \quad \zeta'_T = \sum_{t=7T}^{7T+6} \zeta_t$$

(cf. Exercise 6.1 for a continuous time analogue). The fitting procedure was the standard one of finding a pair of parameters $\alpha \equiv \beta x_0$ (it is impossible to estimate β and x_0 separately) and y_0 which minimized the sum of squares W of the differences between the observed and calculated weekly deaths over a period of T' weeks, namely

$$W = \sum_{T=0}^{T'} (\hat{\zeta}'_T - \zeta'_T)^2, \qquad (6.1.4)$$

where ζ'_T and $\hat{\zeta}'_T$ denote respectively the observed and fitted numbers of deaths in week T. A weighted least squares method was also used.

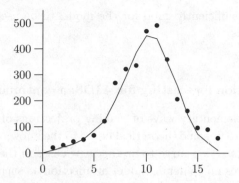

Figure 6.1. Weekly deaths from influenza and influenzal pneumonia
in England and Wales, 1965–66. (Data from Spicer, 1979.)

Spicer fitted his theoretical results to data[1] covering all influenza epidemics in England and Wales for 1958–73 except those that were bimodal. His paper illustrates his results graphically for nine unimodal data sets on deaths in this period, and for seven data sets on deaths in Greater London for 1958–72. To the naked eye, the fits appear reasonably good but with several of the 16 fitted curves being somewhat too high at the beginning and too low at the end of the epidemic. The graph for 1965–66 for England and Wales is reproduced roughly in Figure 6.1; see also the graph of Greater London 1971–72 in Figure 2.12.

One of the two quantities which needs to be estimated is the value $\alpha \equiv \beta x_0$, and this is given, for example, by Spicer for the nine sets of data on deaths in England and Wales mentioned previously, as $3.9 \le \alpha \le 7.7$ (see Table 6.2), and the seven sets of data for Greater London as $4.5 \le \alpha \le 7.7$. The position of the optimum fit was found to be determined more by βx_0 than by κ and y_0.

Table 6.2. *Estimated values of* $\alpha = \beta x_0$ *for England and Wales, 1958–73*

Year	1958–59	60–61	61–62	62–63	65–66	67–68	69–70	71–72	72–73
α	5.2	5.5	6.5	4.7	4.5	5.9	7.7	3.9	5.7

Source: Spicer (1979). Note that these data exclude bimodal cases.

If we take the average value $\bar{\alpha} = 5.51$, this implies that an infective transmits infection to about five susceptibles, which may be an overestimate. The

---

[1]Spicer's calculations were 'based on observations reported by Stuart-Harris *et al.* (1950)'; the data are not otherwise identified; the only data from the 1950 reference matching this description give estimates of $\sum_{j=1}^{5} \varphi_{5d+j}$ $(d = 0, 1, 2)$ and $\sum_{j \ge 16} \varphi_j$ equal to 0.31, 0.41, 0.26 and 0.02 respectively.

fits are, however, sufficiently good for the model to be used for predictions of influenza deaths.

6.2   Extrapolation forecasting for AIDS: a continuous time model

One of the most elementary ways of making projections of new AIDS cases in a population is to fit some theoretical curve to the known data empirically, and then extrapolate this curve to predict new cases in the next one or two years. This involves no epidemic model of infection as such: the theoretical curve is chosen because it seems likely to fit the data; in fact, several curves may do so, as we shall see shortly. Practically speaking, the prediction can only be made for a short period of time ahead, since the conditions which have held in the past for the known data may alter over a longer period.

In a paper on extrapolation forecasting, Wilson (1989) uses AIDS diagnoses D_t by quarter and year in Australia from 1982 to 1988 as the basic data (see Table 6.3).

Table 6.3. *Quarterly AIDS diagnoses in Australia 1982–1988*

Quarter Year	1	2	3	4
1982				1
1983	0	1	2	3
1984	1	5	15	21
1985	26	36	22	29
1986	43	52	60	68
1987	89	93	83	95
1988	101	101	117	132

Note: Table 6.10 contains extended and updated data.

Wilson (1989) fitted several curves to these quarterly data including the three empirical curves listed below, namely the log linear (T), log quadratic (Q) and log log (LT) models with Poisson errors, using the statistical package GLIM. These are

$$\text{T: } \ln D_t = \alpha + \beta t,$$

$$\text{Q: } \ln D_t = \alpha + \beta t + \gamma t^2,$$

$$\text{LT: } \ln D_t = \alpha + \beta \ln t,$$

where the LT curve was originally proposed by Whyte *et al.* (1987). Using $t = 1, \ldots, 25$ to denote the 25 quarters of the data in Table 6.3, Wilson

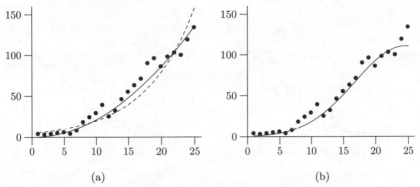

Figure 6.2. 1982–1988 Australian AIDS data (•) with fitted curves:
(a) LT (——) and T (----), and (b) Q (——). (Based on data in
text from Wilson (1989).)

estimated values for these three curves as below:

$$\text{T:} \quad \hat{\alpha} = 1.601, \qquad \hat{\beta} = 0.1386;$$

$$\text{Q:} \quad \hat{\alpha} = -0.446, \qquad \hat{\beta} = 0.421, \qquad \hat{\gamma} = -0.0086;$$

$$\text{LT:} \quad \hat{\alpha} = -1.64, \qquad \hat{\beta} = 2.035.$$

The fit of T gives 159 for the last quarter ($t = 25$) and this was considered
unsatisfactory. The fits of both Q and LT curves were considered adequate
as indicated in Figure 6.2.

The fit was further refined to take account of two events towards the end
of 1987:

(a) the extension of the World Health Organization's (WHO's) definition
of AIDS from its 1985 revision; this may have led to an increase in
AIDS diagnoses; and

(b) the availability of zidovudine (AZT) at about that time in Australia,
with the consequent effect of delaying the onset of AIDS.

Figure 6.3 shows the fitted values taking account of event (b); the disconti-
nuity at $t = 20$ in (6.2.1) reflects (b) also.

Predictions were then made for the next 10 quarters on the basis of these
(and other) models, in the cases where the effect of AZT was considered
or neglected, and for the cases where all the 1982–1988 data were used, or
only the data from 1985–1988. Figure 6.4 gives the predictions based on the
1982–1988 data, with and without the AZT effect. The two LTjZ models
($j = 1, 2$) considered, in which the effect of AZT was taken into account,

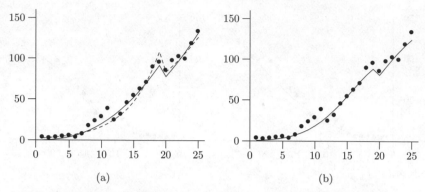

Figure 6.3. 1982–1988 Australian AIDS quarterly data (●) with fitted curves allowing for possible delayed onset of AIDS: (a) LT,Z (——) and T,Z (- - - -), and (b) Q,Z (——). (From Wilson's data, by personal communication.)

though they varied only slightly, yielded very different predictions within two years.

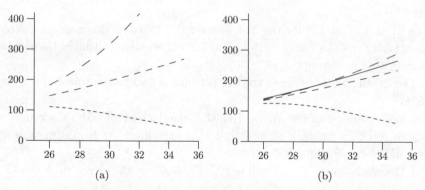

Figure 6.4. Predicted numbers of new cases of AIDS diagnosed in Australia from the first quarter of 1989, using all the data: (a) T (— — —), LT (– – –), Q (- - - -); (b) T,Z (— — —), LT,Z (– – –), LT,Z(2) (——), Q,Z (- - - -). (From Wilson's data, by personal communication.)

The results in Figure 6.5 were obtained using only the last four years of data 1985–1988. These were deemed to be more satisfactory than the models using all the data, and not quite so divergent in their predictions.

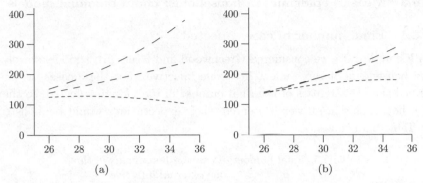

Figure 6.5. Predicted numbers of new cases of AIDS diagnosed in Australia from the first quarter of 1989, using 1985–1988 data only: (a) T (— — —), LT (– – –), Q (----); (b) T,Z (— — —), LT,Z (– – –) and Q,Z (----). (From Wilson's data, by personal communication.)

For yearly predictions up to 1993, the models chosen were

$$\text{TZ(4 years):} \quad \ln D_t = \begin{cases} 1.551 + 0.158t & (t < 20), \\ 2.763 + 0.083t & (t \geq 20); \end{cases}$$

$$\text{LT(4 years):} \quad \ln D_t = -0.978 + 1.814 \ln t; \tag{6.2.1}$$

$$\text{QZ(4 years):} \quad \ln D_t = \begin{cases} 0.764 + 0.272t - 0.004t^2 & (t < 20), \\ 0.521 + 0.272t - 0.004t^2 & (t \geq 20). \end{cases}$$

These models resulted in the annual predictions of D_t for 1989–1993 shown in Table 6.4.

Table 6.4. *Predicted and Actual AIDS diagnoses by year in Australia*

Year Model	1989	1990	1991	1992	1993
TZ (4 years)	600	900	1200	1700	2300
LT (4 years)	600	900	1100	1400	1800
QZ (4 years)	600	700	700	600	500
Actual	568	591	797	793	805

While all models predict the same numbers for 1989, they range widely for 1993, the last year of the predictions. The actual numbers are now known and are shown in the last line of Table 6.4: on this basis the QZ model came closest. These methods of extrapolation forecasting have now been displaced by back-calculation models, described in Section 6.5.

6.3   Measles epidemics in households: chain binomial models

6.3.1   Final number of cases infected

In Example 4.3.1 we considered Greenwood and Reed–Frost models involving households of three infected by one infective. For these cases, we obtained the probabilities of the final number of individuals infected, so that if n households in all were observed, their expectations would be as listed in Table 6.5 below.

Table 6.5. *Final number of cases in households of three infected by one external infective*

Final no. Cases	Expected numbers of households Greenwood model	Reed–Frost model	No. households Observed
0	$n\alpha^3$	$n\alpha^3$	a
1	$3n(1-\alpha)\alpha^4$	$3n(1-\alpha)\alpha^4$	b
2	$3n(1-\alpha)^2\alpha^2(1+2\alpha^2)$	$3n(1-\alpha)^2\alpha^3(1+2\alpha)$	c
3	$n(1-\alpha)^3(1+3\alpha+3\alpha^2+6\alpha^3)$	$n(1-\alpha)^3(1+3\alpha+6\alpha^2+6\alpha^3)$	d
Total no. households	n	n	n

Note: Bailey (1975) regards this as a household of four with one member initially infected; the formulations are identical.

For the Greenwood model, the likelihood L_G of the observed numbers of households is

$$L_G = \alpha^{3a}[3(1-\alpha)\alpha^4]^b[3(1-\alpha)^2\alpha^2(1+2\alpha^2)]^c[(1-\alpha)^3(1+3\alpha+3\alpha^2+6\alpha^3)]^d,$$

from which we can write down $\ln L_G$ and maximize it in α to obtain the equation for the maximum likelihood estimator (MLE) $\hat{\alpha}$

$$\frac{3a+4b+2c}{\hat{\alpha}} - \frac{b+2c+3d}{1-\hat{\alpha}} + \frac{4c\hat{\alpha}}{1+2\hat{\alpha}^2} + \frac{3d(1+2\hat{\alpha}+6\hat{\alpha}^2)}{1+3\hat{\alpha}+3\hat{\alpha}^2+6\hat{\alpha}^3} = 0. \quad (6.3.1)$$

Similarly, for the Reed–Frost model, with the different likelihood function L_{RF} say, the MLE $\hat{\alpha}$ satisfies

$$\frac{3a+4b+2c}{\hat{\alpha}} - \frac{b+2c+3d}{1-\hat{\alpha}} + \frac{2c\hat{\alpha}}{1+2\hat{\alpha}} + \frac{3d(1+4\hat{\alpha}+6\hat{\alpha}^2)}{1+3\hat{\alpha}+6\hat{\alpha}^2+6\hat{\alpha}^3} = 0. \quad (6.3.2)$$

Wilson *et al.* (1939) contains data from Providence RI for the total numbers of infections in 100 households of three infected by one infective (see Table 6.6).

Table 6.6. *Fit of the Greenwood and Reed–Frost models to Providence RI data*

Total no. cases	Data	Fitted values Greenwood model	Reed–Frost model
0	4	2.5	4.2
1	3	1.5	2.8
2	9	14.9	9.0
3	84	81.1	84.0
Total no. households	100	100	100

Using the data values $(a, b, c, d) = (4, 3, 9, 84)$, the values $\hat{\alpha}$ for the probabilities of non-infection in these two models satisfying, respectively, (6.3.1) and (6.3.2) are

$$\hat{\alpha}_G = 0.291, \qquad \hat{\alpha}_{RF} = 0.347. \qquad (6.3.3)$$

The fitted values given by the second and third columns of Table 6.5 with $\alpha = \hat{\alpha}_G$, $\hat{\alpha}_{RF}$ as at (6.3.3) yield the expected numbers shown in the last two columns of Table 6.6. The value for the chi-square goodness-of-fit statistic χ_G^2 for the Greenwood model, combining the categories with 0 and 1 cases because their expectations are both small, equals $3.0^2/4.0 + 5.9^2/14.9 + 2.9^2/81.1 = 4.69$; this is significant at the 5% level but not at the 2.5% level for χ^2 on 1 d.f. For the Reed–Frost model, again combining categories with 0 and 1 cases, the χ^2 statistic on 1 d.f. equals zero, reflecting the perfect fit.

6.3.2 Cases infected for different types of chain

The data from Providence RI provide more information than those in Table 6.6: the numbers of different types of chain as in Table 4.2 are also given. The values of $a, \ldots, h$ for these are listed in Table 6.7.

Table 6.7. *Fit of the Greenwood and Reed–Frost models for specific chain types*

Type of chain	Generic	Providence RI data	Fitted values Greenwood model	Reed–Frost model
$X_t =$ 3 3	a	4	0.9	1.2
3 2 2	b	3	0.4	0.7
3 2 1 1	c	1	0.7	1.0
3 1 1	d	8	8.2	2.2
3 2 1 0 0	e	4	2.7	3.4
3 2 0 0	f	3	6.5	7.3
3 1 0 0	g	10	31.0	38.7
3 0 0	h	67	49.6	45.5
Total no. households	n	100	100	100

For the Greenwood model the log likelihood $\ln L_G$, neglecting a constant term, equals

$$(3a+4b+4c+2d+3e+2f+g) \ln\alpha + (b+2c+2d+3e+3f+3g+3h) \ln(1-\alpha)$$

so the MLE $\hat{\alpha}_G$ is given by

$$\hat{\alpha}_G = \frac{3a + 4b + 4c + 2d + 3e + 2f + g}{3a + 5b + 6c + 4d + 6e + 5f + 4g + 3h}. \tag{6.3.4}$$

Similarly, for the Reed–Frost model, $\ln L_{RF}$ is a linear function of $\ln \alpha$, $\ln(1 - \alpha)$ and $\ln(1 + \alpha)$, and has derivative

$$\frac{\partial L_{RF}}{\partial \alpha} = \frac{3a + 4b + 4c + 3d + 3e + 2f + g}{\alpha_{RF}} + \frac{g}{1 + \alpha_{RF}}$$
$$- \frac{b + 2c + 2d + 3e + 3f + 3g + 3h}{1 - \alpha_{RF}}. \tag{6.3.5}$$

Setting this function equal to zero yields an equation for $\hat{\alpha}_{RF}$.

From the data listed in Table 6.7 we evaluate the MLEs as $\hat{\alpha}_G = 0.209$, $\hat{\alpha}_{RF} = 0.231$ (cf. equation (6.3.3)). The fitted values are given by substituting these MLE values in the algebraic expressions in Table 4.2, each multiplied by the total number of households, $n = 100$, to give the expected numbers for the various types of chain. The chi-square statistics, based on combining chain types 1, 2, 3 and 5 for the Greenwood model, and 1, 2, 3 and 4 for the Reed–Frost model, are $\chi^2_G = 26.2$, $\chi^2_{RF} = 57.4$ on 3 degrees of freedom; since $\Pr\{\chi^2_{(3)} \geq 11.4\} = 0.01$, the fit is very poor for both models.

Several reasons may account for the poor fit, not the least that individuals are heterogeneous (see Exercise 6.3), or that infectivity may vary between households, an issue to which we now turn.

6.4   Variable infectivity in chain binomial models

Becker (1981) generalized the concept of chain binomial models by assuming that, if at time $t \geq 0$ there were $X_t = x$ susceptibles and $Y_t = y$ infectives, then with α_y as the probability of contact between the y infectives and x susceptibles, X_{t+1} would follow the binomial distribution $\mathrm{Bin}(x, \alpha_y)$, i.e.

$$\Pr\{(X, Y)_{t+1} = (u, x-u) \mid (X, Y)_t = (x, y)\} = \binom{x}{u} \alpha_y^u (1-\alpha_y)^{x-u}. \tag{6.4.1}$$

Thus, $\alpha_y = \alpha$ for the Greenwood model and α^y for the Reed–Frost model.

Becker (1981) was concerned with the data collected by Heasman and Reid (1961) on outbreaks of the common cold in families of 5 with 1 initial infective (equivalent to households of 4 infected by 1 external infective). He fitted both the general model, where the α_y were estimated directly from the

Table 6.8. *Reed–Frost chain binomial probabilities for households of size four*

Type of chain	Probabilities*	Expected values of probabilities*
4 4	α^4	$z_q(3)/z(3)$
4 3 3	$4\alpha^6(1-\alpha)$	$4z_q(5)z_p(0)/z(6)$
4 3 2 2	$12\alpha^7(1-\alpha)^2$	$12z_q(6)z_p(1)/z(8)$
4 3 2 1 1	$24\alpha^7(1-\alpha)^3$	$24z_q(6)z_p(2)/z(9)$
4 3 2 1 0 0	$24\alpha^6(1-\alpha)^4$	$24z_q(5)z_p(3)/z(9)$
4 3 2 0 0	$12\alpha^5(1-\alpha)^4$	$12z_q(4)z_p(3)/z(8)$
4 3 1 1	$12\alpha^6(1-\alpha)^3$	$12z_q(5)z_p(2)/z(8)$
4 3 1 0 0	$12\alpha^4(1-\alpha)^3(1-\alpha^2)$	$12z_q(3)z_p(3)(1+q+12z)/z(8)$
4 3 0 0	$4\alpha^3(1-\alpha)^4$	$4z_q(2)z_p(3)/z(6)$
4 2 2	$6\alpha^6(1-\alpha)^2$	$6z_q(5)z_p(1)/z(7)$
4 2 1 1	$12\alpha^5(1-\alpha)^2(1-\alpha^2)$	$12z_q(4)z_p(2)(1+q+13z)/z(8)$
4 2 1 0 0	$12\alpha^4(1-\alpha)^3(1-\alpha^2)$	$12z_q(3)z_p(3)(1+q+12z)/z(8)$
4 2 0 0	$6\alpha^2(1-\alpha)^2(1-\alpha^2)^2$	$6z_q(1)z_p(3)[76z^2+(17+19q)z+(1+q)^2]/z(7)$
4 1 1	$4\alpha^4(1-\alpha)^3$	$4z_q(3)z_p(2)/z(6)$
4 1 0 0	$4\alpha(1-\alpha)^3(1-\alpha^3)$	$4z_q(0)z_p(3)[38z^2+(12+9q)z+(1+q)^2]/z(7)$
4 0 0	$(1-\alpha)^4$	$z_p(3)/z(3)$

*See equation (6.4.5) for definition of p, q, z and $z_p(\cdot)$.

data, and the Reed–Frost model where $\alpha_y = \alpha^y$, to the data. The Reed–Frost probabilities are shown in column 2 of Table 6.8. Both fits proved adequate but not ideal, with that of the Reed–Frost model the better.

Greenwood (1949) had considered possible variations in α, while Bailey (1975) showed that if α is a random variable with a beta distribution, reflecting the variable infectivity of households, then chain binomial models could provide an improved fit for the Providence RI measles data (see Bailey, 1975, Chapter 14, pp. 254–260).

Dietz and Schenzle (1985) reviewed the history of household epidemic statistics and considered the data of Heasman and Reid (1961) who had obtained $\hat{\alpha} = 0.886$ for the probability of no contact in the Reed–Frost model. Becker (1981) found $\hat{\alpha} = 0.884$, and Schenzle (1982), after pooling some of the data (see Table 6.9, column 3), obtained $\hat{\alpha} = 0.893$. Schenzle (1982), following Bailey (1975), also considered the case of a Reed–Frost model in which α is a beta random variable, but did not provide any details; we reproduce his figures in Table 6.9, without having full knowledge of his method of fit.

We now sketch the treatment of Gani and Mansouri (1987), from which paper further details can be obtained. Following Bailey (1975) and Section 4.3 above, we have for the Reed–Frost model

$$p_{ij}(\alpha) = \Pr\{(X,Y)_{t+1} = (j, i-j) \mid (X,Y)_t = (i,y)\} = \binom{i}{j}(1-\alpha^y)^{i-j}\alpha^{yj}.$$

$$(6.4.2)$$

Suppose that α $(0 \le \alpha \le 1)$ varies between households and follows the beta distribution with density function

$$\frac{(1-\alpha)^{a-1}\alpha^{b-1}}{B(a,b)} \qquad (a,b > 0). \tag{6.4.3}$$

Then, integrating $p_{ij}(\alpha)$ over all values of α gives

$$\mathrm{E}[p_{ij}(\alpha)] = \int_0^1 \binom{i}{j} \frac{(1-\alpha)^{a-1}\alpha^{b-1}}{B(a,b)} (1-\alpha^y)^{i-j}\alpha^{yj}\,d\alpha$$

$$= \binom{i}{j} \sum_{k=0}^{i-j} \binom{i-j}{k}(-1)^k \int_0^1 \frac{\alpha^{y[k+j]+b-1}(1-\alpha)^{a-1}}{B(a,b)}\,d\alpha$$

$$= \binom{i}{j} \sum_{k=0}^{i-j} \binom{i-j}{k}(-1)^k \frac{B(y[k+j]+b,a)}{B(a,b)}. \tag{6.4.4}$$

We can simplify the notation by writing

$$\mathrm{E}(\alpha) = \frac{a}{a+b} = q, \qquad p = 1 - q, \qquad s = \frac{1}{a+b},$$

$$z_r(n) = \prod_{k=0}^{n}(r+ks) \quad (0 < r \le 1), \qquad z(n) \equiv z_1(n) = \prod_{k=0}^{n}(1+ks),$$
$$\tag{6.4.5}$$

thereby obtaining the formulae in column 3 of Table 6.8.

Table 6.9. *Common cold data for households of size four with four model fits*

Chain	Observed data	Reed–Frost models variable α	Reed–Frost models fixed α	Becker's general model	Schenzle's model*
$X_t = $ 4 4	423	420.77	405.2	403.9	420.9
4 3 3	131	133.52	147.1	147.3	133.4
4 3 2 2	36	40.17	45.3	45.6	40.1
4 3 2 1 1	14	10.43	10.5	10.7	10.4
4 3 2 1 0 0	4	1.82	1.4	1.4	1.8
4 3 2 0 0	2	1.09	0.8	0.8	1.1
4 3 1 1	8	6.12	6.0	6.2	6.1
4 3 1 0 0	2	2.41	1.7	1.6	2.4
4 3 0 0	2	0.53	0.3	0.3	0.5
4 2 2	24	23.15	25.6	26.9	23.1
4 2 1 1	11	13.34	12.7	12.2	13.4
4 2 1 0 0	3	2.41	1.7	1.6	2.4
4 2 0 0	1	3.21	2.0	1.8	3.2
4 1 1	3	2.84	2.5	3.7	2.8
4 1 0 0	0	2.18	1.1	0.0	2.0
4 0 0	0	0.24	0.1	0.1	0.2
Total	664	664.23	664.0	664.1	663.8
χ^2		2.74	9.1	9.5	5.8

* A Bailey-type variant of the Reed–Frost model; see text for detail.

We now estimate the parameters q and s, and test the goodness-of-fit of the model. From the third column of Table 6.8 and the observed data in column 2 of Table 6.9, we may write the log likelihood function of the chain probabilities as

$$\begin{aligned}
\ln L = {}& C + 664 \ln q + 664 \ln(q + s) + 663 \ln(q + 2s) + 661 \ln(q + 3s) \\
& + 230 \ln(q + 4s) + 217 \ln(q + 5s) + 50 \ln(q + 6s) + 241 \ln p \\
& + 110 \ln(p + s) + 50 \ln(p + 2s) + 14 \ln(p + 3s) + 5 \ln(1 + q + 12s) \\
& + 11 \ln(1 + q + 13s) + \ln(76s^2 + [17 + 19q]s + [1 + q]^2) \\
& - 664 \ln(1 + s) - 664 \ln(1 + 2s) - 664 \ln(1 + 3s) - 241 \ln(1 + 4s) \\
& - 241 \ln(1 + 5s) - 241 \ln(1 + 6s) - 105 \ln(1 + 7s) - 80 \ln(1 + 8s) \\
& - 18 \ln(1 + 9s)
\end{aligned} \tag{6.4.6}$$

for some constant C. Gani and Mansouri (1987) used the ZXMWD subroutine of IMSL to minimize $-\ln L$, and found for the MLEs of q and s

$$\hat{q} = 0.8887 \pm 0.0114, \qquad \hat{s} = 0.0223 \pm 0.0222, \tag{6.4.7}$$

the corresponding information matrix being

$$I = \begin{pmatrix} 31747.4 & -4727.7 \\ -4727.7 & 8535.7 \end{pmatrix}, \tag{6.4.8}$$

and variance-covariance matrix

$$V = \begin{pmatrix} 0.3433 \times 10^{-4} & 0.1901 \times 10^{-4} \\ 0.1901 \times 10^{-4} & 1.277 \times 10^{-4} \end{pmatrix}. \tag{6.4.9}$$

They obtained as the corresponding estimates of a and b

$$\hat{a} = 39.91, \qquad \hat{b} = 4.999.$$

Based on the estimates (6.4.7) of q and s, and the expected probabilities in column 3 of Table 6.8, the fitted values for the Reed–Frost model with variable α were calculated (see Table 6.9, column 3). These were then compared with columns 4–6 of Table 6.9 carried over from results of Becker (1981) and Schenzle (1982).

To obtain chi-square goodness-of-fit statistics, all chains with fitted values less than 5 were combined. For the Reed–Frost model with fixed α (column 4 of Table 6.9), Becker obtained $\chi^2 = 9.1$ with 6 degrees of freedom (P-value $= 0.166$). For Becker's general model (column 5 of Table 6.9), $\chi^2 = 9.5$

with 5 d.f. (P-value $= 0.091$). The Reed–Frost model with variable α gives a closer fit: $\chi^2 = 2.74$ with 5 d.f. (P-value $= 0.728$). Schenzle's variant is likewise closer than the fixed α and Becker's model.

These results lend support to the hypothesis, originally made by Greenwood (1949), that there is variation in the susceptibility to infection between households. Bailey (1975) had already shown in his studies of the Providence RI measles data that both Greenwood and Reed–Frost models with variable α provided improved fits. The present application to common cold data arrives at a similar conclusion.

6.5 Incubation period of AIDS and the back-calculation method

At the end of Section 6.2, we mentioned that simple extrapolation forecasting had now been replaced by the back-projection or back-calculation method as a means of predicting the number of HIV seropositives and AIDS patients in a population. The models used in this method rely on the relation between HIV incidence in the time interval $(s, s + ds)$ and the subsequent AIDS incidence in the time interval $(t, t + dt)$ where $t > s$, following an incubation period of length x whose distribution $f(x)$ is assumed to be known. This incubation period is defined as the time from the instant of infection by HIV to the onset of AIDS, where the onset is evaluated in terms of external clinical symptoms, or by a patient's T-4 cell count (also called CD-4 count). When this count falls below a certain threshold, e.g. below $200/\text{mm}^3$ blood, say, then the patient is said to have AIDS. The expected number $a(t) \, dt$ of new cases of AIDS in $(t, t + dt)$ is given by

$$a(t) = \int_0^t I(s) f(t - s) \, ds$$

where $I(s) \, ds$ is the number of HIV cases reported earlier in $(s, s + ds)$. The integrated form of this equation expresses the cumulative number $A(t)$ of AIDS cases to time t in terms of the distribution function $F(t) = \int_0^t f(u) \, du$ of the AIDS incubation period, namely

$$A(t) = \int_0^t F(t - s) I(s) \, ds. \tag{6.5.1}$$

The distribution $f(u)$ is usually assumed to be of Weibull or gamma type, with an approximate mean of 10 years. On the basis of past HIV infection curves, fitted parametrically or non-parametrically, one can project future numbers of AIDS cases.

Equation (6.5.1) can be used in one of two ways:

(a) assuming $I(s)$ and $F(t)$ are known, one can calculate $A(t)$; and

(b) assuming $A(t)$ and $F(t)$ are known, one can calculate $I(s)$.

It should be noted that data on $A(t)$ are far more reliable than data on $I(s)$, so that case (b) then allows a reasonable estimate of $I(s)$ to be obtained. On the other hand, for predictions of $A(t)$, even an imperfect $I(s)$ can prove useful. The key in both cases is the distribution $F(t)$ of the incubation period, and we begin by considering this.

Several authors have studied the distribution of the incubation period, relying on data from transfusion-associated AIDS patients, for whom the date of initial HIV infection is known. There are for example early papers by Lui, Lawrence *et al.* (1986) and Lui, Peterman *et al.* (1988) in which the data are fitted by a Weibull distribution, with due allowance for truncation at the reporting date (31 December 1984 for the earlier paper). Denoting the 3-parameter Weibull distribution by

$$F(t; \lambda, r, \theta) = 1 - e^{-\lambda(t-\theta)^r} \qquad (t \geq \theta \geq 0), \tag{6.5.2}$$

these authors estimated the parameters λ, r and θ from the data, and concluded, on the basis of 83 adult individuals undergoing transfusions from 1978 to 1983, that the mean incubation period was 54 months = 4.5 yr, with 90% confidence bounds of 2.6 and 14.2 yr. The estimated Weibull density function for this case is shown in Figure 6.6 below. We used the parameters $\hat{\lambda} = 0.000\,044\,5$, $\hat{r} = 2.51$ and $\hat{\theta} = 2.5$ months for this density function, and our time axis is in months. The modal value of the density turns out to be larger than in Lui, Lawrence *et al.* (1986).

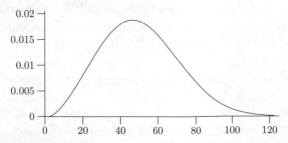

Figure 6.6. Estimated Weibull density function for the transfusion-associated AIDS incubation period in months based on 83 adult patients. (Based on Figure 2 of Lui, Lawrence *et al.* (1986).)

Other authors have used different models for the distribution of the incubation period, such as the gamma density function

$$f(t) = \frac{\lambda(\lambda t)^{\alpha-1}e^{-\lambda t}}{\Gamma(\alpha)} \qquad (t \geq 0). \qquad (6.5.3)$$

Among these are Anderson and Medley (1988), who estimated values of $\alpha = 2.7$, $\lambda = 0.19\,\mathrm{yr}^{-1}$, hence a mean of $2.7/0.19 = 14.3\,\mathrm{yr}$, based on fitting a gamma distribution to data from England and Wales up to April 1988. They also fitted the 2-parameter Weibull distribution $F(t; \rho, \beta) = 1 - e^{-(\rho t)^{\beta}}$, obtaining $\beta = 2.33$, $\rho = 0.12\,\mathrm{yr}^{-1}$ and a mean of $7.4\,\mathrm{yr}$ (cf. the parameters used for Figure 6.6, for the d.f. $1 - \exp\left(-[\rho(t - \theta')]^{\beta}\right)$, which has $\beta = \hat{r} = 2.51, \hat{\theta}' = 0.2\,\mathrm{yr}$, $\hat{\rho} = 12(0.000\,044\,5)^{1/2.51} = 0.221\,\mathrm{yr}^{-1}$). Lawless and Sun (1992) considered in addition a log logistic distribution function

$$F(t) = \frac{(\alpha t)^{\beta}}{1 + (\alpha t)^{\beta}}. \qquad (6.5.4)$$

Each of these distributions for the incubation period provides an adequate fit to various transfusion associated data sets. On the other hand, Bacchetti, Segal and Jewell (1992), who estimated the incubation distribution from similar data on haemophiliacs using two different parametric models (including the Weibull distribution as a special case), concluded that their analysis showed significant evidence against the Weibull distribution. We would comment simply that *fitting* any particular distribution without having a model-based rationale for doing so, provides no assurance of the propriety of the chosen distribution.

An excellent survey of methods used in the estimation of the AIDS incubation period, and the back-calculation method, may be found in Section 1 of Jewell, Dietz and Farewell's book (1992) on *AIDS Epidemiology*. Further details are also available in some of the early papers (Brookmeyer and Gail, 1988; Centers for Disease Control, 1990; Brookmeyer, 1991; and Solomon *et al.*, 1991).

We now give some detail of the methods in Lui, Peterman *et al.* (1988) for paediatric patients, as an example of the procedures commonly used. Their data consisted of the incubation periods t_i of 32 patients ($i = 1, \ldots, 32$) in the period 1979–1984, while the AIDS diagnoses were made in the period 1982–1985. For patient i let R_i denote the number of months between transfusion and 31 December 1985, L_i the number of months between transfusion and 1 January 1982 (the month of the first diagnosed case of AIDS). Then

assuming (6.5.2) holds, the likelihood of the observed data can be written
as

$$L = \prod_{i=1}^{32} \frac{\lambda r (t_i - \theta)^{r-1} e^{-\lambda(t_i - \theta)^r}}{e^{-\delta_i \lambda (L_i - \theta)^r} - e^{-\lambda(R_i - \theta)^r}}, \tag{6.5.5}$$

where $\delta_i = 1$ if the critical transfusion date for i was before January 1982,
$\delta_i = 0$ otherwise. Thus, when $\delta_i = 1$,

$$F(R_i) - F(L_i) = e^{-\lambda(L_i - \theta)^r} - e^{-\lambda(R_i - 0)^r} = \Pr\{L_i \leq t_i \leq R_i\}$$

and when $\delta_i = 0$,

$$F(R_i) = 1 - e^{-\lambda(R_i - \theta)^r} = \Pr\{t_i \leq R_i\}.$$

The maximum likelihood estimates of r and λ can now be obtained, assuming the value $\theta = 3$ months which is found to maximize L for the values of
r and λ derived from the equations

$$\frac{\partial \ln L}{\partial \lambda} = 0, \qquad \frac{\partial \ln L}{\partial r} = 0. \tag{6.5.6}$$

Writing these out in full detail, we have

$$\frac{\partial \ln L}{\partial \lambda} = \frac{32}{\lambda} - \sum_{i=1}^{32} (t_i - \theta)^r$$

$$- \sum_{i=1}^{32} \frac{-\delta_i (L_i - \theta)^r e^{-\lambda(L_i - \theta)^r} + (R_i - \theta)^r e^{-\lambda(R_i - \theta)^r}}{e^{-\delta_i \lambda (L_i - \theta)^r} - e^{-\lambda(R_i - \theta)^r}},$$

$$\frac{\partial \ln L}{\partial r} = \frac{32}{r} + \sum_{i=1}^{32} \ln(t_i - \theta) - \sum_{i=1}^{32} \lambda (t_i - \theta)^r \ln(t_i - \theta)$$

$$- \sum_{i=1}^{32} \frac{-\delta_i \lambda (L_i - \theta)^r \ln(L_i - \theta) e^{-\lambda(L_i - \theta)^r} + \lambda (R_i - \theta)^r \ln(R_i - \theta) e^{-\lambda(R_i - \theta)^r}}{e^{-\delta_i \lambda (L_i - \theta)^r} - e^{-\lambda(R_i - \theta)^r}}.$$

The results obtained were $\hat{r} = 1.418$, $\hat{\lambda} = 0.008\,56$ with $\hat{\theta} = 3$, giving a
mean incubation period of 29 months or 2.4 yr with an approximate 90%
confidence interval of 18 to 86 months. The mean is smaller than the equivalent mean for adults (4.5 yr) quoted earlier. The estimated Weibull density
function for the 32 paediatric patients is given in Figure 6.7, with the time
axis in months as before. Note that this differs considerably from Figure
6.6, both in its range and its shape.

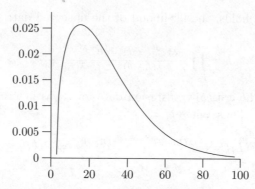

Figure 6.7. Estimated Weibull density function for the AIDS incubation period in months based on 32 paediatric patients. (Based on data in text from Lui, Peterman *et al.* (1988).)

An alternative approach is to use death or birth-and-death processes for modelling the associated T-4 cell count process as in Gani (1991) and Rossi (1991). Whatever model is used, one may assume that the distribution function $F(t)$ of the incubation period of AIDS is adequately estimated. We now proceed with the back-calculation method itself.

6.5.1   The distribution of the AIDS incubation period

Solomon *et al.* (1991) used AIDS data for Australia from 1982 to 1990 to reconstruct HIV prevalence; these data are reproduced in Table 6.10 and thereby bring Table 6.3 up to date to 1990, including revisions of the data given previously.

Table 6.10. *Quarterly AIDS diagnoses in Australia, 1982–1990*

Year \ Quarter	1	2	3	4
1982				1
1983	0	1	2	3
1984	1	6	16	23
1985	26	37	29	30
1986	42	51	63	70
1987	86	96	87	102
1988	112	112	143	155
1989	142	121	153	152
1990	150	131	167	143

Using the 2-parameter Weibull distribution in the form

$$F(t; \lambda, r) = 1 - e^{-\lambda t^r} \qquad (6.5.7)$$

with $r = 2.55$ and $\lambda = 0.002\,078\,\mathrm{yr}^{-2.55} = (0.0887)^{1/2.55}\,\mathrm{yr}^{-2.55}$ for the AIDS incubation period distribution, and adopting a parametric approach in which the HIV infection curve is assumed to be either
(a) quadratic exponential, $I(t) = a_0 \exp(a_1 t - a_2 t^2)$, or
(b) linear logistic, $I(t) = (b_0 + b_1 t)/(1 + e^{b_2 - b_3 t})$,

then the AIDS diagnoses in a particular quarter (t_j, t_{j+1}) are predicted by

$$A(t_{j+1}) - A(t_j) = \int_{t_j}^{t_{j+1}} I(s)F(t-s)\,\mathrm{d}s \qquad (j = 0, \ldots, 33).$$

Here the increments in $A(\cdot)$ are known from Table 6.10, $F(t)$ is given by (6.5.7) with $(r, \lambda) = (2.55, 0.002\,078)$, and $I(t)$ has one of the two parametric forms mentioned; it is, of course, possible to reconstruct $I(t)$ nonparametrically.

Given these conditions, assuming the epidemic to have begun in 1981, Solomon et al. (1991) obtained the following estimates of $\int_y^{y+1} I(s)\,\mathrm{d}s$ for the years $(y, y+1)$ in the period 1981–1990.

Table 6.11. *Estimated annual HIV infection incidence in Australia*

Model	Year	1981	'82	'83	'84	'85	'86	'87	'88	'89	'90
(a) Quadratic	(i)	34	912	4046	4380	1160	73	1			
exponential	(ii)	34	912	4046	4380	1374	1000	1000	1000	1000	1000
(b) Linear	(i)	62	678	4032	5522						
logistic	(ii)	62	678	4032	5690	1000	1000	1000	1000	1000	1000

The values at i) for both the quadratic exponential and linear logistic curves are calculated without adjustment, while at ii) they include various adjustments, such as an allocation of 1000 new HIV cases annually from 1986 in A and 1985 in B, or the effects of various treatments, in order to achieve greater realism. From these scenarios, HIV infection curves can be reconstructed under different assumptions.

These HIV infection curves can then be used to make short-term projections of new AIDS diagnoses from (6.5.1). Table 6.12 sets out these for the years 1991–1995 for Australia as given in Solomon et al. (1991).

Table 6.12. *Estimated annual HIV infection incidence in Australia*

Year	1991	'92	'93	'94	'95
Quadratic exponential $I(t)$	765	830	863	863	831
Linear logistic $I(t)$	756	816	844	840	804

Note: No actual numbers are available for comparison

6.6   Exercises and Complements to Chapter 6

6.1 As a setting for a continuous time analogue of (6.1.2) and (6.1.3), let $X(t)$, $Y(t)$, $Z(t)$ denote the number of susceptibles, the (analogue of the) number of infectives at time t, and the number of deaths by time t. Develop the following relations:

$$Y(t) = Y(0)\psi(t) + \int_0^t \psi(t-u)\,|\mathrm{d}X(u)|,$$

$$\dot{X}(t) = -\beta X(t)Y(t), \quad \text{i.e.} \quad \frac{\mathrm{d}}{\mathrm{d}t}\ln X(t) = -\beta Y(t),$$

$$\dot{Z}(t) = \kappa\Big[Y(0)\int_0^t \varphi(u)\,\mathrm{d}u + \int_0^t \varphi(t-u)\,|\mathrm{d}X(u)|\Big],$$

where $\psi(u)$ denotes the probability that an infected individual is still infectious (and mixing in the population) time u later, and $\kappa\varphi(u)\,\mathrm{d}u$ is the probability that an infected individual dies in the interval $(u, u + \mathrm{d}u)$ after infection. Observe that, from an algorithmic viewpoint, the discrete time model is easily implemented, but not so the continuous time model.

6.2 Table 1.6 presents data of En'ko (1889) recording the daily numbers of measles cases for several years from records at the Smolnyi Institutions. Find estimates of the variance of the dates of identification of cases within each generation, (a) for each year as tabulated, (b) for the pooled data. Is there any evidence for a model like $s_m^2(j) = \alpha_m + \beta_m j$, for $m = $ a, b according as data are from (a) or (b) and $j = $ generation number. How would you interpret $\alpha_b = 2\alpha_a$, $\beta_b = \beta_a$?

6.3 Consider a chain binomial model in which the probability p_t of pairwise infection is no longer constant but is monotonically non-increasing in t. This can reflect the propensity of individuals who are more gregarious or more infectious or more susceptible, to be infected ahead of others. Investigate the estimation of $\{p_t\}$ and the fit of such models to data like Aycock's measles epidemic (Table 1.5) or En'ko's data (Tables 1.6 and 4.1).

Remark: This discrete time model attempts to reproduce the effects of heterogeneous mixing or infectivity and susceptibility as done for continuous time models in Cane and McNamee (1982) and Daley, Gani and Yakowitz (2000).

7

The Control of Epidemics

One of the purposes of modelling epidemics is to provide a rational basis for policies designed to control the spread of a disease. This aim was already evident in Macdonald's pioneering work on malaria. In his Presidential address to the Royal Society of Tropical Medicine and Hygiene (Macdonald, 1965), he referred to the development of a prevention strategy for epidemics, malaria in particular, stating that

> there is only one way of doing this—through a working model ... made by assembling all we know, or more aptly, all that we believe to be significant, of the factors involved in transmission ... in a form describable in mathematical terms.

A major contribution of Macdonald compared with his predecessors (he mentions Farr, Brownlee, Ross, Lotka, Kermack and McKendrick) was to pursue this approach to its

> logical conclusion—of final interpretation of mathematical reasoning into non-mathematical explanations of epidemiological happenings such as could be readily understood by most practising epidemiologists.

In this spirit we consider three models for epidemics to illustrate possible prevention policies of control by (a) education, (b) immunization, and (c) screening and quarantine. We could add that modelling is of vital importance in evaluating the likely effects of spreading a disease deliberately as a means of biological control, as with myxomatosis or the calicivirus to reduce the rabbit population in Australia.

Often the data available to decision makers are inadequate, as for example in the case of HIV/AIDS in Africa or South East Asia. Yet policies need to be formulated, if only on the basis of rough qualitative measures. One

175

may, for example, need to know the likely effects of spending funds on two alternative policies, or the optimal method of immunizing a population. Here, exact models may not be easy to formulate, though one usually tries to make all modelling as realistic as possible. Accurate data may be impossible to obtain, but one should always be in a position to minimize the cost of a policy or to compare the effects of policy A against those of policy B, however approximately. Examination of the control methods discussed in this chapter shows that they use and extend the simple models discussed in previous chapters.

When a policy depends only on a single variable, it is relatively easy to minimize the cost. If two policies are to be compared, one can examine their respective costs and choose the cheaper policy. Alternatively, if the criterion is not cost, one can rank the policies with respect to the criterion selected.

The control methods we describe in this chapter can be understood in terms of the general epidemic model of Chapters 2 and 3, with pairwise transmission rate β and removal rate γ, or of more complex models that include this as the simplest case. We present strategies aimed at one or more of the following results:

(a) depressing the number of susceptibles in the population, and, where possible, to below the threshold level $\rho \equiv \gamma/\beta$ described earlier in the Kermack–McKendrick criticality theorem (Theorem 2.3.1 above);

(b) accelerating the rate of removal of infectives to reduce their mixing with the population of susceptibles (i.e. increasing γ, hence ρ also);

(c) lowering the pairwise rate of infectious contact between infectives and susceptibles (i.e. decreasing β, thereby increasing ρ).

For example, immunizing some or all of the population reduces the initial number X_0 of susceptibles; operating a screening program or raising public awareness of higher disease prevalence may raise γ or lower β (or both); discouraging the assembly of large crowds reduces β.

7.1   Control by education

The AIDS epidemic has spread rapidly throughout the world. But its effect has been more limited in countries where a campaign for information and education has been sponsored by the state, or by a foundation, as for example in Switzerland.

In February 1987 a 'STOP-AIDS' advertising campaign was launched by the Swiss AIDS Foundation to provide the population with detailed knowledge of the AIDS infection and its spread, and to discourage risk-prone

Table 7.1. *Annual expected increase* $32\,000(1 - m - pr)n\alpha$
in the number of infectives

	Before advertising ($m = 0.08$, $p = 0.25$)						After advertising ($m = 0.17$, $p = 0.45$)					
	$r = 0.25$			$r = 0.50$			$r = 0.25$			$r = 0.50$		
n	1	3	5	1	3	5	1	3	5	1	3	5
α												
0.05	1372	4116	6860	1272	3816	6360	1148	3444	5740	968	2904	4840
0.10	2744	8232	13729	2544	7632	12720	2296	6888	11480	1936	5808	9680
0.15	4116	12348	20580	3816	11448	19080	3444	10332	17220	2904	8712	14520

behaviour by recommending (a) the use of condoms in sexual contacts with multiple or casual partners, (b) mutual faithfulness between sexual partners, and (c) the use of clean needles in drug usage (i.e. no exchanges between users).

It emerged that between January and October 1987, the number of occasional sexual contacts of those aged 17–30 years in Switzerland declined from 18 to 14% of the population, and among these the number always using condoms in sexual contacts increased from 8 to 17%, while those using them sometimes increased from 25 to 45%. The number of condoms (about 9.2 million) placed on the market in this nine-month period increased about 60% over the same period in 1986 (see Hausser *et al.*, 1988).

We can calculate roughly the effect of such greater sexual caution on the development of an AIDS epidemic as follows, using illustrative numbers for the land of Erehwemos with a population of 6.4 million where before a campaign like STOP-AIDS begins, we assume that the number of HIV carriers is 0.5% or 32,000 infectives. If on average each infective has n sexual partners in a year, with each of these partners being infected with probability α, where $0.05 \leq \alpha \leq 0.15$, then the number of new infectives to be expected would be about $32\,000n\alpha$. If as a result of a STOP-AIDS type campaign a proportion $m < 1$ of these infectives always use condoms, and a further proportion $p < 1 - m$ use condoms for a proportion r of the time, then the number of new infectives expected in a year would be about

$$32\,000(1 - m - pr)n\alpha. \tag{7.1.1}$$

This assumes that condoms provide total protection from HIV infection.

Table 7.1 lists the number of new infectives expected in a year for different values of the proportions m of regular and p of occasional condom users, the latter using them a proportion r of the time. The values of m and p in the table are assumed to be similar to those reported in Switzerland. The infection rate is set at $0.05(0.05)0.15$, and the number of sexual partners

$n = 1$, 3 or 5. Depending also on whether $r = 0.25$ or 0.50, the number of new infectives computed by the model would decline between 16.3% and 23.9%. This indicates the extent to which a STOP-AIDS type campaign could be expected to modify the course of the epidemic.

One could imagine that a government might wish to minimize the total cost C of (a) the annual expenditure y on pamphlets, advertisements and other educational material, and (b) the cost of medical treatment of HIV patients, each of whom requires the sum c per annum. The total expenditure C at the end of the year, starting with N HIV seropositives, would be

$$C = [N + N(1 - m - pr)n\alpha]c + y. \qquad (7.1.2)$$

Suppose now that plausible equations for m and p are

$$m = \tfrac{1}{3}(1 - e^{-ky}), \qquad p = \tfrac{2}{3}(1 - e^{-ky}), \qquad (7.1.3)$$

where $k > 0$ is some constant, and the maximum proportions of regular and occasional condom users, whatever sum y is spent on education, are $\tfrac{1}{3}$ and $\tfrac{2}{3}$ respectively. Then the expression for C at (7.1.2) becomes

$$C = Nc + Nn\alpha c[\tfrac{2}{3}(1 - r) + \tfrac{1}{3}(1 + 2r)e^{-ky}] + y. \qquad (7.1.4)$$

This function is concave in y, so differentiation yields an equation for the value of y giving the least cost C, with solution

$$y = \frac{1}{k} \ln \left(\tfrac{1}{3}k(1 + 2r)Nn\alpha c \right). \qquad (7.1.5)$$

As an example, suppose we take $r = 0.25$, $N = 32\,000$, $\alpha = 0.10$ and $n = 3$, while $c = 1$ is the financial unit. Then $y = k^{-1}\ln(4800k)$. Depending on the value of k, the value of y rises from 0 to a maximum of 1765.8 before decreasing to 0 as $k \to \infty$, as shown in Table 7.2 and Figure 7.1. In the optimal scenario, the budget y for educational material will be 1765.8, leading to a minimal cost $C = 44\,451.9$ where $y/C = 3.97\%$. Choosing some smaller y, say $y = 61.7$ for $k = 0.1$, yields minimal cost $C = 36\,895.1$ so that $y/C = 0.17\%$.

Table 7.2. *Values of y for different k*

k	0.0002083	0.0003	0.000566309	0.001	0.01	0.1	1.0	10
$\ln k$	−8.48	−8.11	−7.48	−6.91	−4.61	−2.30	0	2.30
y	0	1215.48	1765.82	1568.62	307.12	61.74	8.48	1.08

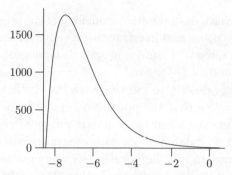

Figure 7.1. Graph of y as a function of $\ln k$.

While there is no claim that these are realistic figures, the calculations we have given indicate the type of decision that policy makers can attempt to make in the allocation of funds. In this example, spending on education a sum that is approximately 4% of the cost of medical treatment, results in a minimal cost C.

A recent paper of Kaplan (1995) on the merits of needle exchange for intravenous drug users provides an alternative example of HIV control by education. O'Neill (1995) has also studied epidemic models in which behavioural change plays a role.

7.2 Control by immunization

Immunization has long been used as a method for controlling the spread of an epidemic; in the case of smallpox, a worldwide vaccination campaign succeeded in eradicating the disease totally (see Fenner *et al.*, 1988). The fact that parents are sometimes lax in ensuring that their children are immunized against preventable diseases like measles and poliomyelitis for example, has resulted in their random recurrence. Accounts of animal and human immunization schemes may be found in Knox (1980), Dietz (1981) and Anderson (1982), among other authors. Readers should, however, note the cautionary remarks on Knox and Dietz's work in Anderson and May (1991, pp. 152–153).

In considering immunization as a technique for controlling the spread of a disease, at least two policy questions arise, both subsumed in the pursuit of maximum effect with minimum effort:

(a) how widespread can (or, should) the immunization be, and

(b) which susceptibles should be immunized for this effort to produce the best effect (e.g. should individuals be immunized at random, or should groups such as schools or families be targeted)?

These questions involve us in detailed modelling of the population where the immunization takes place, and in estimating its effect given some description of how the disease spreads. If infection spreads homogeneously through the population then question (b) is void.

Any quasi-realistic description of the spread of contagious infection usually requires recognition that the population in which the process occurs is inhomogeneous. Yet even when the population is subdivided into groups of individuals belonging to different strata (however defined), those in a given stratum are assumed to mix homogeneously amongst themselves, and to behave similarly towards individuals of other strata. In other words, homogeneity is not entirely dispensed with, for it is this very similarity that underlies the statistical approach. As in Section 3.5, we use the neutral term 'stratum' to describe such sub-populations within which individuals are regarded as identical apart from their disease status, noting that it may cover spatial variability, or distinct social behaviour, for example. Anderson and May (1991, Chapter 12) describe an optimal immunization strategy within a spatially heterogeneous population; Becker and Dietz (1995, 1996) have considered a population consisting of a number of smaller units (households, clubs or schools), and computed the effects of different strategies determined by the characteristics of these units. The four particular strategies they discussed were

  (i) random immunization of individuals;

 (ii) households chosen at random and all their members immunized;

(iii) preferential selection of large households for immunization;

(iv) immunization of a fixed fraction of members in every household.

Suppose for the moment that immunization is to be administered uniformly and at random in a population that is susceptible to a disease which is characterized by a Basic Reproduction Ratio R_0 (see Section 3.5). Recall that the threshold criterion can be stated in terms of this as

the disease can spread if $R_0 > 1$, whereas it cannot if $R_0 < 1$.   (7.2.1)

Then, a result dating back at least to Gordon Smith (1964, Figure 3) states that v^*, the minimum fraction of the population that should be immunized so as to prevent a major outbreak, is given by

$$v^* = 1 - 1/R_0. \qquad (7.2.2)$$

If immunization is carried out randomly and uniformly in a stratified population, then equation (7.2.2), first established for a single homogeneously mixing population, also holds for stratified populations with the general definition of R_0. To see this, recall that R_0 is defined as the dominant eigenvalue of a linear mapping between strata determined by the mean number m_{ij} of j-stratum infectives produced by an i-stratum infective during its entire period of infectivity. Now a random uniform immunization programme at level v reduces the expected number of susceptibles uniformly by the constant factor $(1 - v)$. The m_{ij} are therefore reduced similarly, and thus all eigenvalues are reduced by the same factor. In particular the Reproduction Ratio is $(1 - v)R_0$, and when (7.2.2) holds, this equals the critical level of unity (see (7.2.1)).

That this relation fails to provide the *optimum* immunization strategy in a genuinely heterogeneous population, where pairwise infection transmission rates β within groups are typically higher than between groups, is intuitively understandable (Anderson and May (1991), p. 307). Immunizing the same fraction in all strata results in relatively too many immunes in small groups and too few in large groups; the deficit in the latter is not made up by the excess in the former because the overall rate of infectious contacts is quadratic in the group size. Thus a uniform immunization rate, to be effective in the population as a whole, must produce more immunes than would be needed for uniform immunity within the separate strata. Using a deterministic model, Anderson and May showed that, if the pairwise infection rates β_{ij} for an i-stratum infective to transmit the disease to a specified j-stratum susceptible are β_H or β_C depending only on whether $i = j$ or $i \neq j$ respectively, then the optimal policy (i.e. requiring the minimum total amount of immunization) is such that the non-immunized susceptible numbers in each stratum are identical. Again, this is understandable, for such an immunization program reduces the susceptible populations to a collection of identical sub-population units.

In more detail and in a stochastic setting, consider a population of m strata with N_i susceptibles, $i = 1, \ldots, m$, as in Example 3.5.1, in which the pairwise infectious contact rates are β_H within each stratum and β_C between strata. We saw at (3.5.14) (recall also Exercise 3.10) that when no N_i is small,

$$R_0 \geq \frac{[\beta_H + (m - 1)\beta_C]\overline{N}}{\gamma}, \qquad (7.2.3)$$

where $\overline{N} = \sum_{i=1}^{m} N_i/m$; equality holds, when $\beta_H \neq \beta_C$, if and only if all N_i are identical. Suppose that as a result of an immunization programme the N_i susceptibles are reduced to N_i^*, say. Then the resulting Reproduction Ratio R_0^*, say, would satisfy (7.2.3) with $\overline{N}$ replaced by $\overline{N^*}$, and the equality would now hold if and only if all N_i^* are equal. Consequently, among those immunization programmes that reduce R_0 to $R_0^* = 1$, the programme requiring the smallest number of people to be immunized (i.e. the programme for which $m(\overline{N} - \overline{N^*})$ is least), is the one for which each N_i is reduced to

$$N_i^* = \overline{N^*} = \frac{\gamma}{\beta_H + (m-1)\beta_C} \quad (i = 1, \ldots, m). \tag{7.2.4}$$

This analysis depends on none of the N_i being small, a condition which is not generally met when each stratum is a household; in this case an alternative setting is needed, such as was discussed in Example 3.5.2. There we showed that when $\beta_H \gg \gamma$, $R_0 \approx \frac{1}{2}(A + \sqrt{A^2 + 4B})$, where

$$A = \frac{\sum_{i=1}^m N_i \beta_C}{\gamma + \beta_C}, \qquad B = \frac{\sum_{i=1}^m N_i(N_i - 1)\beta_C \gamma}{(\gamma + \beta_C)(\gamma + 2\beta_C)}. \tag{7.2.5}$$

Here A, but not B, is independent of the detailed household structure.

Suppose that under an immunization strategy, the N_i are reduced to N_i^*, so that A, B and R_0 reduce to A^*, B^* and R_0^* respectively, where these are given by

$$A^* = \frac{(\sum_{i=1}^m N_i^*)A}{\sum_{i=1}^m N_i}, \qquad B^* = \frac{[\sum_{i=1}^m N_i^*(N_i^* - 1)]B}{\sum_{i=1}^m N_i(N_i - 1)},$$
$$R_0^* = \frac{1}{2}(A^* + \sqrt{(A^*)^2 + 4B^*}). \tag{7.2.6}$$

Inspection of the expression for B^* shows that it is a convex increasing function of each N_i^*. Hence a maximal reduction in R_0^* is achieved for a given overall reduction $\Delta N \equiv \sum_{i=1}^m (N_i - N_i^*)$ in the number of susceptibles, when $\max_i N_i$ is reduced maximally subject to this given total reduction. Thus the conclusion immediately above (7.2.4) continues to hold in this changed setting.

Specifically, given the number ΔN of susceptibles to be immunized, R_0^* is reduced maximally by finding d for which $N_i^* = \min(N_i, d)$ and $\Delta N = \sum_{j=i}^m (N_i - d)_+$, with $0 \leq N_i^* \leq N_i$. This is a discrete analogue of the continuous variable result of Anderson and May (1991, Chapter 12 and Appendix G) referred to above (7.2.3). In fact, unless d is an integer, to attain the optimum exactly we must further adjust the N_i^* for those i for which $0 \leq d - N_i^* < 1$ so that all the adjusted N_i^* are integers.

Administratively, this optimal policy may not be as convenient as the uniform fraction (i.e. strategy (i)), or the targeting of specific households (either (ii) or (iii)), and so may prove more costly. But knowing the nature of an optimal strategy, provides a rational basis for the assessment of

Table 7.3. Values of the reproduction ratio and immunization fractions for different strategies in the case $\beta_H \gg \gamma$

k	1	2	3	4	5	6
n_k	300	400	200	75	20	5
			Quasi-optimal strategy			
R_0^*	0.4998	1.3626	1.7439	1.8933	1.9379	1.9485
v_{opt}	0.5305	0.2019	0.0610	0.0141	0.0023	0.0000
v_{unif}	0.7435	0.3007	0.1050	0.0283	0.0054	0.0000
			All-or-none in households $> k$			
R_0'	0.1499	0.9640	1.5106	1.8027	1.9114	1.9485
$v_{all/none}$	0.8592	0.4836	0.2019	0.0610	0.0141	0.0000

other policies. For example, if instead one were to immunize the largest households completely, how much more immunization would be needed? We discuss such questions in Example 7.2.1 and Exercises 7.1 and 7.2.

Example 7.2.1. Consider a population of $m = 1000$ households consisting of n_k households with k susceptibles ($k = 1, \ldots, 6$) as shown in Table 7.3; let $\gamma = 1$, $\beta_C = 0.0005$. Suppose first that $\beta_H \gg \gamma$ so that all the analysis of Example 3.5.2 is applicable. From equation (3.5.20) the Basic Reproduction Ratio R_0 of the population equals 1.9485 as shown in the last column. The rest of the entries in the table show the effects of three immunization strategies.

The effect of the *Quasi-optimal* strategy, when immunization is carried out to reduce all households to a maximum of j susceptibles, is shown via the reproduction ratio R_0^* that would then be realized. This entails immunizing a fraction $v_{opt} \equiv \sum_{k>j} (k-j)n_k / \sum_{k \geq 1} k n_k$ of the population; of course, $v_{opt} < v_{unif} = 1 - R_0^*/R_0$, the fraction needing immunization under a random strategy to reduce the reproduction ratio by the same amount.

Consider next the effect of an *all-or-none* strategy in which all members in every household of more than k members are immunized (strategy (iii)). Then the reproduction ratio R_0' and fraction immunized $v_{all/none}$ are as shown. The population numbers in the households were chosen so as to make some of the $v_{all/none}$ fractions coincide with fractions v_{opt} under the quasi-optimal strategy but for smaller k. Observe that the ratios under the quasi-optimal strategy are smaller than the ratios under the all-or-none strategy when $v_{all/none} = v_{opt}$.

We can draw at least two conclusions from this table, for this particular distribution of households. First, to reduce the value of the reproduction ratio to below 1, requires the immunization of about 50% more individ-

Table 7.4. *Values of the reproduction ratio and immunization fractions for different strategies in the case* $\beta_H = 0.2\gamma$

k	1	2	3	4	5	6
n_k	300	400	200	75	20	5
Quasi-optimal strategy						
R_0^*	0.4998	0.9697	1.1933	1.2802	1.3065	1.3131
v_{opt}	0.5305	0.2019	0.0610	0.0141	0.0023	0.0000
v_{unif}	0.6194	0.2615	0.0912	0.0250	0.0050	0.0000
All-or-none in households $> k$						
R_0'	0.1499	0.6518	1.0235	1.2184	1.2892	1.3131
$v_{\mathrm{all/none}}$	0.8592	0.4836	0.2019	0.0610	0.0141	0.0000

uals under a random strategy than under the optimal one. Second, the all-or-none strategy is marginally more efficient than the random strategy. Strategies (ii) and (iv) are considered in Exercises 7.1 and 7.2.

Suppose now that $\beta_H \gg \gamma$ does not hold. The analysis we have given must then be reworked starting from the matrix $\mathbf{M}$ at (3.5.18) and finding its eigenvalue of largest modulus, much as in the concluding paragraph of Section 3.5. We illustrate this approach in the context of Example 7.2.1 except that now $\beta_H = 0.2\gamma$ while the other parameter values are unchanged. We computed the dominant eigenvalue by reduction of $\mathbf{M}$ to upper Hessenberg form via Gaussian elimination and use of the QR algorithm as in Press *et al.* (1987, Chapter 11). This leads to Table 7.4 in place of Table 7.3.

Qualitatively, what is an optimal immunization strategy for an epidemic that may spread in a community of households, for which the conditions justifying the approximations do not hold? Intuitively, since the optimal strategy described earlier is a function of the graph-theoretic structure of the infectious path of the disease, then, assuming the same homogeneity within households and the same infectivity relation between households, we would expect the same strategy to remain optimal. In other words, the quantitative details may change, but the qualitative principle would remain.

7.3   Control by screening and quarantine

A third method of controlling the spread of a disease is by screening suspected infectives and quarantining those who are thought to pose a risk. This is a procedure often adopted in countries free of malaria (e.g. Australia) when a returning tourist is suspected of carrying the disease. In California, prisoners known to be HIV seropositive (i.e. HIV+) are interned in a separate correctional facility at Vacaville, but in general HIV screening

Table 7.5. *Numbers of AIDS cases among US correctional inmates, 1985–1992*

Survey period	Number of cases	Per cent increase from preceding survey
November 1985	766	–
October 1986	1 232	61%
October 1987	1 964	59%
October 1988	3 136	60%
October 1989	5 411	72%
October 1990	6 985	29%
November 1992	11 565	66% [= 29% p.a.]

Source: Thomas and Moerings (1994), p. 139.

is not compulsory. The fact that HIV is more prevalent in prisons than in the community at large, suggests that HIV may spread more rapidly in confinement than in the free community (see Exercise 7.2).

HIV is spread in prisons by sexual contacts and by needle sharing among intravenous drug users (Brewer *et al.* 1988). The US Department of Justice (1993) reports that there were 11 500 known cases of AIDS in Federal prisons for the five months from November 1992 to May 1993, with an average growth of over 50% annually during the past several years (see Table 7.5). This was considerably greater than the rate of increase in the total number of prisoners (roughly, 75% between 1985 and 1992), and represented an incidence rate of over 1% (cf. less than 0.1% in the wider population then). Thomas and Moerings's book (1994) has documented worldwide concern about the spread of HIV/AIDS in prisons.

Blumberg and Langston (1991) raised the question of mandatory HIV testing of prisoners on entry into jail, but such a procedure is not currently acceptable. However, voluntary reporting or testing for HIV is possible (Stevens, 1993; see also Hsieh, 1991), and both medical and educational help then becomes available to HIV+ prisoners; Siegal *et al.* (1993) state that HIV+ prisoners who do not report their status do not receive medical help. Hsieh (1991) considered a model of HIV screening that incorporates the quarantine of infectives.

We consider in turn models for a single isolated prison, and for a prison interacting with the outside world. Then in Section 7.3.3, we discuss a screening and quarantine procedure for which the overall medical costs over a fixed period of time T, including costs of treating undiagnosed HIV+ prisoners, are minimized.

While only deterministic models are used here, their stochastic equivalents can also be analysed (see Yakowitz, Gani and Blount (1996), Gani, Yakowitz and Blount (1997) for details, and Section 4.4 above for a related model).

7.3.1   The single prison model

Suppose that a prison containing N inmates, allows a simultaneous inflow and outflow of $n < N$ prisoners at time t $(t = 0, 1, \ldots)$, after which there are y_t prisoners who are HIV+ and $N - y_t$ susceptibles. During the interval $(t, t + 1)$, which we take to be relatively short so that y_t does not vary greatly in it, assume that homogeneous mixing occurs with an infection rate β, so that $\beta y_t(N - y_t)$ new infectives are produced. This is a discrete time approximation based on the continuous time simple epidemic; for details see Bailey (1975, Chapter 5) or Section 6.1 above (Daley and Gani (1999a) discuss another model analogous to a simple epidemic). Thus at time $t+1-$ there are

$$z_{t+1} = y_t[1 + \beta(N - y_t)] \tag{7.3.1}$$

infectives. In the outflow of $n \equiv rN$ prisoners at time $t + 1$, there are

$$v_{t+1} = r z_{t+1} = r y_t[1 + \beta(N - y_t)] \tag{7.3.2}$$

infectives, and amongst the inflow of n new prisoners we can expect a proportion μ_t to be infectives, where $0 < \mu_t < 1$, so at time $t + 1+$ there are

$$y_{t+1} = \mu_t n + (1 - r)y_t[1 + \beta(N - y_t)] \equiv f(y_t, \mu_t) \tag{7.3.3}$$

infectives amongst the N prisoners.

Are there stable scenarios for this model? We could ask whether a stable regime is reached starting from y_0 infectives at time $0+$ under the assumption that $\mu_t = \mu$ (all t). To this end we examine the transformation $y \mapsto f(y, \mu)$ for any fixed points lying in $[0, N]$. Observe that the function $g(y) \equiv f(y, \mu) - y$ is concave, with $g(0) = n\mu > 0$ and $g(N) = n(\mu - 1) < 0$ under our assumptions on μ. Thus, a unique stable scenario $y_t = y_s$ (all t) exists, namely

$$
\begin{aligned}
y_s &= \frac{(1 + \beta N)(1 - r) - 1 + \sqrt{[(1 + \beta N)(1 - r) - 1]^2 + 4n\mu\beta(1 - r)}}{2\beta(1 - r)} \\
&= \frac{\beta(N - n) - r + \sqrt{[\beta(N - n) - r]^2 + 4\mu r\beta(N - n)}}{2\beta(1 - r)} .
\end{aligned}
$$
$$\tag{7.3.4}$$

In the limiting case $\mu = 0$, $y_s = 0$ is also a fixed point and further argument is needed to decide which of these roots of $g(y_s) = 0$ equals $\lim_{t \to \infty} y_t$. The matter is easily decided: equation (7.3.4) always represents the larger root, and is zero (hence, the only root in $[0, N]$) if and only if

Table 7.6. *Stable infective sizes in the single prison model for different* n, μ, βN

n	μ	0.0	0.05	0.075	0.1	0.125	0.15	βN 0.2	0.25	0.5	5
25	0.01	5.0	39.8	160.1	242.3	293.1	327.2	370.2	396.1	448.0	494.8
	0.005	2.5	25.4	154.8	239.6	291.3	325.9	369.3	395.4	447.7	494.8
50	0.01	5.0	9.0	14.5	31.8	82.5	142.6	228.3	281.7	390.3	489.0
	0.005	2.5	4.5	7.5	18.7	71.2	136.4	225.3	279.8	389.6	489.0

$(1 + \beta N)(1 - r) \leq 1$. In other words, (7.3.4) always gives the required root: when $\mu = 0$ it simplifies to

$$y_s = \begin{cases} 0 & \text{if } \beta N \leq r/(1 - r), \\ N - r/[\beta(1 - r)] & \text{otherwise.} \end{cases} \qquad (7.3.5)$$

We interpret this equation as indicating that infection is contained to small levels within the prison if the former case holds, i.e. if $n \geq \beta N^2/(1 + \beta N)$.

Example 7.3.1. Suppose that $N = 500$. Table 7.6 indicates the stable values y_s under a range of values for β for $n = 25$ and 50, and $\mu = 0.01$ and 0.005. The time taken to attain these stable values depends on both the initial infection intensity y_0 and the contact rate β (see Exercise 7.3). Note that when βN exceeds the threshold $r/(1 - r)$ the endemic level rises appreciably above the endemic level μ of the new prisoners, though the threshold does depend on interplay of all of μ, βN and n. For βN below the threshold, $y_s \approx n\mu/[r - \beta N(1 - r)]$, $\approx \mu N$ for $\beta \to 0$.

7.3.2 Interaction of a prison with the outside world

Consider a city of fixed population size M with Y_t infectives at time $t = 0, 1, \ldots$, in which there is a single prison with N inmates of whom y_t are infectives. We make the same assumptions as in the previous section concerning the prison, so that in $(t, t + 1)$ there are $\beta y_t(N - y_t)$ new prison infectives. The same proportion of infectives leaves as before.

For the city population, homogeneous mixing and an infectivity rate β_0 per susceptible–infective pair produces $\beta_0 Y_t(M - Y_t)$ new infectives. Suppose also that deaths occur at rate γ, and that the number of births, all healthy, equals the number of deaths, thus keeping the city population size constant. Then at time $t + 1-$, before exchange with the prison occurs, the city has

$$(1 - \gamma)Y_t + \beta_0 Y_t(M - Y_t)$$

infectives, so with $r = n/N$, $R = n/M$,

$$Y_{t+1} = (1 - R)Y_t[1 - \gamma + \beta_0(M - Y_t)] + ry_t[1 + \beta(N - y_t)] \equiv f_1(Y_t, y_t),$$
$$y_{t+1} = RY_t[1 - \gamma + \beta_0(M - Y_t)] + (1 - r)y_t[1 + \beta(N - y_t)] \equiv f_2(Y_t, y_t).$$
$$(7.3.6)$$

Write $f(Y, y)$ for the vector-valued function $(f_1(Y, y), f_2(Y, y))$. For a realistic model we require that for (Y, y) in the rectangle $[0, M] \times [0, N]$, $f(Y, y)$ should also lie within the rectangle. Since f is continuous, and the rectangle is a compact set, there is at least one fixed point $(Y_s, y_s) = f(Y_s, y_s)$ which we interpret as a vector of stable values for Y and y. Then (Y_s, y_s) satisfies

$$\begin{pmatrix} Y_s \\ y_s \end{pmatrix} = \begin{pmatrix} (1 - R)[1 - \gamma + \beta_0(M - Y_s)] & r[1 + \beta(N - y_s)] \\ R[1 - \gamma + \beta_0(M - Y_s)] & (1 - r)[1 + \beta(N - y_s)] \end{pmatrix} \begin{pmatrix} Y_s \\ y_s \end{pmatrix}.$$
$$(7.3.7)$$

Addition of these two equations gives

$$Y_s + y_s = Y_s[1 - \gamma + \beta_0(M - Y_s)] + y_s[1 + \beta(N - y_s)], \qquad (7.3.8)$$

and hence

$$\beta_0 Y_s(M - Y_s) + \beta y_s(N - y_s) = \gamma Y_s. \qquad (7.3.9)$$

Equivalently, the number of new infectives in $(t, t + 1)$ equals the number of infectives removed in $(t, t + 1)$. Substitution in (7.3.7) so as to eliminate one or other of the quadratic terms yields

$$\begin{aligned} ry_s &= R(1 - \gamma)Y_s + (1 - R - r)\beta y_s(N - y_s) \\ &= RY_s + (1 - r)\gamma Y_s - (1 - R - r)\beta_0 Y_s(M - Y_s), \end{aligned} \qquad (7.3.10)$$

showing that $(0, 0)$ and (M, N) are always fixed points, and that they are the only fixed points when $\gamma = 0$, i.e. when the city population has no births and deaths.

Equation (7.3.9) shows that for the disease to be confined to a small number, ϵM say, of the city population, the various parameters must satisfy both $\beta_0 M(1 - \epsilon) < \gamma$, i.e. the infection rate β_0 must lie below a threshold level determined by the relative removal rate γ/M, and the endemic infection level in prison y_s must likewise be contained by a function, namely $\beta y_s(N - y_s) < (\gamma - \beta_0 M)\epsilon M$. Ideally, having $\beta < 4(\gamma - \beta_0 M)\epsilon M/N^2$ would contain the incidence in the city population irrespective of the incidence rate in prison. See also Exercise 7.4.

Rewrite (7.3.7) as $0 = g_1(Y_s, y_s) \equiv f_1(Y_s, y_s) - Y_s$, and $0 = g_2(Y_s, y_s) \equiv f_2(Y_s, y_s) - y_s$. For given y, $g_1(Y, y)$ is concave in Y, with stationary point $Y(y)$ equal to

$$Y(y) \equiv \frac{A + \sqrt{A^2 + 4\beta_0(1 - R)ry[1 + \beta(N - y)]}}{2\beta_0(1 - R)}, \qquad (7.3.11)$$

where $A = (1 - R)[1 - \gamma + \beta_0 M] - 1$. Similarly, for given Y, $g_2(Y, y)$ is concave in y with stationary point

$$y(Y) \equiv \frac{B + \sqrt{B^2 + 4\beta(1-r)RY[1 - \gamma + \beta_0(M-Y)]}}{2\beta(1-r)}, \qquad (7.3.12)$$

where $B = (1 - r)\beta N - r$. Alternatively, the first expression in (7.3.10) shows that y_s and Y_s are related by $y_s = y_2(Y_s)$ where

$$y_2(Y) = \frac{B_2 + \sqrt{B_2^2 + 4\beta(1-f)R(1-\gamma)Y}}{2\beta(1-f)}, \qquad (7.3.13)$$

with $f = R + r$ and $B_2 = \beta N(1 - f) - r$.

Example 7.3.2. Suppose we take $M = 50\,000$, $N = 1\,000$, $\beta_0 = 1.5 \times 10^{-7}$, $\beta = 1.5 \times 10^{-3}$. Recall that γ and n define the equivalents of immigration–emigration rates for the city and prison respectively. For the four pairs of values of γ and n shown in Table 7.7 the stable values Y_s and y_s are as shown; note that the infection rate in prison, which is almost 100%, is little affected by γ, whereas the infection rate in the city is affected by both γ and n, reflecting respectively the removal rate and rate of introduction of infectives 'new' to the city population.

Table 7.7. *Stable infective sizes in a prison-and-city model*

n	γ	Y_s	y_s
100	0.03	4096.3	932.3
	0.015	9404.3	940.6
50	0.03	2132.3	966.4
	0.015	5446.9	968.8

7.3.3   A quarantine policy in prison

Gani, Yakowitz and Blount (1997) studied a cost effective model for a prison in which prisoners may be screened regularly, and quarantined if found to be HIV+. We follow the single prison model of Section 7.3.1 with the difference that at time $t = 0, 1, \ldots$, the prison population of size N is now subdivided into three groups: susceptibles x_t, infectives not in quarantine y_t, and quarantined prisoners q_t, where

$$x_t + y_t + q_t = N. \qquad (7.3.14)$$

Assuming homogeneous mixing between susceptibles and infectives in $(t, t+1)$, there are

$$z_{t+1} = y_t + \beta x_t y_t = y_t(1 + \beta x_t) \qquad (7.3.15)$$

infectives at time $t + 1-$. At this epoch we suppose there is an inflow of $n = rN$ new prisoners of whom a proportion μ_{t+1} are HIV+, so that

$$u_{t+1} = n\mu_{t+1} \tag{7.3.16}$$

infectives are added. At the same time, n prisoners leave, among them

$$v_{t+1} = rz_{t+1} \qquad \text{and} \qquad w_{t+1} = rq_t \tag{7.3.17}$$

non-quarantined and quarantined infectives. Thus before a new screening and quarantine of prisoners, the total numbers of non-quarantined and quarantined infectives, at $t + 1-$, are, respectively,

$$z_{t+1} + u_{t+1} - v_{t+1} = y_t(1 + \beta x_t)(1 - r) + n\mu_{t+1} \tag{7.3.18a}$$

and

$$q_t - w_{t+1} = (1 - r)q_t. \tag{7.3.18b}$$

Let us now screen a proportion σ (with $0 \leq \sigma \leq 1$) of the non-quarantined prison population, and quarantine those who test HIV+. Then at $t+1+$ the numbers of non-quarantined and quarantined infectives, and susceptibles, are respectively

$$y_{t+1} = (1 - \sigma)[\mu_{t+1}n + y_t(1 + \beta x_t)(1 - r)], \tag{7.3.19a}$$
$$q_{t+1} = q_t(1 - r) + \sigma[\mu_{t+1}n + y_t(1 + \beta x_t)(1 - r)], \tag{7.3.19b}$$
$$x_{t+1} = N - y_{t+1} - q_{t+1}. \tag{7.3.20}$$

Suppose the costs involved per prisoner in such screening, quarantining and medical treatment of prisoners are

$$\begin{array}{ll} a & \text{for the HIV test,} \\ b & \text{for quarantining and associated treatment,} \\ c & \text{for treating an unquarantined infective.} \end{array} \tag{7.3.21}$$

Then the cost C_t for the time interval $(t - 1, t)$ is

$$C_t = a\sigma(N - q_t) + bq_t + cy_t, \tag{7.3.22}$$

and the cost over the time interval $(0, T)$ is

$$J(\sigma, T) \equiv \sum_{t=1}^{T} C_t. \tag{7.3.23}$$

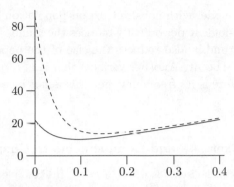

Figure 7.2. Cost of an epidemic in prison as a function of the screening rate σ, for finite (——) and infinite (- - - -) time horizons.

Example 7.3.3 (cf. Gani, Yakowitz and Blount (1997)). Assume that $b > c > a > 0$, so we can expect the optimal screening rate $\sigma' < 1$. We confirm this expectation for the parameter values N, μ, n and β much as in Example 7.3.1, under the two scenarios of stability, and of a finite time horizon $T = 50$. In general the optimal screening rate differs for these conditions. It is arguable that the screening rate should be chosen according to the worse scenario which, in the case of a low initial incidence rate, is always the stationary case.

Figure 7.2 shows the average cost $J(\sigma, T)/T$ and its limit for $T \to \infty$ as functions of the screening rate σ in the case $\mu = 0.005$, $n = 25$, $\beta N = 0.15$ with $y_0 = 0$. It shows that the optimal screening rate is about 10% or 15% depending on whether a finite $(T = 50)$ or infinite time horizon is used. Table 7.8 shows the optimal screening rates for the two scenarios for the range of parameter values considered.

Table 7.8. *Optimal prison population screening rates for isolated prison model*

					βN				
n	μ	0.05	0.075	0.1	0.125	0.15	0.2	0.25	0.5
25	0.01	0.0	0.027	0.065	0.100	0.129	0.182	0.228	0.396
		0.038	0.082	0.119	0.151	0.180	0.231	0.276	0.440
	0.005	0.0	0.0	0.032	0.065	0.094	0.146	0.191	0.357
		0.008	0.051	0.086	0.116	0.144	0.194	0.237	0.396
50	0.01	0.0	0.0	0.026	0.063	0.095	0.151	0.200	0.378
		0.0	0.036	0.075	0.108	0.139	0.193	0.240	0.412
	0.005	0.0	0.0	0.0	0.026	0.057	0.112	0.159	0.334
		0.0	0.003	0.040	0.073	0.102	0.154	0.199	0.367

For each (n, μ), the upper (lower) rows correspond to finite (infinite) time horizon.

In terms of our model with constant prison population size N, the effect of screening is two-fold: it periodically reduces the number of infectives who may infect others, and it also reduces the size of the population where infectious contact can occur. Another variable that is of concern in managing a screening procedure is its frequency, but this is not investigated here (see Exercise 7.6).

7.4   Exercises and Complements to Chapter 7

7.1 *(Community of m households with $\beta_H \gg \gamma$).* In Example 7.2.1, the assumption $\beta_H \gg \gamma$ implies that either none or all of the members of any given household become infected in the course of an epidemic. Regard such a community of m households as consisting of n' strata, where stratum k consists of the n_k households with j susceptibles initially and $n' = \max\{k : n_k > 0\}$. The probability that a household with j infectives would infect a specific kth stratum household of susceptibles (assuming no other households have any effect in the meantime) equals

$$1 - \prod_{i=1}^{j} \frac{i\gamma}{i\gamma + ik\beta_C} = 1 - \left(\frac{\gamma}{\gamma + k\beta_C}\right)^j \approx \frac{jk\beta_C}{\gamma} = \frac{jk}{\rho_C},$$

where $\rho_C = \gamma/\beta_C$ and the approximation is valid for $\beta_C \ll \gamma$. Then m_{jk}^H, the mean number of kth stratum households infected by a household of j infectives, is given by

$$m_{jk}^H = n_k \left[1 - \left(\frac{\gamma}{\gamma + k\beta_C}\right)^j\right] \approx \frac{jkn_k}{\rho_C},$$

and the Basic Reproduction Ratio R_0^H in terms of household units is the largest eigenvalue of the matrix $\mathbf{M}^H = (m_{jk}^H)$. Verify that

$$\det(\mathbf{M}^H - \lambda) \approx (-\lambda)^{n'-1}\left(\sum_{k=1}^{n'} \frac{k^2 n_k}{\rho_C} - \lambda\right)$$

(cf. (3.5.19)), so that

$$R_0^H \approx \sum_{k=1}^{n'} \frac{k^2 n_k}{\rho_C}.$$

In the context of Table 7.3, conclude that in order to reduce R_0^H below 1, about two-thirds of the households would need to be immunized if Becker and Dietz's strategy (ii) were followed; alternatively, since $0 < \rho_C - (n_1 + 4n_2) < 9n_3$, it would suffice to immunize all members of households with three or more susceptibles under a quasi-optimal all-or-none strategy (iii).

7.2 Consider a community of 1000 households as in Example 7.2.1. Suppose that in a randomly chosen proportion p of these households, all members are immunized, leaving an expected number $(1 - p)n_k$ households with k susceptibles. Assuming $\beta_H \gg \gamma$, show that R_0 is reduced to $R_0'(1 - p)$ given by

$$R_0'(1 - p) \approx (1 - p)\tfrac{1}{2}\left(A + \sqrt{A^2 + 4B/(1 - p)}\right) > (1 - p)R_0,$$

where A, B are given at (7.2.5). By way of contrast, immunizing the same proportion of randomly chosen members of the population yields $R_0''(1 - p)$ given by

$$R_0''(1 - p) \approx (1 - p)R_0 < R_0'(1 - p).$$

7.3 For the prison model of Section 7.3.1 investigate numerically the rate of attainment of equilibrium values with $N = 500$, different β and y_0.

7.4 In the context of the model of Section 7.3.2, show that when $M \gg N$, the stationary solution (Y_s, y_s) cannot have $Y_s/M \ll y_s/N$ if $\beta_0 = \beta$.

7.5 In Example 7.3.2 investigate the rate of convergence to equilibrium (cf. Exercise 7.3).

7.6 In Example 7.3.3, investigate the effect on the optimal screening rate σ of screening only every d time units.

References and Author Index

At the end of each reference entry is the page number or numbers where it is cited. For other than first-named authors there is a cross-reference to the first-named author.

Abbey, Helen (1952). An examination of the Reed–Frost theory of epidemics. *Hum. Biology* **24**, 201–233.   [11, 14–15, 105, 115, 154]

Allen, J. R. *See* Lui, Peterman *et al.*

Allen, M. *See* Wilson *et al.*

Anderson, R. L. and Medley, G. F. (1988). Epidemiology, HIV infection and AIDS: the incubation and infectious periods, survival and vertical transmission. Quoted by Isham, V. (1988), Appendix 4. In *Short-Term Prediction of HIV Infection and AIDS in England and Wales*, HMSO, London, 53–55. [170]

Anderson, R. M. (1982). Fox rabies. In *The Population Dynamics of Infectious Diseases: Theory and Applications*, R. M. Anderson (Ed.), Chapman and Hall, London, 242–261.   [179]

Anderson, R. M. and May, R. M. (1991). *Infectious Diseases of Humans: Dynamics and Control.* Oxford Univ. Press, Oxford. (Oxford paperback edition, 1992.)   [xii, 1, 8, 11, 16–17, 46, 85, 154, 179–182]

Arita, I. *See* Fenner *et al.*

Athreya, K. B. and Ney, P. E. (1972). *Branching Processes.* Springer-Verlag, New York.   [87]

Attewell, R. G. *See* Solomon *et al.*

Aycock, W. L. (1942). Immunity to polyomyelitis. Heterologous strains and discrepant neutralization tests. *Amer. J. Med. Sci.* **204**(3), 455–467.   [14, 154, 174]

Bacchetti, P. R., Segal, M. R. and Jewell, N. P. (1992). Uncertainty about the incubation period of AIDS. In Jewell, Dietz and Farewell (1992), 61–80.   [170]

Bailey, N. T. J. (1953). The total size of the general stochastic epidemic. *Biometrika* **40**, 177–185.   [77]

Bailey, N. T. J. (1955). Some problems in the statistical analysis of epidemic data (with Discussion). *J. Roy. Statist. Soc. Ser. B* **17**, 35–68.   [21, 107, 115]

Bailey, N. T. J. (1963). The simple stochastic epidemic: a complete solution in terms of known functions. *Biometrika* **50**, 235–240.   [60, 66]

Bailey, N. T. J. (1964). *The Elements of Stochastic Processes with Applications to the Natural Sciences.* John Wiley, New York. [56]

Bailey, N. T. J. (1975). *The Mathematical Theory of Infectious Diseases and its Applications.* Charles Griffin, London. [xii, 1, 16, 21, 60, 77, 99, 107, 117–118, 154–155, 162, 165, 168, 186]

Bailey, N. T. J. (1982). *The Biomathematics of Malaria.* Charles Griffin, London. [46]

Ball, F. (1985). Deterministic and stochastic epidemics with several kinds of susceptibles. *Adv. Appl. Probab.* **17**, 1–22. [53]

Ball, F. (1986). A unified approach to the distribution of total size and total area under the trajectory of infectives in epidemic models. *Adv. Appl. Probab.* **18**, 289–310. [126, 132]

Ball, F. and Clancy, D. (1993). The final size and severity of a generalized stochastic multitype epidemic model. *Adv. Appl. Probab.* **25**, 721–736. [38]

Ball, F., Mollison, D. and Scalia-Tomba, G. (1997). Epidemics with two levels of mixing. *Ann. Appl. Probab.* **7**, 46–89. [94]

Barbour, A. D. (1972). The principle of diffusion of arbitrary constants. *J. Appl. Probab.* **9**, 519–541. [84, 145]

Barbour, A. D. (1974). On a functional central limit theorem for Markov population processes. *Adv. Appl. Probab.* **6**, 21–39. [84, 145]

Barbour, A. D. (1994). Threshold phenomena in epidemic theory. In *Probability, Statistics and Optimization: A Tribute to Peter Whittle*, F. P. Kelly (Ed.), John Wiley, Chichester, 101–116. [85]

Baroyan, V. O. and Rvachev, L. A. (1967). Deterministic epidemic models for a territory with a transport network. *Kibernetika* **3**, 67–74. (In Russian.) [155]

Baroyan, V. O., Rvachev, L. A., Basilevsky, U. V., Ermakov, V. V., Frank, K. D., Rvachev, M. A. and Shashkov, V. A. (1971). Computer modelling of influenza epidemics for the whole country (USSR). *Adv. Appl. Probab.* **3**, 224–226. [155]

Baroyan, V. O., Rvachev, L. A. and Ivannikov, Yu. G. (1977). *Modelling and Prediction of Influenza Epidemics in the USSR.* Moscow: Gamelei Institute of Epidemiology and Microbiology. (In Russian). [155]

Bartholomew, D. J. (1973). *Stochastic Models for Social Processes*, 2nd Edn. John Wiley, London. (1st Edn, 1967; 3rd Edn, 1982). [17, 58, 133, 136, 138]

Bartlett, M. S. (1947). *Stochastic Processes* (mimeographed notes of a course given at the University of North Carolina in the Fall Quarter, 1946). [21]

Bartlett, M. S. (1949). Some evolutionary stochastic processes. *J. Roy. Statist. Soc. B* **11**, 211–229. [13]

Bartlett, M. S. (1960). *Stochastic Population Models in Ecology and Epidemiology.* Methuen, London. [85]

Bartlett, M. S. (1978). *An Introduction to Stochastic Processes*, 3rd Edn. Cambridge University Press, Cambridge. [57, 73]

Basilevsky, U. V. *See* Baroyan, Rvachev, Basilevsky *et al.*

Becker, Niels G. (1981). A general chain binomial model for infectious diseases. *Biometrics* **37**, 251–258. [164–168]

Becker, Niels G. (1989). *Analysis of Infectious Disease Data*. Chapman and Hall, London.   [107, 115, 154]

Becker, N. G. and Dietz, K. (1995). The effect of the household distribution on transmission and control of highly infectious diseases. *Math. Biosci.* **127**, 207–219.   [180]

Becker, N. G. and Dietz, K. (1996). Reproduction numbers and critical immunity levels for epidemics in a community of households. In *Athens Conference on Applied Probability and Time Series* (Springer Lecture Notes in Statistics, Vol. 114), C. C. Heyde, Yu. V. Prohorov, R. Pyke and S. T. Rachev (Eds), Springer-Verlag, New York, 267–276.   [180, 192]

Bennett, C. *See* Wilson *et al.*

Bernoulli, Daniel (1760). Essai d'une nouvelle analyse de la mortalité causée par la petite vérole et des avantages de l'inoculation pour la prévenir. *Mém. Math. Phys. Acad. Roy. Sci., Paris,* 1–45. In *Histoire de l'Académie Royale des Sciences* (1766).   [2–4, 6, 154]

Blount, M. *See* Gani, Yakowitz and Blount; Yakowitz, Gani and Blount.

Blumberg, M. and Langston, D. (1991). Mandatory HIV testing in criminal justice settings. *Crime and Delinquency* **37**, 5–18.   [185]

Bregman, D. J. *See* Lui, Lawrence *et al.*

Brewer, T. F., Vlahov, D., Taylor, E., Hall, D., Munoz, A. and Polk, F. (1988). Transmission of HIV1 within a statewide prison system. *AIDS* **2**, 363–367. [185]

Brookmeyer, R. (1991). Reconstruction and future trends of the AIDS epidemic in the United States. *Science* **253**, 37–42.   [170]

Brookmeyer, R. and Gail, M. H. (1988). A method of obtaining short-term projections and lower bounds on the size of the AIDS epidemic. *J. Amer. Statist. Assoc.* **83**, 301–308.   [170]

Brownlee, J. (1906). Statistical studies in immunity: the theory of an epidemic. *Proc. Roy. Soc. Edinburgh* **26**, 484–521.   [8, 175]

Brownlee, J. (1915). Historical note on Farr's theory of the epidemic. *Brit. Med. J.* **1915(2)**, 250–252.   [8]

Burke, M. H. *See* Wilson and Burke.

Burnet, M. and White, D. O. (1972). *The Natural History of Infectious Disease* (4th Edn). Cambridge University Press, Cambridge.   [1]

Cane, V. and McNamee, R. (1982). The spread of infection in a heterogeneous population. *J. Appl. Probab.* **19A**, 173–184.   [174]

Carlson, R. G. *See* Siegal *et al.*

Centers for Disease Control. (1990). HIV prevalence estimates and AIDS case projections for the United States: Report based on Workshop. *Morbidity and Mortality, Weekly Report* **39** (RR–16) 1–31.   [170]

Clancy, D. (1994). Some comparison results for multitype epidemic models. *J. Appl. Probab.* **31**, 9–26.   [38]

Clancy, D. *See also* Ball and Clancy.

Cooper, D. A. *See* Whyte *et al.*

Cox, D. R. and Miller, H. T. (1965). *The Theory of Stochastic Processes*. Methuen, London.   [56]

Creighton, C. (1894). *A History of Epidemics in Britain*, Vol. One: A.D. 664–1666, and Vol. Two: A.D. 1666–1893. Cambridge University Press, Cambridge. (Reprinted 1965, Frank Cass & Co., London.)   [1]

Daley, D. J. (1967a). Concerning the spread of news in a population of individuals who never forget. *Bull. Math. Biophys.* **29**, 373–376.   [40]

Daley, D. J. (1967b). *Some Aspects of Markov Chains in Queueing Theory and Epidemiology*, Ph.D. thesis, University of Cambridge.   [43]

Daley, D. J. (1990). The size of epidemics with variable infectious periods. Technical Report SMS-012-90, Statistics Research Section, School of Mathematical Sciences, Australian National University.   [125]

Daley, D. J. and Gani, J. (1994). A deterministic general epidemic model in a stratified population. In *Probability, Statistics and Optimisation: A Tribute to Peter Whittle* (F. P. Kelly, Ed.), John Wiley, Chichester, 117–132.   [17, 37, 103]

Daley, D. J. and Gani, J. (1999). Models for the spread of infection via pairing at parties. In *Advances in Applied Probability and Stochastic Processes: Festschrift for Julian Keilson* (G. Shantikumar and U. Sumita, Eds), Kluwer: Boston. (95–113).   [105, 126, 186]

Daley, D. J., Gani, J. and Yakowitz, S. (1999). An epidemic with individual infectivities and susceptibilities. *Math. Computer Modelling* (155–167).   [63, 174]

Daley, D. J. and Kendall, D. G. (1964). Epidemics and rumours. *Nature* **204**, 1118.   [133]

Daley, D. J. and Kendall, D. G. (1965). Stochastic rumours. *J. Inst. Math. Applns.* **1**, 42–55.   [84–85, 133, 135–137, 139, 141–146, 149–153]

Daniels, H. E. (1967). The distribution of the total size of an epidemic. *Proc. Fifth Berkeley Symp. Math. Statist. Probab.* **4**, 281–293. University of California Press, Berkeley.   [84]

Darroch, J. N. and Seneta, E. (1965). On quasi-stationary distributions in absorbing discrete-time finite Markov chains. *J. Appl. Probab.* **2**, 88–100.   [122]

de Hoog, F., Gani, J. and Gates, D. (1979). A threshold theorem for the general epidemic in discrete time. *J. Math. Biol.* **8**, 113–121.   [52]

Diekmann, O., Heesterbeek, J. A. P. and Metz, J. A. J. (1990). On the definition and the computation of the basic reproduction ratio R_0 in models for infectious diseases in heterogeneous populations. *J. Math. Biol.* **28**, 365–382.   [89]

Dietz, K. (1981). The evaluation of rubella vaccination strategies. In *The Mathematical Theory of the Dynamics of Biological Populations II*, R. W. Hiorns & D. Cooke (Eds), Academic Press, London, 81–97.   [179]

Dietz, K. (1988). The first epidemic model: a historical note on P. D. En'ko. *Australian J. Statist.* **30A**, 56–65.   [11, 55]

Dietz, K. and Schenzle, D. (1985). Mathematical models for infectious disease statistics. In *A Celebration of Statistics*, A. C. Atkinson and S. E. Fienberg (Eds), Springer-Verlag, New York, 167–204.   [13, 165]

Dietz, K. *See also* Becker and Dietz; Jewell, Dietz and Farewell.

Dobson, A. J. *See* Whyte *et al.*

Dubois-Arber, F. *See* Hausser *et al.*

Dunstan, R. (1982). The rumour process. *J. Appl. Probab.* **19**, 759–766.   [43]

En'ko, P. D. (1889). On the course of epidemics of some infectious diseases. *Vrach. St. Petersburg.* **X**, 1008–1010, 1039–1042, 1061–1063. [Translated by K. Dietz, *Internat. J. Epidemiology* **18** (1989), 749–755.]   [1, 17–18, 55, 105, 113, 154, 174]

Ermakov, V. V. *See* Baroyan, Rvachev, Basilevsky *et al.*

Falck, R. *See* Siegal *et al.*

Farewell, V. T. *See* Jewell, Dietz and Farewell.

Farr, W. (1840). Progress of epidemics. In *Second Annual Report of the Registrar-General of Births, Deaths and Marriages in England*, 91–98.   [7–8, 175]

Feller, W. (1957). *An Introduction to Probability Theory and its Applications*, Vol. 1, 2nd Edn. John Wiley and Sons, New York. (1st Edn, 1950; 3rd Edn, 1968).   [133]

Fenner, F., Henderson, D. A., Arita, I., Jažek, Z. and Ladnyi, I. D. (1988). *Smallpox and its Eradication*. WHO, Geneva.   [1, 179]

Flannery, B. P. *See* Press *et al.*

Foster, F. G. (1955). A note on Bailey's and Whittle's treatment of a general stochastic epidemic. *Biometrika* **42**, 123–125.   [77]

Frank, K. D. *See* Baroyan, Rvachev, Basilevsky *et al.*

Franks, Z. *See* Stuart-Harris, Franks and Tyrrell

Freeman, E. B. *See* Solomon *et al.*

Gail, M. H. *See* Brookmeyer and Gail.

Gani, J. (1965). On a partial differential equation of epidemic theory, I. *Biometrika* **52**, 613–616.   [67]

Gani, J. (1967). On the general stochastic epidemic. *Proc. Fifth Berkeley Symp. Math. Statist. Probab.* **4**, 271–279. University of California Press, Berkeley.   [67, 71]

Gani, J. (1978). Some problems of epidemic theory (with Discussion). *J. Roy. Statist. Soc. Ser. A* **141**, 323–347.   [4, 48]

Gani, J. (1991). A note on a stochastic model for the incubation of transfusion associated AIDS. *Discrete Maths.* **92**, 89–94.   [172]

Gani, J. and Jerwood, D. (1971). Markov chain methods in chain binomial epidemic models. *Biometrics* **27**, 591–603.   [105]

Gani, J. and Mansouri, H. (1987). Fitting chain binomial models to the common cold. *Math. Scientist* **12**, 31–37.   [117–118, 165, 167]

Gani, J. and Yakowitz, S. (1993). Modelling the spread of HIV among intravenous drug users. *IMA J. Maths. Appl. Med. Biology* **10**, 51–65.   [118, 122]

Gani, J., Yakowitz, S. and Blount, M. (1997). The spread and quarantine of HIV infection in a prison system. *SIAM J. Appl. Math.* **57**, 1510–1530.   [185, 189, 191]

Gani, J. *See also* Daley and Gani; Daley, Gani and Yakowitz; Yakowitz, Gani and Blount; de Hoog, Gani and Gates.

Gart, J. J. (1968). The mathematical analysis of an epidemic with two kinds of susceptibles. *Biometrics* **24**, 557–566.   [53]

Gart, J. J. (1972). The statistical analysis of chain-binomial epidemic models with several kinds of susceptibles. *Biometrics* **28**, 921–930.   [53]

Gates, D. *See* de Hoog, Gani and Gates.

Giesecke, J. (1994). *Modern Infectious Disease Epidemiology*. Edward Arnold, London.   [87]

Glasstone, S. (1948). *Textbook of Physical Chemistry* (2nd Edn). Macmillan, London.   [6]

Goffman, W. (1965). An epidemic process in an open population. *Nature*, **205**, 831–832.   [136]

Goffman, W. and Newill, V. A. (1964). Generalization of epidemic theory—an application to the transmission of ideas. *Nature* **204**, 225–228.   [136]

Goffman, W. and Newill, V. A. (1967). Communication and epidemic processes. *Proc. Roy. Soc. Ser. A* **298**, 316–334.   [136]

Gold, J. *See* Whyte *et al.*

Graunt, John (1662). *Natural and Political Observations Made Upon the Bills of Mortality*. John Martin, London. [Reprinted in facsimile in *The Earliest Classics: John Graunt and Gregory King* (1973), Gregg International Publishers, Farnborough.]   [1–3, 6]

Greenwood, M. (1931). On the statistical measure of infectiousness. *J. Hyg. Cambridge* **31**, 336–351.   [105–119, 162–164]

Greenwood, M. (1949). The infectiousness of measles. *Biometrika* **36**, 1–8.   [165, 168]

Gutzwiller, F. *See* Hausser *et al.*

Hall, D. *See* Brewer *et al.*

Halley, E. (1693). An Estimate of the Degrees of the Mortality of Mankind, drawn from curious Tables of the Births and Funerals at the City of Breslaw; with an Attempt to ascertain the Price of Annuities upon Lives. *Phil. Trans. Roy. Soc. Lond.* **17**, No.196, 596–610.   [4–6]

Hamer, W. H. (1906). The Milroy Lectures on Epidemic disease in England— the evidence of variability and persistency of type. Lecture III *Lancet* **1**, 733–739.   [8–9. 29]

Hausser, D., Lehmann, P., Dubois-Arber, F. and Gutzwiller, F. (1988). Effectiveness of the AIDS prevention campaigns in Switzerland. In *The Global Impact of AIDS*, A. F. Fleming, M. Carballo, D. W. FitzSimmons, M. R. Bailey & J. Mann (Eds.), Alan R. Liss Inc., New York, 219–228.   [177]

Haverkos, H. W. *See* Lui, Lawrence *et al.*

Heasman, M. A. and Reid, D. D. (1961). Theory and observation in family epidemics of the common cold. *Brit. J. Prevent. Soc. Med.* **15**, 12–16. [164–165]

Heesterbeek, J. A. P. *See* Diekmann, Heesterbeek and Metz.

Henderson, D. A. *See* Fenner *et al.*

Hethcote, H. W. (1994). A thousand and one epidemic models. In *Lecture Notes in Biomathematics* **100**, 504–515.   [13, 56]

Hoppensteadt, F. *See* Waltman and Hoppensteadt.

Hsieh, Y.-H. (1991). Modelling the effects of screening in HIV transmission dynamics. In *Differential Equations Models in Biology, Epidemiology and Ecology*, S. Busenberg & M. Martelli (Eds), Lecture Notes in Biomathematics **92**, Springer-Verlag, Berlin, 99–120. [185]

Hudson, H. P. *See* Ross and Hudson.

Isham, V. and Medley, G. (Eds) (1996). *Models for Infectious Human Diseases: Their Structure and Relation to Data.* Cambridge University Press: Cambridge. [xii, 16]

Ivannikov, Yu. G. *See* Baroyan, Rvachev and Ivannikov.

Jažek, Z. *See* Fenner *et al.*

Jerwood, D. *See* Gani and Jerwood.

Jewell, N. P., Dietz, K. and Farewell, V. T. (Eds.) (1992). *AIDS Epidemiology: Methodological Issues.* Birkhäuser, Boston. [170]

Kaplan, E. H. (1995). Probability models of needle exchange. *Oper. Res.* **43**, 558–564. [179]

Karlin, S. and Taylor, H. M. (1975). *A First Course in Stochastic Processes* (2nd Edn). Academic Press, New York. [56]

Karlin, S. and Taylor, H. M. (1984). *An Introduction to Stochastic Models.* Academic Press, New York. [56]

Kendall, D. G. (1948). On the generalized "birth-and-death" process. *Ann. Math. Statist.* **19**, 1–15. [99]

Kendall, D. G. (1956). Deterministic and stochastic epidemics in closed populations. *Proc. Third Berkeley Symp. Math. Statist. Probab.* **4**, 149–165. University of California Press, Berkeley. [31–32]

Kendall, D. G. (1957). La propagation d'une épidémie ou d'un bruit dans une population limitée. *Publ. Inst. Statist. Univ. Paris* **6**, 307–311. [62, 101, 133]

Kendall, D. G. *See also* Daley and Kendall.

Kermack, W. O. and McKendrick, A. G. (1927). A contribution to the mathematical theory of epidemics. *Proc. Roy. Soc. Lond.* A **115**, 700–721. [9–11, 13, 28–29, 37–38, 52, 73, 105, 112, 123–124, 155, 175–176]

Knox, E. G. (1980). Strategy for rubella vaccination. *Inter. J. Epidemiology* **9**, 13–23. [179]

Ladnyi, I. *See* Fenner *et al.*

Langston, D. *See* Blumberg and Langston.

Lawless, J. and Sun, J. (1992). A comprehensive back-calculation framework for the estimation and prediction of AIDS cases. In Jewell, Dietz & Farewell (1992), 81–104. [170]

Lawrence, D. N. *See* Lui, Lawrence *et al.*; Lui, Peterman, *et al.*

Lehmann, P. *See* Hausser *et al.*

Lefèvre, C. and Picard, P. (1994). Distribution of the final extent of a rumour process. *J. Appl. Probab.* **31**, 244–249. [145]

Lui, K.-J., Lawrence, D. N., Morgan, W. M., Peterman, T. A., Haverkos, H. W. and Bregman, D. J. (1986). A model-based approach for estimating the mean incubation period of transfusion-associated acquired immunodeficiency syndrome. *Proc. Nat. Acad. Sci. USA* **83**, 3051–3055. [169]

Lui, K-J., Peterman, T. A., Lawrence, D. N. and Allen, J. R. (1988). A model-based approach to characterize the incubation period of paediatric transfusion-associated acquired immunodeficiency syndrome. *Statist. Med.* **7**, 395–401. [169–170, 172]

Macdonald, G. (1952). The analysis of equilibrium in malaria. *Trop. Dis. Bull.* **49**, 813–829. [Reprinted in Macdonald (1973), 131–145.]   [47]

Macdonald, G. (1965). On the scientific basis of tropical hygiene. *Trans. Roy. Soc. Tropical Med. Hyg.* **59**, 611–620. [Reprinted in Macdonald (1973), 18–27.] [175]

Macdonald, G. (1973). *Dynamics of Tropical Disease* (Selected papers of the late George Macdonald, L. J. Bruce-Chwatt and V. J. Glanville (Eds.)). Oxford University Press, London.   [46]

McKendrick, A. G. (1926). Applications of mathematics to medical problems. *Proc. Edinburgh Math. Soc.* **14**, 98–130.   [11]

McKendrick, A. G. *See also* Kermack and McKendrick.

McNamee, R. *See* Cane and McNamee.

Mansouri, H. *See* Gani and Mansouri.

Maki, D. P. and Thompson, M. (1973). *Mathematical Models and Applications.* Prentice–Hall, Englewood Cliffs NJ.   [135, 140, 142–144, 149–151, 153]

Mautner, A. J. *See* Rushton and Mautner.

May, R. M. *See* Anderson and May.

Medley, G. F. *See* Anderson and Medley; Isham and Medley.

Metz, J. A. J. *See* Diekmann, Heesterbeek and Metz.

Miller, H. T. *See* Cox and Miller.

Miner, J. R. (1933). Pierre-François Verhulst (1804–49), the discoverer of the logistic curve. *Hum. Biol.* **5**, 673 689.   [2]

Moerings, M. *See* Thomas and Moerings

Mollison, D. (Ed.) (1995). *Epidemic Models: Their Structure and Relation to Data.* Cambridge University Press: Cambridge.   [xii, 16]

Mollison, D. *See also* Ball, Mollison and Scalia-Tomba.

Morgan, W. M. *See* Lui, Lawrence *et al.*

Munoz, A. *See* Brewer *et al.*

Nagaev, A. V. (1971). Asymptotic methods for problems in the mathematical theory of epidemics. *Adv. Appl. Probab.* **3**, 222–223.   [85]

Nagaev, A. V. and Startsev, A. N. (1970). The asymptotic analysis of a stochastic model of an epidemic. *Teor. Veroyat. Primen.* **15**, 97–105 (transl. *Theory Probab. Appl.* **15**, 98–107).   [85]

Newill, V. A. *See* Goffman and Newill.

Ney, P. E. *See* Athreya and Ney.

O'Neill, P. (1995). Epidemic models featuring behaviour change. *Adv. Appl. Probab.* **27**, 960–979.   [179]

Pearce, C. E. M. (2000). The exact solution of the general stochastic rumour. *Math. Computer Modelling* **31**, 289–298.   [150]

Perlin, T. *See* Siegal *et al.*

Peterman, T. A. *See* Lui, Lawrence *et al.*: Lui, Peterman *et al.*

Picard, P. *See* Lefèvre and Picard.

Pittel, B. (1990). On a Daley–Kendall model of random rumours. *J. Appl. Probab.* **27**, 14–27.   [141, 144–145]

Polk, F. *See* Brewer *et al.*

Press, W. H., Flannery, B. P., Teukolsky, S. A. and Vetterling, W. T. (1987). *Numerical Recipes: The Art of Scientific Computing.* Cambridge University Press, Cambridge.   [184]

Puri, P. S. (1975). A linear birth and death process under the influence of another process. *J. Appl. Probab.* **12**, 1–17.   [95, 99–100]

Razzell, P. (1977). *The Conquest of Smallpox: The Impact of Inoculation on Smallpox Mortality in Eighteenth Century Britain.* Caliban Books: Firle, Sussex BN8 6NY.   [1]

Reece, R. D. *See* Siegal *et al.*

Reid, D. D. *See* Heasman and Reid.

Reinert, G. (1995). The asymptotic evolution of the general stochastic epidemic. *Ann. Appl. Probab.* **5**, 1061–1086.   [85]

Ross, R. (1916). An application of the theory of probabilities to the study of *a priori* pathometry, I. *Proc. Roy. Soc. Lond.* A **92**, 204–230.   [9, 46–47, 175]

Ross, R. and Hudson, H. P. (1917). An application of the theory of probabilities to the study of *a priori* pathometry, II; III. *Proc. Roy. Soc. Lond.* A **93**, 212–225; 225–240. [Reprinted together with Ross (1916) as Ross and Hudson (1931), *A priori pathometry*, Harrison: London.]   [9, 46]

Ross, S. M. (1983). *Stochastic Processes*, John Wiley, New York.   [57]

Rossi, C. (1991). A stochastic mover/stayer model for an HIV epidemic. *Math. Biosciences* **107**, 1–25.   [172]

Rushton, S. and Mautner, A. J. (1955). The deterministic model of a simple epidemic for more than one community. *Biometrika* **42**, 126–132.   [23]

Rvachev, L. A. *See* Baroyan and Rvachev; Baroyan, Rvachev and Ivannikov; Baroyan, Rvachev, Basilevsky *et al.*

Rvachev, M. A. *See* Baroyan, Rvachev, Basilevsky *et al.*

Sakino, S. (1968). On the solution of the epidemic equation. *Ann. Inst. Statist. Math. Suppl.* **V**, 9–19.   [67]

Saunders, I. W. (1980). A model for myxomatosis. *Math. Biosciences* **45**, 1–15.   [50, 52, 154]

Scalia-Tomba, G. *See* Ball, Mollison and Scalia-Tomba.

Schenzle, D. (1982). Problems in drawing epidemiological inferences by fitting epidemic chain models to lumped data. *Biometrics* **38**, 843–847.   [165–168]

Schenzle, D. *See also* Dietz and Schenzle.

Sellke, T. (1983). On the asymptotic distribution of the size of the stochastic epidemic. *J. Appl. Probab.* **20**, 390–394.   [84]

Seneta, E. (1981). *Non-negative Matrices and Markov Chains* (2nd Edn). Springer-Verlag, New York.   [103, 123]

Seneta, E. *See also* Darroch and Seneta.

Shashkov, V. A. *See* Baroyan, Rvachev, Basilevsky *et al.*

Siegal, H. A., Carlson, R. G., Falck, R., Reece, R. D. and Perlin, T. (1993). Conducting HIV outreach and research among incarcerated drug abusers. *J. Substance Abuse Treatment* **10**, 71–75.   [185]

Siskind, V. (1965). A solution of the general stochastic epidemic. *Biometrika* **52**, 613–616.   [67]

Smith, C. E. Gordon (1964). Factors in the transmission of virus infections from animals to man. In *The Scientific Basis of Medicine Annual Reviews 1964*, London, Athlone Press, 125–150.   [180]

Solomon, P. J., Attewell, R. G., Freeman, E. B. and Wilson, S. R. (1991). *AIDS in Australia: reconstructing the epidemic from 1980 to 1990 and predicting future trends in HIV disease*. National Centre for Epidemiology and Public Health Working Paper **29**, Australian National University, Canberra.   [170, 172–173]

Soper, H. E. (1929). The interpretation of periodicity in disease prevalence. *J. Roy. Statist. Soc.* **92**, 34–73.   [11]

Spicer, C. C. (1979). The mathematical modelling of influenza epidemics. *Brit. Med. Bull.* **35**, 23–28.   [49–50, 155–157]

Spitzer, F. (1964). *Principles of Random Walk*. Van Nostrand, Princeton. (2nd Edn, 1976, Springer-Verlag, New York.)   [125]

Startsev, A. N. *See* Nagaev and Startsev.

Stevens, S. (1993). HIV prevention programs in a jail setting: educational strategies. *The Prison J.* **73**, 379–390.   [185]

Stuart-Harris, C. H., Franks, Z. and Tyrrell, D. (1950). Deaths from influenza—a statistical and laboratory investigation. *Brit. Med. J.* **1950, I**, 263–266. [157]

Sudbury, A. (1985). The proportion of the population never hearing a rumour. *J. Appl. Probab.* **22**, 443–446.   [145]

Sun, J. *See* Lawless and Sun.

Taylor, E. *See* Brewer *et al.*

Taylor, H. M. *See* Karlin and Taylor.

Teukolsky, S. A. *See* Press *et al.*

Thomas, P. A. and Moerings, M. (Eds.) (1994). *AIDS in Prison*. Dartmouth: Aldershot, Hants.   [185]

Thompson, M. *See* Maki and Thompson.

Todorovic, P. (1992). *An Introduction to Stochastic Processes and Their Applications*. Springer-Verlag, New York.   [79]

Tyrrell, D. *See* Stuart-Harris, Franks and Tyrrell.

US Department of Justice (1993). *1992 Update: HIV/AIDS in Correctional Facilities*. US Department of Justice, Washington DC.   [185]

Verhulst, P.-F. (1838). Notice sur la loi que la population suit dans son accroissement. *Corr. Math. Phys. (Bruxelles)* (publ. par A. Quételet) **10**, 113–121. [20]

Vetterling, W. T. *See* Press *et al.*

Vlahov, D. *See* Brewer *et al.*

Waltman, P. and Hoppensteadt, F. (1970). A problem in the theory of epidemics, I. *Math. Biosciences* **9**, 71–91.   [56]

Waltman, P. and Hoppensteadt, F. (1971). A problem in the theory of epidemics, II. *Math. Biosciences* **12**, 133–145.   [56]

Watson, G. N. *See* Whittaker and Watson.

Watson, R. K. (1972). On an epidemic in a stratified population. *J. Appl. Probab.* **9**, 659–666.   [37]

Watson, R. (1988). On the size of a rumour. *Stoch. Proc. Appl.* **27**, 141–149. [136, 144–145]

Waugh, W. A. O'N. (1958). Conditioned Markov processes. *Biometrika* **45**, 241–249.   [102]

White, D. O. *See* Burnet and White.

Whittaker, E. T. and Watson, G. N. (1927). *A Course of Modern Analysis* (4th Edn). Cambridge University Press, Cambridge.   [63]

Whittle, P. (1955). The outcome of a stochastic epidemic—a note on Bailey's paper. *Biometrika* **42**, 116–122.   [74, 76, 83, 86–87]

Whyte, B. M., Gold, J., Dobson, A. J. and Cooper, D. A. (1987). Epidemiology of acquired immunodeficiency syndrome in Australia. *Med. J. Australia* **146**, 65–69.   [158]

Williams, T. (1965). The simple stochastic epidemic curve for large populations of susceptibles. *Biometrika* **52**, 571–579.   [58]

Williams, T. (1971). An algebraic proof of the threshold theorem for the general stochastic epidemic. *Adv. Appl. Probab.* **3**, 223.   [77]

Wilson, E. B., Bennett, C., Allen, M. and Worcester, J. (1939). Measles and scarlet fever in Providence, R. I. 1929–1934 with respect to age and size of family. *Proc. Amer. Phil. Soc.* **80**, 357–476.   [14, 162]

Wilson, E. B. and Burke, M. H. (1942). The epidemic curve. *Proc. Nat. Acad. Sci., Washington*, **28**, 361–367.   [11]

Wilson, E. B. and Burke, M. H. (1943). The epidemic curve, II. *Proc. Nat. Acad. Sci., Washington*, **29**, 43–48.   [11, 19, 33, 154]

Wilson, S. R. (1989). Extrapolation forecasting. In *Predicting the Course of AIDS in Australia and Evaluating the Effect of AZT: A First Report*, by Solomon, P. J., Doust, J. A. and Wilson, S. R., National Centre for Epidemiology and Public Health, Working Paper **3**, Australian National University, Canberra, 33–41.   [158–159]

Wilson, S. R. *See also* Solomon *et al.*

Worcester, J. *See* Wilson *et al.*

Yakowitz, S., Gani, J. and Blount, M. (1996). Computing marginal expectations for large compartmentalized models, with application to AIDS evolution in a prison system. *IMA J. Maths. Appl. Med. Biology* **13**, 223–244.   [185]

Yakowitz, S. *See also* Daley, Gani and Yakowitz; Gani and Yakowitz; Gani, Yakowitz and Blount.

Subject Index

Winners' Competition Series, Volume 3

~ ~ ~

Award-winning 60-Second Comic Monologues Ages 13 to 18

A Smith and Kraus Book
Published by Smith and Kraus, Inc.
177 Lyme Road, Hanover, NH 03755
www.smithandkraus.com

First Edition: October 2008
Manufactured in the United States of America
10 9 8 7 6 5 4 3 2 1

Book production by Julia Gignoux, Freedom Hill Design
Text design by Kate Mueller, Electric Dragon Productions
Cover design by Alex Karan, www.alexkarancreative.com
Cover photo by Alex Karan, featuring Elizabeth Cheney

ISBN-13: 978-1-57525-614-6 / ISBN-10 1-57525-614-2
Library of Congress Control Number: 2008935717

WINNERS' COMPETITION SERIES, VOLUME 3

Award~winning 60~Second Comic Monologues

Ages 13 to 18

~ ~ ~

JANET B. MILSTEIN

YOUNG ACTORS SERIES

A Smith and Kraus Book

CONTENTS

FEMALE MONOLOGUES

MALE MONOLOGUES

ACKNOWLEDGMENTS

The monologue workshop and this resulting book would not have been possible were it not for the unflinching support, unfathomable generosity, endless creativity, and invaluable advice of Eric Kraus. He is one of the kindest people I have ever met, and the fact that he not only will offer me guidance and suggestions, but will listen and consider mine (and other authors) as well, makes him even more amazing and ultimately adds to the success of Smith and Kraus. Of course, it is no surprise that Marisa Smith is just as generous, creative, supportive, and wise. Thank you both for everything. I would also like to thank the following people for their support, hard work, assistance, and belief in me:

Everyone at Smith and Kraus
Everyone at JRP Atlanta
Karen "Kovy" Milstein
Alex Karan
Julia Gignoux
The Howells
Amethyst Milstein
Shemetra Carter
Barbara Lhota
Ellen Crabill
Chadwick Ford
Kate Mueller
Margaret Milstein
Natalie "Novy" Milstein
Donald Milstein
John "Tom" Miller

Karen Milstein
Joshua Milstein
Kathyrn Milstein
Melissa Milstein
Freda Milstein
Soledad Milstein
Jennifer MacLeod
Erin Mary
Jane Hoffman
Birgit Neuhaus
Ann Cheney
Cindy Cheney
Elizabeth Cheney
Carol Garner
Cody

ACKNOWLEDGMENTS OF
WORKSHOP PARTICIPANTS

I would like to thank each and every student who participated in the monologue workshops. It was wonderful getting to know all of you and going through this exciting new process with you! I want to thank you all for trusting me and sharing your experiences, ideas, and desires with me. The monologues in this book would not exist without you because all of you were the inspiration. You guys rock!

Taylor Adkins

(Britni) Chole' Arrington

Alejandro Avina

Tu Cam Bach

Heather Bailey

Bryant Baptiste

Erin Barnes

Karli Barnett

Sarah Bell

Keely Bilthouse

Krystin Bitoy

David Boughton

Brittany Braswell

Drew Carlos

Seth Cartledge

Kathryn Caswell

Joshua Cliatt

Tyreece Cole

Cassie Cope

Mark Couch

Kimberly Coulton

Raven Cox

Juliana Daniell

Victoria Diaz

Meredith Doody

Greyson Dover

Tiffany Dunlap

(Brian) Keith Durham

Brooke Edwards

Emily Ellis

Kristen Feyt

Lauren Fishman

Chelsea Ryan Fletcher

Chakier Francis

Claire Fredericks

Amanda Freeman

Dillon Greene

Brianna Groves

Beatrice Harrod

Kaelyn Hawley

Anna Hou

Marlon Hulett

Celeste Iglesias

Tamara Jelici

Jade Jones

Copelyn Jue

Thomas Justusson

Ruth Kahsay

Divya Kannegenti

Kelly Kay

Young Kim
Diana Lam
Katie Lawhorne
Angela Lee
Kyle Lewis
A'Olyian Lindsey
Olivia Lodise
Courtney Lowery
Rachel McDonal
Carleigh McLerran
Louie Medick
Megan Megahee
Mackenzie Moody
Nikeia Moore
Nahla Muhammad
Jenna Newstrom
Diana Nguyen
Kathy Nguyen
Destiny Nickelsen
Alexandria Ogletree
Sevana Ohanian
Ezinne Okpareke
Amanda Olewicz
Andrew Olewicz
Jessica Palmer
Nicole Parry
Alexis Phillips

Taylor Pullen
Bianca Reyes
Bethany Rountree
Deja Rush
Karen Ryan
Rachel Sale
Naomi Sharma
Taylor Shope
Cameron Singleton
Austin Smith
Samantha Solomon
Anna Stabler
Albert Stephenson
Joshua Stephenson
Trish Strain
Shatnee Thomas
Levi Thompson
Darby Walker
Shenell Watts
Silken Weinberg
Brandon White
Georgia White
Heather White
Jewel Wilcox
Roddas Workneh
Tempest Young

Introduction

In one long week and a half that spanned late January to early February, I was hospitalized, had gall bladder surgery, was diagnosed with sarcoidosis, totaled my car, and celebrated my birthday in the hospital. Then I was housebound for a month to recover (thus, unable to work). There's nothing like a frightening health incident to make you reevaluate your priorities. I am blessed to have such a wonderful family and friends.

During my recovery, I thought about what I really wanted to do, what would be realistic given my condition, and how I'd make money. My three main creative passions—acting, teaching acting, and writing—whirled around in my mind. It would probably be a while before I'd be healthy enough to perform in a show. Writing seemed to make the most sense, but after so much time spent at home alone, I was craving a social setting.

I thought about the times I most enjoyed writing, and they were usually when I was writing for my students. I wanted to write for students again, but where and how? I had taught intensive weekend workshops for students who were going to compete at acting conventions, such as iPOP! (International Presentation of Performers) and IMTA (International Model and Talent Association) in New York and Los Angeles. In fact, my first two monologue books were written primarily for such students. Perhaps I could design a longer monologue class to help students prepare for auditions.

I decided to call Dale Howell, owner of John Robert Powers (JRP), Atlanta (where I'd been hired several times for training). Fortunately, he was interested in my idea of offering his students a special monthlong monologue class, but the objective and end result were still a bit unclear.

So I called Eric Kraus. When in doubt, call Eric Kraus. We threw ideas around and decided that I should go to Atlanta and write monologues for the students. They'd inspire my writing, I'd provide them with personalized monologues, and the whole experience would culminate in a book with the participating students thanked within. Smith and Kraus would publish the monologue book, and hopefully it would lead to a great new series. Dale liked the idea and decided to offer the workshop to his new group of iPOP! students. It seemed we'd created a win-win situation for everyone involved: the students, the school, Smith and Kraus, and myself.

The undertaking was huge, exciting, scary, and coming up fast. I'd have to do a lot of teaching, learning about the students, writing, and editing in a short amount of time—one month.

Off to Atlanta I went.

It was great meeting and getting to know the students I'd be working with over the next month. Class time was limited, so I had to quickly find out about each person's interests, likes, dislikes, personality, and style of speech. From games to questionnaires to one-on-one exchanges, I gathered enough information to sit down and write their monologues.

This process was more difficult than I anticipated due to the short time we had to work together, balancing writing time with teaching time and the time it later took me to hear, time, and cut the monologues with the students. To make it more challenging, the students were all in different steps of the process. Some students had received the monologues I had written for them, and we had timed and edited them; other monologues needed to be heard and cut. While several students were waiting for me to finish writing their monologues, a number of students had not gotten to discuss ideas. And last, there were a few I had not even met yet! Somehow within this unusually hectic environment, I managed to get everyone's monologue completed.

It's amazing how quickly a month can go by. I would've loved another week to just work the pieces. However, I did manage to schedule a long evening at the end of the month to work each monologue, give final notes and time, and discuss how the acting competitions at iPOP! would work. This proved to be

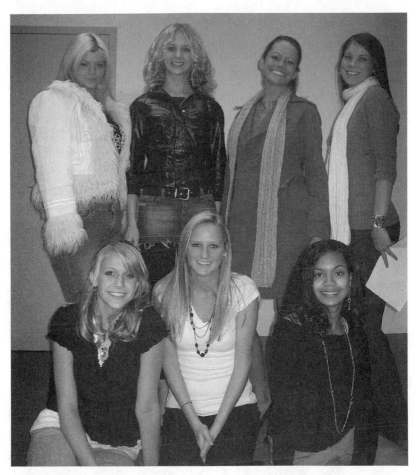

Acting class.

very valuable (as I was told by the students and parents), and it was fun presenting the results of our hard, monthlong work to the parents and JRP staff.

As usual, ending is always sad due to the wonderful bonds and friendships formed. I wanted to stay and coach them all the way through iPOP! Ahhh, letting go.

I told the students that they could write a brief essay or letter about their experience, and I'd select a handful or two to include in the published book (please see the essays on page 75).

I returned to Chicago and wondered if I had done my best. About two months later, I got a call from Dale. The students had done fantastically well—they all received awards, callbacks, or both. In addition, they swept the monologue awards and wound up winning School of the Year! This was far beyond the results I was hoping for. The workshop had turned out to be unbelievably successful, and I couldn't have been happier. I was so proud of the students—all of our hard work (including the JRP staff) had paid off. In this book, you'll find the award-winning monologues created for this talented group of students.

Eric Kraus and I have decided to turn this experience—this living, breathing thing—into a new monologue workshop and book series! I've made some improvements to the process, and I'm looking forw a rd to visiting more schools and working with new acting students. Please see page 89 for information about holding a workshop at your school.

Looking back, I realize what a unique and exciting experience this has been. I can't wait to do it again!

—*Janet B. Milstein*

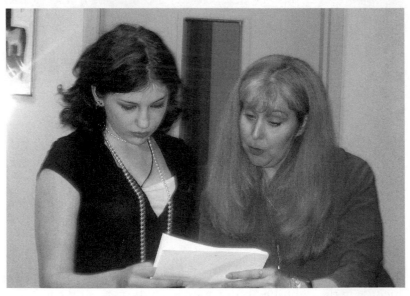

Janet works with Destiny Nickelsen on her monologue.

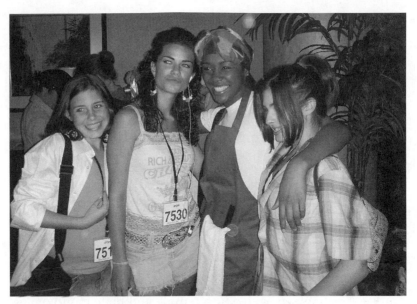

Students pose before going to compete.

P.S. I went back to JRP Atlanta in the fall to do another month-long monologue workshop with a new, even larger group of iPOP! students. It was a pleasure getting to know all the students and crafting personalized monologues for them. You will find both groups' monologues in this book and *Winners' Competition Series, Volume 1: Award-winning 60-Second Comic Monologues, Ages 4 to 12.*

Tips on Using This Book and Choosing a Monologue

When writing and organizing this book, I tried to make it as easy to use as possible. Here's what you should know:

- The monologues in this book are original and self-contained—they are not from plays.

- All the monologues are comedic.

- The monologues are one minute and under—perfect for most auditions.

- The book is divided into female and male monologues.

- The book contains more female than male monologues to better meet the needs of acting teachers and students.

- The pieces were written for teens aged thirteen to eighteen.

- Age ranges are not indicated for the monologues since teens mature at a varied pace and often look older or younger than they actually are.

- For easier searching, the monologues are arranged in each section from youngest to oldest.

- A brief description of the situation precedes each monologue and quickly sets the scene.

When choosing a monologue, consider your age range, personality, the nature and language of the piece, and the audition situation. For example, a monologue that mentions going to the prom or driving would not be believable if performed by a twelve-year-old. Sometimes a piece simply sounds too young or old for the person who's performing it. Choosing a character that you could realistically be cast as will increase your audi-

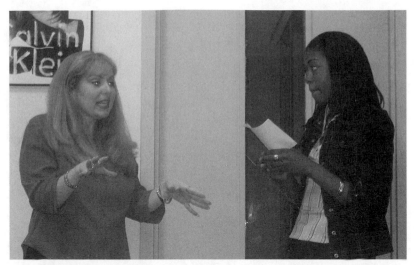

Janet challenges Shenell Watts to go further with her monologue.

tioning success. Use your best judgment and ask your acting teacher or coach if you need help.

Also, pick a monologue that you like! I can't tell you how many times I ask students, "Do you like this monologue?" and they say "not really." "Why are you doing it then?" I ask. "My mom (or teacher) picked it for me" or "I couldn't find any I liked," they respond. If your mother, father, teacher, or best friend want to help you pick a monologue, great, but it is still your responsibility to choose a piece you like. After all, you're the one who will spend a lot of time working on it and auditioning with it. So, regardless of what others recommend, remember it is your job to pick your monologue. Since you get to choose, pick a piece that excites you—one that makes you laugh or think "I can totally relate to this!" If you're not having fun performing it, chances are the people auditioning you are not having fun watching it. If you *are* having fun, they will be enjoying it much more.

Pick your monologue(s) far in advance of your upcoming auditions. It can sometimes take a lot of searching before you find a monologue you really like, but the benefits of finding that perfect piece more than make up for the time spent searching

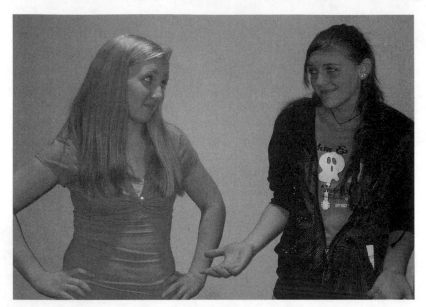

Jenna Newstrom and Heather White improvise a scene.

for it. Also realize that choosing a monologue that fits you well, and working and memorizing the piece all take time. If you wait until the last minute, you will not be adequately prepared. Unlike cold readings, monologues give you the chance to show what you're capable of when you have time to prepare a piece. So, don't make excuses, don't expect your parents or acting teacher to find your monologue, and don't put it off until the last minute—start looking today!

The monologues in this book are one minute and under. You may encounter auditions that ask for two-minute monologues, two monologues to be performed in three minutes, or one-minute monologues. You can always go under the time limit—leave them wanting more! However, it is not professional to run overtime. In some cases you may even be timed. Therefore, it is best to keep your monologue at least ten seconds shorter than the allotted time. Also, keep in mind when you are reading and timing your monologue(s) that performing time will run longer than reading time. So, to get a more accurate assessment, time your monologue while performing it, not just reading it.

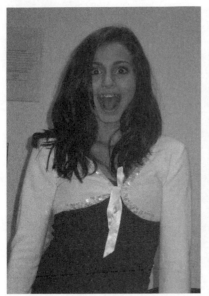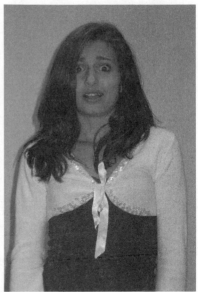

Listening exercise: left, marvelous surprise; right, disgusting surprise.

You will see *(Beat)* in many of the monologues. A beat is a pause and is usually included to indicate that the "invisible other character" is speaking. However, a beat is occasionally taken simply because the character paused. Either way, it is the actor's job to decide what happened during each beat and to keep those moments alive. Since the lines of the other person are not given, you must figure out exactly what he or she said to you. Be a detective and examine the lines surrounding each beat for clues. Then choose specific lines or physical actions for the "invisible other person." Do this for each beat in your monologue. Make strong, clear choices that will definitely cause you to respond in a manner that makes logical sense with the text and the circumstances. Write these lines or actions on your monologue in pencil for each beat. Imagine the other person saying and doing the lines and actions you chose each time you rehearse your monologue. This will help you to stay connected to your invisible partner and make your performance at auditions much more genuine, powerful, and successful!

Female Monologues

In order of age,
younger to older

An Awkward Attempt

Erin has a major crush on Angelo, a cute Greek boy who goes to her church. Erin is extremely shy around him and finally musters up the courage to try to tell him how she feels.

Hey Angelo, I was wondering . . . um, maybe if you . . . I think you know . . . or maybe notice that I . . . always sit closer and closer to you on the pew each Sunday? And so I was wondering . . . ya know, I always wanted to be your, um, when everyone's doing the Greek dances that, uh . . . I ask you in my mind to dance with me. Um, because you're so *(She looks at him, melts, and makes a sound meaning hot.)* uhhhhhhhh! I mean, I mean, oh gosh! Um, do you want to maybe, perhaps, like possibly, go out with me? *(Beat.)* Really? Cool! Uh, so I guess I'll call you—or you call me—or we can call—yeah. OK, bye! *(She turns to walk away, looks back enamored, and trips.)*

Casting Miss Cooper

Dawn accidentally ran into her gym teacher, Miss Cooper, and knocked her down last gym class. Noticing Miss Cooper's casts and attitude toward her today, Dawn approaches Miss Cooper to apologize.

Miss Cooper, I noticed that I was the only one in gym class that you made run an extra ten laps. And every time I look at you, you give me this evil death stare. And I was thinking that maybe it has to do with me breaking your leg last class? I'm not sure though. But if that's it, that was a total accident! I was running too fast when you suddenly sprung out of nowhere and landed right in my path. Do you think I wanted to smack into you and eat dirt? No! I stubbed my baby toe! I know it's not broken like your leg . . . and your wrist . . . and middle finger—but it still hurts! I guess what I'm trying to say is, I want to apologize. Personally, sincerely, and formally. Can I sign your cast?

Bitter About the Bee

Salena finally stands up to Danielle, a girl on her cheerleading squad who is always mean to her.

Danielle, why do you have to be obnoxious and mean to me all the time? Why can't you be nice like the other cheerleaders? And please quit flinging your pom-poms in my face! I know what this is really about. You're rude to me because you're jealous that I beat you in the kindergarten spelling bee! Don't deny it! In first grade, you stomped on my lunch every day. In third grade, you spread rumors that I was married! In fourth grade, you pushed me off the stage in *A Christmas Surprise*! Get over it already! It's not my fault I'm an excellent speller and you're, um, NOT! Get Hooked on Phonics, eat alphabet soup, date Webster! Just back off and stop harassing me, or I'll suggest a cheer with your favorite word: we rule the ball, we rule the field, we rule the stands, we're the HOME TEAM, H-O-A-M! *(Making of fun of Danielle's misspelling.)* Home.

Fashion Is My Forté

Shawna tries to convince her best friend, Missy, not to wear the pants she has on.

Missy, listen to me. Watch my lips. You cannot wear those pants. They are wrong. In fact, they are so wrong, if you wear them out in public, I will not be caught dead with you! I'm telling you this because I'm your best friend. Would you want me to tell you they look hot and let you walk around the mall looking like a color-blind person who got dressed in their brother's closet then got run over by a lawn mower after slipping in a puddle of neon pink mud? *(Beat.)* I didn't think so. You are lucky to have me around to stop the crisis before it happens. Thank God fashion is my forté. Hey, now those pants are so cute. Can I wear them? I'll let you wear my pants. *(Beat.)* What do you mean they're ugly?! What a cruel thing to say to your best friend!

Kindly Cruel

Emma's best friend, Kyra, accuses her of being too nice. Here, Emma tries to prove her wrong.

Kyra. What do you mean I'm too nice? I'm not nice. I'm . . . I'm . . . well, I do a lot of crazy, mean things. I do! Once, I stole a lollipop from CVS! That was so not nice—or legal. How about that, huh? And one time, I stuck my tongue out at Mrs. Walker in math class behind her back! I am a rebel. I'm fierce, I'm cruel, I'm ruthless! When I was four, I threw a mud pie at my mother! I'm a sinner. *(Beat.)* Nice?! You still think I'm nice? You're my best friend and you so don't know me! *(Jumping up and down.)* I am mean! I'm an evil, brutish person! Kyra, you know how you've been in love with Sebastian since last summer? I have a date with him Friday night! *(Beat.)* I'm sorry! He just asked me and, and—I'll cancel if you want? *(Beat.)* I know, you're right! I'm so mean!

"Just Friends"

Holly tries to tell Trent that she just wants to be friends.

Wait. Before you say anything, I really feel like I need to tell you something, Trent. It was really nice of you to invite me to your party. Even though your band friends went a little overboard with the school songs. And wow, your mom really loves Scrabble. And the movie Friday was, um . . . I know you didn't mean to spill the popcorn all over me. Or the Coke. Or the Raisinets. We probably shouldn't have seen a scary movie. Anyway, before you ask me out this weekend, I want to . . . what I'm trying to say is, I think you're really nice and all, but I just want to be friends. No offense. What do you say? *(Beat.)* What do you mean that's what you were gonna tell me?! That's not possible! Don't you realize how cool and nice and, and, and pretty I am? How dare you just want to be friends with me?!

Perfectly Sickening

Jessie's mother is good friends with Meredith's mother. Jessie and Meredith go to the same school. Meredith is the perfect, straight-A student, while Jessie is average. Jessie is sick and tired of hearing how wonderful Meredith is, so she decides to confront her.

Meredith, I need to talk to you. You know how your mom and my mom are really good friends, even though we're not? Well, all I hear all the time now is "Why can't you be more like Meredith? She has perfect grades. She's so well-behaved. She's Beta Club president." Blah, blah, blah. You're making my life miserable. Do you even have a life outside of school, Miss Prima Ballerina? Don't you ever cheat, lie, talk in class? *(Beat.)* Well, you better start. Take a risk and pass a note. Get an A-minus, don't give it 100 percent. How about a little eff o rt on your part to mess up once in a while, huh? You're raising the standards in class so much that you're making enemies day by day. People hate you. I'm doing you a favor! Trust me, you'll be much more popular if you start screwing up!

Oh My Atheist!

Corky has a major crush on Trey and seeks advice from her friend Donna.

Oh my atheist, Donna, did you see how cute Trey looked in his new Q. T. shirt? He's such a hottie, it's sickly not right. All I want is for him to give me his jersey to wear and beg me to m a rry him in front of the whole school. That's not soooo much to want, is it? Don't answer. I know you think I'm Oscarly dramatic, but I swear he was flirting with me in science. It was at least four full minutes of eye tag! That's a new record for us! What do you think it means, Donna? Think he's gonna ask me out? Think he's playing games? Think he had a bug in his eye? *(Beat.)* I know there were fruit flies in the science lab! Thanks, Donna! Thanks a lot for your—oh my atheist! Don't look but Trey's heading this way. Don't look! Donna—does my hair look OK? How's my makeup? Anything in my teeth? Don't leave me! No, leave me—he might be shy. Wait—don't go! I'm wigging, I'm freaking, I— *(Cool, chill, and calm.)* Oh, hey, Trey, I didn't see you there. What's up?

The Math Chef

*Jane just received her report card and got all A's and a C in math.
Here, Jane confronts her math teacher.*

Mr. Campbell, I can't believe you gave me a C in your math
class. This is the only class that I didn't get an A in. Doesn't
that tell you something? Like maybe the reason I'm not doing
well in your class is because you can't teach? No offense, but
HELLO! All you talk about in math are your kitchen appliances!
Your blender that's "more than a blender." Do you talk about
fractions and decimals? No! Just your George Foreman Grill
and your Cuisinart Breadmaker! How am I supposed to make
bread if I don't get into college? Mr. Campbell, I need an A and
I think it's only fair that you change my grade since it's clearly
not my fault, OK? *(Beat.)* No?! Well then I'm going to report
you to the superintendent! I'm gonna show you a pressure
cooker like you've never seen! You crock pot!

Mixing with the Deejay

Angela has a big crush on Joel. Here she asks him to go out with her and her friends.

(Nervously talks without letting him get a word in.) Hey Joel, how was practice? Good, I hope—or more like fantastic. Well, some of my friends and I are thinking about going to Garfield's Saturday night—just to hang, listen to some tunes, and read all about the gossip in *The Daily Word*. Which, by the way, I read the article saying how mind-blowing your deejaying was at Monica's party. And now you're getting so "rock star" popular! You're quiet—you don't talk much—me either—it's cool—so what I was saying is that I was wondering if you wanted to go with me. To Garfield's. Saturday night. If you're not busy. But if you are I completely understand. So what do you say? *(Beat.)* Oh. Well, it's cool. No biggie. *(Starts to turn away and turns back.)* By the way, I was at Monica's party that night, and your deejaying sucked!

Obsessed

Charlotte, a huge fan of Eminem, spots him eating dinner in a local restaurant.

(She runs over to Eminem's table and trips, but catches herself. She breathes heavily and stares at him, unable to speak. She tries to talk again but nothing comes out. Finally she speaks.) I just want you to know I'm obsessed with you. I know everything about you. Eminem, I've been in love with you since I was like five. Every inch of my bedroom walls are plastered with posters of you. I have an Eminem bedspread on my bed at all times. Even my favorite candy is M&M's. You just don't even know! Do you wanna play basketball with me? I know that's your favorite sport. I'm not very good, but who cares! Oh, hey, they serve Cheerios here and even though it's dinnertime, I could go and make them get some for you. *(Beat.)* Wait, you can't leave! *(She tries to block his exit path from the table. Maybe she kneels on the floor.)* Now that you're finally here, right in front of me, I cannot let you go. *(Beat.)* I'm not moving, so if you really aren't fascinated by me yet, you're going to have to walk away knowing that you're breaking my heart! And throwing away your one true love. *(Beat. She calls after him as he walks away.)* Eminem! Don't go! You'll meet me again one day! *(She sighs and sort of collapses on the floor.)*

Demanding Approval

Brittany has just been asked out by a cute boy at school. However, she's been burned before and wants to make sure he understands that she needs to be accepted for who she is.

What? Will I be your girlfriend? Well, my last boyfriend, he didn't accept me for who I am. And I'm not gonna change for anybody. Nobody. So don't even think that just because I'm pretty that I'm gonna be this weak, little groupie and do whatever you want. Uh-uh. I am strong, I know what I want, and I do what I want! I might have a quiet personality, but I won't let anybody—including you—push me around! This is me! You need to accept me for me! I'm never gonna change just because—what? *(Beat.)* You do? You like me for who I am? You don't want me to change? Well, I like you too, for who you are. But if you want me to go out with you, you seriously need to cut your hair and stop wearing sandals! Your toes are hideous!

Mickey D's

Kirsten has just arrived at her friend Samantha's house. As she walks into the kitchen, she sees Samantha preparing to eat McDonald's.

Hey, Samantha, your mom said— *(She sees what she's about to eat.)* Oh my God! You've got McDonald's. Samantha, that's McDonald's on your table. Please tell me you are not going to eat McDonald's. Sam, didn't you hear about that movie they made where they had some guy eat only McDonald's for every meal for like a year and he got so sick that . . . well, I can't even really talk about it without getting queasy. *(She shudders.)* Uhhh. Do you know there's more grease in those fries than a L'Oréal hot-oil treatment? I'm talking two whole hair repairs. Think about that. And that so-called burger? I saw a box of frozen ones being delivered to the McDonald's on Forest Lane and ya know what the box said? "Grade D." That means dog. Dog meat. There's dog meat in there. *(She makes a pathetic puppy whine.)* Tell me you are so not gonna eat that. *(Beat.)* Good. Cause I'm starving!

Stalking Up Friends

A weird girl named Marlene always follows Sarah around at school and tells her all the things she knows about her. Sarah can't take it anymore, so she finally confronts Marlene.

Marlene, stay away from me. Every day at school, you follow me around like I'm your best friend. I'm not your friend. And I'm not your mom. You're like a groupie and I'm not even famous—yet! I'll give you money if you'll go away? Maybe if you didn't dress like Elvis, people would talk to you. And it's really creepy that you know everything about me. You're like total stalker material. I wouldn't be surprised to see you on the news. " C reepy Elvis stalker breaks into popular girl's bedroom to steal a handful of her hair!" Not to give you any ideas! How do you know so much about me, anyway? Are you one of those brainy internet spyware dorks? *(Beat.)* You forge report cards? Wanna go to the mall Saturday?

Inventing the Truth

Faith has a crush on her good friend Dave. The problem is that he is going out with Rachel. Faith tells Dave a lie about Rachel so he'll break up with her and go to the dance with Faith.

Oh my God, Dave, I'm so sorry about Rachel! What a two-faced witch! *(Beat.)* You didn't hear? Oh Dave, I hate to break it to you because I'm your good friend, and I know you really like Rachel, God knows why, and you've been going out with her for three weeks and five days, but she's not what you think. Friday at the football game she was seen kissing Robbie Hoffman! In front of everyone! She obviously has no respect for you, and as your true friend, I think you should dump her as soon as you see her! I know that sucks and it's such bad timing with the dance coming up this weekend. But since I'd hate to see you have to go alone, I'll go with you. Of course, just as friends, ya know. Good friends. Very good friends. *(Beat.)* Cool! Oh, by the way, she'll probably deny it, but don't believe a word she says! It's a fact! So, what time are you picking me up?

Dressing Up the Code

Christina is always getting in trouble for breaking the dress code at her school. Today her teacher sends her to the principal's office because her skirt is too short.

Miss Pickett, I would stick to the dress code if it made any sense but it doesn't. I mean, OK, we have to wear closed-toe shoes with backs. I understand you want us to look alike. But socks? How is not wearing socks a "safety hazard"?! And the rule about our skirts not being more than three inches above the knee? You can't find skirts these days that long! All the skirts are like three inches below the waist! And it's not like I'm trying to attract boys. It just gets hot wearing almost knee-length skirts all the time. *(Beat.)* Miss Pickett, I think you're just jealous because I have great legs and you don't! I shouldn't be punished for that! Maybe if you put on some makeup and seriously hemmed your skirt, you'd get a date and you wouldn't take your lonely, old, crotchety regrets out on me! *(Beat.)* Detention?! How ungrateful! That's the last time I try to improve your love life!

Flirting with Phonics

Vanessa tries to convince her mom that she needs a tutor because she has a crush on Mr. Goodman, the student teacher in her English class.

Ya know, Ma, every time we go somewhere and you ask me to read something to you, I screw the words all up and it's really embarrassing. Like when we went to Red Lobster and you forgot your glasses and made me order, and I ordered espresso instead of escargot. I need reading and phonics help! I need a private tutor, Mom. Do you want me to fail middle school and work at Burger King for the rest of my life? Mom, I need serious help! *(Beat.)* Great! I know the perfect tutor. Mr. Goodman—you know, the student teacher in my English class? He is so smart . . . and funny . . . and cute . . . and— *(Beat.)* He has a girlfriend?! *(Beat.)* You know what, Mom, I changed my mind. Tutors are so overrated.

Got Game?

Leslie just beat the boy she likes at basketball. She is offended when he refers to her as a tomboy.

What do you mean I'm a tomboy? I'm a girlie-girl. Look at me, Jeff. I'm a hottie. Are tomboy's sexy? I don't think so! Just because I play basketball better than you doesn't mean I'm all boyish. Maybe you need to work on your game. Don't hate me because I've got skill and you don't. You're such a sore loser. Shake it off! Stop being such a wuss. God. You're worse than my little sister. *(Beat.)* What do you mean I just got lucky?! You didn't score once! Face it, Jeff, you could never beat me. I could whip your butt blindfolded with one arm tied behind my back. *(Beat.)* Oh, really? You wanna see me try? Let's go! Bring it on, little girl!

The Klutz and
Danny Smallwood

Paige is clumsy and she accidentally ran into Danny Smallwood and knocked him down. She got called down to the dean's office because of her behavior. Here she defends herself to Dean Armstrong.

Dean Armstrong, it was an accident! I didn't mean to smack into Danny Smallwood and send him flying into the lockers! He's the shortest boy in the whole school—I didn't even see him! Plus I have really bad depth perception! I was rushing to English because I was running late because I spilled juice on Claire Bradford's sweater, and I was trying to help wash it out. And the tardy bell rang and I dropped my books and didn't get all the juice out, but I'm such a serious student that I, of course, didn't want to be late! So I ran and wham! Danny Smallwood should watch where he steps! And three detentions is a little extreme for an accident, don't you think? *(Beat.)* Dean Armstrong, this is discrimination! I shouldn't be punished because I was born clumsy and Danny was born puny! That's our parents' fault! You should give the detentions to them, not me!

So Not Cool

Skylar lets Carson know why she won't date him.

OK. If you really wanna know why I won't go out with you, Carson, I'll tell you. It's because nothing about you is cool. Look at your pants! They're plaid! And maybe if you pulled the belt down from the middle of your chest they wouldn't be floods. And your hair is scary! Ever hear of Little Orphan Annie? Cause with that hair, you could be her twin! And you don't have any pierings or tattoos—none! That's not just uncool, it's like frightening. And you listen to dorky music instead of cool bands like Fall Out Boy and Evanescence. *(Beat.)* What?! Your dad can get backstage passes to Evanescence?! Ya know, I think cool is totally overrated.

Formally Best Friends

Scarlet has a secret crush on her best friend, Brandon. Scarlet decides to ask him to go to the formal "as friends."

Hey, Brandon. Ya know how there's the formal coming up and you don't have a date and I don't have a date? Well, I was thinking—cause we're such good friends—that maybe we should go together? Just as friends. Cause it's not like I like you or anything. I mean, I know everything about you, and we sit together at lunch every day, and you call me every night. So if we were to date, it would be kinda like . . . ya know? Don't you agree? *(Beat. Brandon doesn't say anything.)* Cause it's almost like we're this old married couple. Except we're not married. Or old. But I mean if we were. Ya know? *(Beat.)* Say something! *(Beat.)* Well, do you wanna go to the formal as like best friends slash old married couple? *(Beat.)* Really?! Uh, cool. So I'll, um, I'll like see you at lunch. Bye! *(Beat. He leaves.)* YESSSSSSSS! *(She does some crazy dance or poses of triumph.)*

Pants Off!

Karli just had an extremely embarrassing experience during break at school and seeks help and revenge from her friend Rusty.

Oh my God, Rusty, you will not believe what just happened to me! I was outside during break and "Miss Hair" Michelle Evans was right behind me. So, of course, I wanted to get away from her. So I decided I'll go to the picnic table and I take a step and— whoosh—my pants hit the floor! *(Beat.)* Stop laughing! I was mortified! Michelle Evans was standing on the hem of my pants! I know she did it on purpose. You've never seen somebody pull their pants up so fast! Too fast, because they ripped! *(Beat.)* It's not funny! Patrick was there, and I know he saw! He's never gonna ask me out now! And it's all Michelle's fault! I need your help, Rusty. Ya know how you sit behind her in geometry? Well, I have a pack of gum and a pair of scissors. Your choice.

A Punchy Predicament

Diana has secretly had a crush on her good friend Tommy for quite some time. Diana just went to give Tommy a hug in the hallway at school and accidentally punched him in the nose.

Oh my gosh, Tommy, I'm so sorry! I was just trying to give you a hug. How was I supposed to know you'd turn your nose into my fist? Are you OK? Ooh, you're bleeding. Does it hurt? *(Beat.)* I'm so, so, so, so sorry! It was an accident! I swear I didn't mean to punch you! I never realized how strong I am when I go to hug someone. But hey, ya know, that shows how much I really like you. Otherwise I would have just gone in for a half-hug. I know you wouldn't be bleeding then, but at least you finally know how much I care. There, I said it, it's true. I've liked you all this time. It just never seemed like the right moment to tell you. Ooh, you better pinch your nose and tilt your head back. Anyway, now that you know how I really feel, do you wanna go out Friday night?

Eyeing You Eyeing Me

Megan is a bit paranoid about a group of girls at her school. She is sure they are talking about her all the time, and today she finally confronts them. She is agitated and speaks quickly without letting them get a word in.

(She starts down the hall, eyes a group of girls suspiciously, and comes back.) Say it why don't you—come on, say it! I know you're talking about me. All of you— *(Cutting them off.)* don't try to deny it! I can feel you watching me—glaring at me like salivating rottweilers! You all do that eye-tag thing with each other. I see you—I'm not blind. You just don't like me because you're jealous that I've been cheering for five years, and you all suck! You can't even spot a pompom when you see one, touch your toes, spell TEAM! Well, it's not my fault I'm talented and you are mean, gossiping wanna-be's! So if you have something to say about me, just say it already! *(Beat.)* You like my shirt? Oh my God, thanks! I got it on sale at Hollister. They have the totally cutest stuff!

A Note of Surprise

Phoebe found a note shoved in her locker from Jonathan, the boy she likes, asking her to the football game. Phoebe approaches Jonathan with newfound confidence to accept his offer. But she's in for a little surprise.

Hi, Jonathan. So about Friday night. I'd love to go to the football game with you. And I was thinking afterwards we could go to the Waffle House and get some . . . waffles. So why don't you pick me up at my house—in your dad's Cadillac—at seven o'clock? You didn't say what time in the note, so I just figured seven would be good. And I'm really glad you finally wrote to me. *(Beat.)* "What note?" Your note asking me to the game that was shoved in my locker. Stop messing around. *(Beat.)* You didn't write me a note? *(Beat.)* Oh, well, uh, my mistake. It must have been Jonathan Ramsey. He's been in love with me forever. I gotta go! *(She quickly walks off looking totally humiliated.)*

The Zit

Donna has a big date with a cute boy tonight. She's panicking because she has a zit. She calls her friend Angie and begs her to come over. Angie's just arrived.

Look at me, Angie. There is no way I can go dancing with Scott tonight! *(Beat.)* What do you mean "why?" I have a zit! Don't act like you can't see it! It's taking over my face! *(Beat.)* "Not so bad?" Sure, it's not so bad, because it's on my face! If it were on your face, it would be a catastrophe! 911—SOS—emergency surgery needed! What am I supposed to do when he gets here? *(Cupping her hands around her mouth and calling loudly.)* "Hey, Scott, it's me— *(Waving for him to see her.)* back here behind my zit!" *(Realizing.)* Oh, God. What if he wants to slow dance? We'll need a good ten feet between his cheek and mine! It's ruined, it's over, it's done with. I look like a lopsided chipmunk. *(Beat.)* It's not funny! Angie, help me! What am I gonna do? *(Beat.)* Make it a beauty mark? Do they come that big?

Pet-Peeve Provoked

Vicky's parents sent her to a therapist because they think she's overly particular.

Look I'm only here because my parents think I need therapy because I get a little irritated about things. I really don't think I need—could you not crack your knuckles while I'm talking? Or like ever again? It's beyond annoying. Anyway, I was saying that—my gosh! Did you know you flare your nostrils almost nonstop? *(Beat.)* Uh, yeah you do. You're like. *(She imitates.)* And your eyebrows arch up really freakin' high when you do it. Like this. *(She imitates.)* I can't believe you're a therapist! You're supposed to be helping me, not traumatizing me! Can I have some water please, it's really hot in here. Not the red Dixie cup—the blue one! Ya know what—forget it! Listen, just tell my parents I'm completely normal and I don't need therapy. And STOP CLICKING YOUR TONGUE!

Dumb It Up

Abigail is a straight-A student with the highest GPA in her class. She recently started going out with Jacob, a football player at school. Jacob has just told Abigail that he wants to break up. She tries to change his mind.

Jacob, let me get this straight. You're breaking up with me because your friends think I'm a brainy nerd? *(Beat.)* So you're going to listen to your dense friends instead of listening to your heart? *(Beat.)* You think I'm a brainy nerd too?! Oh my heavens! I can't believe you think such an atrocious thing! Just because I have straight A-pluses and the highest GPA in the ninth grade, does not mean I'm a brainy nerd! I can't help it that I was born smart! And I don't know why I like to study, but that's just a hobby—like how you like to play football. *(Beat.)* Jacob, wait! I can try to be dumb! I can get an A-minus—I know I can! Just give me another chance! I'll throw out my Encyclopedia Britannica collection? I'll stop studying on Saturday nights?! Jacob, Come back! I want to be stupid for you!

Heads Will Roll

In the hall after class, Nicole finally gathers up the courage to talk to James, a cute boy in her biology class.

Hey, James, um, I don't know exactly how to say this but, well, I kind of watch you a lot, and I've known you for a long time even though you probably don't know who I am, do you? I'm Nicole? I sit behind you in biology class? I was the one who dissected the frog the wrong way and his head bounced over and fell in your lap? *(Beat.)* Yeah! That was me! Not one of my better moments. Well, anyway, I think if you would get to know me, we could have a lot of fun together . . . and I promise not to behead anything that might roll in your direction. So, I was wondering—if you're not busy—like after school Friday, we could hang out—if you want to? *(Beat.)* You have a girlfriend?! Why didn't you tell me like way back at "Hey, James"?! I wouldn't have stood here and embarrassed myself in front of you! Or do you think that's funny or something?! God, you're such a jerk. I can't believe I actually liked you! Oh, and the frog head? Did it on purpose!

A Sticky Situation

Felicia's sister April put glue in Felicia's body lotion before gym class. Felicia used the lotion, and now her pants are stuck on her. She frantically finds her sister as next period's classes are about to start and calls her over to the bathroom.

(Whispering harshly.) April, get over here! I'm gonna kill you! I know it was you who put the glue in my lotion! *(Beat.)* I'm serious—it's not funny! I put lotion on my legs after gym and now I can't get my pants off! *(Sarcastically.)* Yeah, ha ha ha, April fools, you're the funniest sister ever. I knew it was you! You're jealous because Ryan asked me to prom and not you! Well, it's not my fault you're socially inept! You better help me get my pants off right now! I mean it! If you don't help me April, not only am I gonna tell Dad, I'm gonna tell Principal Parker! Then you'll be the one in the sticky situation! *(Beat.)* OK, I won't tell! Now come on, April, grab a leg and start pulling! Hurry up, I have to pee!

Rocky Road Man

Lindsay is infatuated with John, the singer of an up-and-coming rock band. After watching their concert, she sees John come out of the backstage area near the band's tour bus.

John! Great show! What's up? *(Beat.)* It's Lindsay. Don't you remember me? I wrote to you on MySpace? I took a picture with you and your drummer? I tripped over all the wires and knocked out the sound? *(Beat.)* Yeah, that was me! I was wondering if you wanted to go out sometime—like now? Cause I like you— a lot—and I truly think we were meant to be together. Get this—we both love Rocky Road ice cream, and Jim Carrey, and, the color blue! Freaky, huh? Plus, we're both weird— in a good way. Also, you might not know this, but I'm a singer too! I wrote a song just for you. *(She sings.)* "I'm so in love with you, I don't know what to do. If you don't ask me out, I think I'll have to shoot you. My Rocky Road man." *(Beat. Calling after him.)* Hey, where are you going?

Rewarding Rumors

Connor has a big crush on Heather and spread a rumor that she cheated on her boyfriend with him. Heather secretly likes Connor and just broke up with her boyfriend for him, though she does not want to admit that to Connor.

Connor, I cannot believe you told everyone that I cheated on my boyfriend with you when you know that's not true! Me hook up with you? As if! I don't care if you were the chubby kid at school last year and now you're not and think you're so hot. You're not that amazing, tall guy! I could probably kick your butt! And your ears are colossal! The only reason people are believing your tall tale is because I just broke up with Tyler yesterday. Even his mom thinks I left him for you, you oversized leprechaun! Well let me assure you, it had nothing to do with you! I'd never go out with you! Not in a million years, you lying, jumbo elf! *(Beat.)* Friday night? I thought you'd never ask!

Lighting Up Mom's Birthday

Carissa was making a special dinner for her mother's birthday and accidentally started a fire in the kitchen. She goes upstairs to wake her mom and break the news.

Um, Mom, are you awake? *(Beat.)* Good. About your special birthday dinner that I'm cooking . . . Well, I had a little accident. I put a sturdy metal bowl in the microwave, and something must have been wrong with the microwave because it sort of blew up. And it started smoking so I opened it, and it somehow caught the paper towel roll on fire, which burned the cabinets above it and kind of moved on to the drapes, which are pretty much gone. Oh, and Fluffy won't need a shave for a while. But the good news is I didn't get hurt! But what I really wanted to say was . . . Happy birthday, Mom! I love you. Wanna go to Taco Bell? I'll buy?

Festive Flaunting

Kimmy was just humiliated by a girl she hates during lunch at school. She finds her friend Laura at her locker and begs her to help get revenge.

Laura, oh my gosh, I can't believe what just happened to me! I was in lunch and Tina Jordan and her friends start singing "Rudolph the Red-Nosed Reindeer." And they're pointing at me and laughing. And Nick was there. I'm like, "What's going on—it's not even Christmastime and why would they be singing that anyway?" Well, suddenly Tina points at me and screams really loud, "Love the Rudolph undies!" I almost died! I bet Nick was laughing with them at my red-nosed butt! Ooh, I hate Tina Jordan! She should be hung up by her toenails and forced to read a novel! You've got to help me get her back! *(Beat.)* She's in cosmetology with you? That's perfect! Offer to do her hair, and accidentally give her a buzz cut!

The Depths of Friendship

*Lacey has just dropped her cell phone into the toilet. She tries
to convince her friend Alexis to get it out.*

Alexis, thank God you just walked in! I need your help! Quick!
I just dropped my cell phone in the toilet! Could you not laugh?
This is serious! My mom will kill me if you don't get it out.
Yes, you! *(Beat.)* No, I didn't go! It's perfectly clean toilet water.
I can't do it because . . . because I just got my nails done. I heard
toilet water instantly dissolves nail polish. Anyway, it's your
fault! Remember how you begged me to call Derek and hint
about how you "maybe" like him and he should ask you out?
Well, I called him—like the good friend I am—right before my
phone dropped and plunged to the bottom of the toilet! I was
helping you, Alexis, and you won't even get your hands a little wet to help me?! God, that's really—hey, listen—it's ringing
under the water! *(Perhaps she looks in toilet.)* It's Derek, I just
know it! Alexis, this is your chance! Go get 'em, girlfriend!

It's All About You

Fiona likes Logan even though he can often be conceited. At the school dance, she puts him in his place.

Hey, Logan, I'm surprised to see you here at the dance. Did you come by yourself? *(Beat.)* Me, too. *(Beat.)* What do you mean, "It figures"? Are you implying that I couldn't get a date? Because let me tell you, Logan, fifteen guys asked me to this dance. I chose to come alone. Unlike you, I'm sure. As if any girl would want to dance with you! They'd be trying to dance, listening to you going on and on about you! *(Imitating him.)* "The football team is so lucky to have me. Aren't my biceps looking hot? I am in love with myself!" Logan, Logan, Logan! And it's not like you're all that. You just convince yourself you are. And ya know what? You have a monstrous nose and you look like a Neanderthal! I bet you can't even dance anyway! *(Beat.)* Oh, really? Prove it! Go ahead, dance with me!

Oh, Brother!

Ashley is fed up with her younger brother, Ricky, for constantly embarrassing her in front of her boyfriend, Andrew.

Ricky, I can't believe you did that! Thanks a lot for telling Andrew that I still suck my thumb! I just . . . bite it sometimes because I'm dieting, and I'm trying not to overeat! I do not suck my thumb! And why is it that every time Andrew comes over you sneak around the corner and spy on us?! You're always embarrassing me in front of my boyfriend! Like last Saturday when we were watching Gilmore Girls and he kissed me, and suddenly we heard strange smooching noises coming from behind the couch! You're lucky I didn't kill you instantly! Don't you have anything better to do than pester me and Andrew?! Why don't you go pluck your unibrow, hairball! I think you're just jealous because I have a boyfriend and you don't! *(Beat.)* I meant girlfriend, stupidhead! But what girl would want to go out with you when you're thirteen and you still wet your bed?! *(Beat.)* I am not a thumb sucker, you bed wetter! *(Beat.)* Sesame Street lover?! You're so dead!

A New, Blue You

Cassandra just finished dying her friend Janelle's hair. Unfortunately, it turned blue and most of her long locks burned off.

Janelle, calm down! Your hair doesn't look so bad. I followed the instructions—I don't know what happened! But hey, short hair is in. Halle Berry has short hair, and it's so cute on her. I know hers isn't blue, but that just shows how unique you are. Look at Pink. She's famous and her hair is never a normal color. Not that your hair isn't normal! Actually, now it matches your eyes! Hair-eye coordination is totally stylish. *(Beat.)* I know you liked your hair smooth, but those burnt ends make you look . . . fierce. It's bold and sexy. *(Beat.)* Janelle, I followed the instructions! It's not my fault your hair didn't! You should have warned me you have bad hair. I never would have volunteered my expertise. *(Beat.)* Don't cry! Come on, Janelle. It's really not that . . . I mean your hair looks . . . Oh! You know what is so in? Hats!

Driving Each Other Crazy

Taylor is taking driver's ed at school with Mr. Dickey. He also gives her driving lessons. Mr. Dickey is loud, bitter and yells a lot. His yelling, today, caused Taylor to crash the car, though no one got hurt. She has had it with him.

Mr. Dickey, it's not my fault I crashed the car! As usual, you were barking at me in that overbearing tone! I can't believe you ever got hired as a driver's ed teacher! All you do is yell at us and call us "you people" just because we're teenagers! I have a name! And you're always blaming us for all the fatalities on the road. "You people cause 90 percent of all car crashes, you inexperienced drivers!" Of course, we're inexperienced—that's why we're in driver's ed! Did you ever stop to think that if we're causing all those crashes it's because you didn't train us well? And how am I supposed to understand you with that lisp? "You people need to thhop terrorithing our thstweets." And when we're driving, screaming "Minimize!" every time I get close to the dividing line doesn't help! Look where you got us—crashed! Not crathed—crashed! You scared the living daylights out of me! You're fired! You're not a driver's ed teacher, you're a menace to society!

Dating Mr. Daybreak

Cassidy does not do mornings. Especially Saturday mornings. Unfortunately, the guy she is dating keeps showing up Saturday mornings to see if she wants to do something. This morning she has had it.

Keith, it's really nice that you want to see me so much that you come over every Saturday morning. But this is the limit! It's only eleven o'clock in the morning, and I do not function at this ungodly hour! And you want me to go to the gym?! Have you lost your mind?! Do you realize you've done this every Saturday since we've been together? And how did I respond the last three times? *(Beat.)* Not good. Riiight. Normal people don't wake up before noon on Saturdays. Ya know, I think there's something seriously mentally wrong with you! You're like an AM addict! You need therapy. Keith, I'm sorry, but this is not gonna work between us. I don't do morning people! If you ever get the urge to knock on my door again before noon, restrain yourself, or I will knock you out!

Baiting the Boy

Tara's friend Stephanie paid her to talk Aaron into going to the prom with Stephanie. Here, Tara attempts to win him over.

Hey Aaron, could I talk to you for a minute? So who are you going to prom with? *(Beat.)* No one? Excellent! I know someone perfect for you. She's very beautiful—all the guys want to go to prom with her—but she wants to go with you! She's adventurous like you, and she loves football! How about that, huh? Hard to come by. Plus she's smart, outgoing, and extremely fun to be with. She's perfect for you! *(Beat.)* It's Stephanie Hart! *(Beat.)* What's wrong with her? She's a good friend of mine. She's cute! Look, she paid me fifty bucks to convince you to ask her! I'll split it with you? *(Beat.)* Fine. Be that way. *(Beat.)* How about going with me?

Unusual Impact

Raven has only had her driver's license for a week. She is a very impatient driver. She just caused a crazy accident with an old lady who was driving too slowly for her tastes. Raven defends herself to the police officer.

Officer, this is so not my fault! There I was driving along, following the rules of the road very carefully since I just started driving a week ago, and suddenly I'm stuck behind this old lady here who's driving like thirty miles an hour below the speed limit! So I tried to pass her, but her big boat of a car was like blocking both lanes! So I blew my horn like five million times, but she still didn't move! So, I thought she might need some help getting to her destination a little faster. And I took it upon myself to help push her along. But how was I suppose to see what was ahead of us with her handicap sign dangling in the way? It's not my fault we went up the curb and crashed into that adult bookstore! If she had just followed the law—like me—we wouldn't have been in a pornographic accident!

A Second Chance

Shannon attempts to win back her ex-boyfriend, Jackson, now that he is going out with her archenemy.

Look, Jackson, I know I dumped you and you cried a lot and you're hurting right now. But going out with Heidi Buckmaster is not gonna make your wounds heal any faster. I know I broke your heart. I mean, I'm gorgeous and popular and—what? I didn't break your heart? Right. ANYWAY! I'm just trying to help you from making a ginormous mistake! Did you know Heidi Buckmaster has really bad gas? I sit behind her in biology and it's tort u re! It's a good thing no one's lit a Bunsen burner too close to her! Cause I'm talkin' KA-BOOM! And nobody likes her. Why do you think they let her fall off the top of the cheerleading pyramid? They want her gone! Too bad she only dislocated her thumb. Anyway, I've decided to give you a second chance. I couldn't bear seeing you with that gassy gargoyle. So, here's your chance. *(Beat.)* What do you mean, "You'll pass"?! OK, clearly you're confused. Let's start over.

Way Too Cheesy

Bianca hates cheese and her new boyfriend, Eddie, hasn't even noticed. Here, Bianca fills him in and then some.

Eddie, remember two weeks ago when we went on our first date? You took me out to eat at Barry's? You got a cheeseburger and cheese fries and I got a regular burger and regular fries? *(Beat.)* Good, stay with me. Then last week we went to Tony's Pizzeria where you ordered us a cheese pizza. Did you notice how I didn't eat anything? So today you bring me to this buffet and what do they have? Cheese sticks, macaroni and cheese, cheesy bread, and cheese ravioli! And what did I put on my plate? Nothing! Rinnnggg! *(Mimes answering a phone.)* It's for you, Eddie. It's the Get-A-Clue phone! I despise cheese! I can't believe you didn't even notice that I hate it! I'm sorry, Eddie, but it's over between us. I cannot date a cheese-aholic. Now please get me outta this cheese nightmare. *(Beat.)* Don't give me that cheesy smile! I feel sick enough as it is!

Sitting Smashed

Trisha got drunk while babysitting little Cassie tonight. Cassie's parents just came home and found the empty vodka bottle. Trisha attempts to get out of trouble.

Mr. and Mrs. Strickland, I don't know what you're talking about. I'm wasn't drinking. I've been busy watching little Cassie perform her Tinker Bell show. I don't know how your vodka bottle got empty. Maybe Ruffy knocked it over and . . . and . . . licked it up. Or not. I can't believe you would think that I would jeopardize your child's well-being by getting smashed! I'm so offensneded! I'm a serious babysitter! I came with references! Call 'em up! They know how responsive I am! Ya know what? I don't need to stand here *(Staggers.)* and be insulted like this by bad parents like you! I quit! Give me my money and I'm outtie! And by the way . . . your vodka sucks!

Downing Carbs

Calista is on a low-carb diet. She is at the counter in a pizzeria checking out the menu on the wall when the pizza guy comes over to take her order.

Um, I think I'm ready to order. Ohhh. OK, I'm on a low-carb diet so I need something healthy. And I see you have a lot of salads, which is great, but I just don't feel like salad. Do ya'll have any low-carb pizza? *(Beat.)* What about extra-extra thin crust? *(Beat.)* Oh, man. Well, I did go to the gym today so I deserve a little something. Why don't you give me the extra-small, thin-crust plain-cheese pizza. Wait a second! If I'm gonna eat pizza, you might as well make it a medium. Hold on! If I'm gonna get a medium, I might as well just go for a large. With pineapple. And sausage. And bacon. Oh hell, just give me the extra-jumbo deluxe family-size everything pizza! That should do it. Oh, and a Diet Coke with lemon. Please.

The Hyper Hygienist

Kathryn's dorm roommate, Jillian, is obsessive-compulsive and is driving Kathryn crazy with her cleaning rituals. Kathryn finally loses it.

Jillian, I've been putting up with your "interesting quirks" since the school year started. But I can't take it anymore! I'm your roommate—I live here too! I shouldn't have to leave the room just because you feel the need to sanitize it from top to bottom. Look at that mask you're wearing! This is not a hospital! And I'm sick of you compulsively scrubbing my desk. My papers keep sticking to the residue of your Clorox Ultra-Power disinfectant wipes! And your obsessive cleaning doesn't help. Hello! If you wash the walls and leave them damp, they grow mold! It festers, it breeds, it sends toxic spores into the air, which linger in our room for you to inhale! Oh God, you're looking pale! You might have TB! You should be quarantined and moved out of this bacteria-infested room! Or maybe, you could just STOP CLEANING!

Bonding Roommates

Haley just moved into her new dorm room and found a knife in her new roommate's stuff. She is excited because she also collects knives. Here, Haley greets her new roommate.

Hey, I'm Haley! It looks like we're roommates this semester. Nice to meet you. I hope you don't mind, but I was going through some of your stuff, and I noticed you've got a switchblade in your desk drawer. Which is so cool because I have about twenty different knives. I collect them. Not just knives, of course. I collect tasers, nunchucks, and nightsticks too. Basically anything that can inflict severe pain. I'm obsessed with all things sharp and shiny. I can't believe we got matched up as roomies! We're so gonna get along! I know we'll be best friends. So bust out your switchblade and let me play with it. *(Beat.)* A nail file? But can you really draw blood with that? *(Beat.)* Are you all right? You look sick!

Screwball Relatives

Amber's boyfriend, Ray, is bringing his parents over to Amber's house to meet her parents and have dinner. Amber finished cooking, got dressed, and is now outside her parents' bedroom door, checking to make sure they are ready.

(Sideways, talking through the door.) Momma, Daddy, are ya'll ready? Ray and his parents are gonna be here any minute. Are you dressed yet? And you better not be wearing anything embarrassing like when you wore those hideous luau costumes on Christmas! Open the door and let me approve what you're wearing. *(The door opens. She looks.)* Oh my God, Mom! What are you doing on the floor in your underwear?! *(Beat. She gasps.)* Uhhh! You're schnockered! Daddy, Mom's totally drunk! Do something—straighten her up! *(Silence.)* Dad? *(Beat.)* Holy crap! You're plastered too! What's wrong with ya'll?! Who let you be parents?! Oh my God, they'll be here any second! Be quiet, Momma, I'm trying to think! *(Hears door.)* Aaahh! They're here! That's it. I'm locking ya'll in for the night! I'll tell them, you had some emergency. So I don't want to hear a single word out of you two. Now go to bed, and when you wake up, I hope you have the worst hangovers ever!

The Pickup Line

Janessa is at a party when a guy hits on her with a terrible pickup line. Janessa responds.

You've got to be kidding me. "Am I a cartoon, cause I look too good to be real?"! You think that's gonna make me wanna go home with you? You think I'm all hot and bothered by your sexy, romantic words? Are you on crack?! That has got to be the worst pickup line I've ever heard in my entire life! I mean, I thought "Are you tired? Cause you've been running through my mind" was bad, but yours definitely takes the cake! Honey, please, don't say another word. Look, you seem like you're probably a decent guy—don't speak— so let me give you some advice. Women don't like clichéd, cheesy, fake lines. They like men who are confident enough to just come over and say, "Hey, how are you doing?" It's that simple. Trust me, women will respond much better to that. *(Beat.)* How am I doing? Oh, honey, no, not me! Use it on someone else!

A Match Made in Heaven

Patty was set up on a date with Randy by her friend Cheryl. On the date, Randy's cigarette caught her hair on fire, and it all burned off. Here, she shows up at Cheryl's house, angry and wearing a wig.

What's up with my hair? I'll tell you what's up with my hair— you! You just had to set me up with Randy, didn't you? It wasn't just a bad date, Cheryl, it was beyond bad! Why didn't you tell me that he smoked? You know I hate smokers. And I went to all the trouble of getting my hair fixed and bought a hot outfit. Well Randy definitely liked it cause he moved in close and his cancer stick met my hairspray and KABOOM! My hair went up in flames! I mean my hair is gone! This is a wig! *(Imitating her friend.)* "You'll be a match made in heaven." You weren't kidding! It's not funny! You need to buy me whatever wigs I pick out until my hair grows back! And none of that cheap synthetic hair! I want the real stuff! Let's go. Oh, by the way, I got you a date with Damien. He's an amateur dart player.

Male Monologues

In order of age,
younger to older

The Bad Influence

Michael just got a referral. Here, he confronts Willis, who he blames for getting him in trouble.

Thanks a lot for ruining my day, Willis! Just what I need—another referral on my record on top of all the other stuff I've gotten in trouble for. Only, for once, it wasn't my fault! Why were you trying to hang around me and my friends in the first place, when you're just a goody-goody-gumdrop-suck-up?! Why don't you go polish your apples and count up your A's? Just cause I sat next to you in pre-algebra to copy your answers doesn't mean we're friends. And now, for the first time in your life, you get in trouble and you bring me down with you! *(Beat.)* Don't act innocent! When Miss Linwad said it's not like you to talk in class and made you name the bad influence on you, you wrote down me! That's not gonna make me wanna hang out with you. It might make me wanna kill you! *(Beat.)* You didn't write down my name? Yeah, right. Why else would I get a referral? *(Beat.)* Oh, yeah, I forgot about the explosion. That was pretty good, huh?

Bust a Move

Jordan tries to charm Tiffany into dancing with him.

What's up, Tiffany? Did you come to the dance alone today? *(Beat.)* Yeah? Me too. Well I came with Chelsea, but she can't dance, so would like to dance with me? *(Beat.)* Come on, just one dance? You know you want to. How can you resist? Look how stylish I am. Not to mention hot. And I've got the sexiest smile in history. *(Smiles at her.)* Come on, you know you like this song. I'm not taking no for an answer. Let's go. *(He starts dancing.)* Don't make me have to bust a move. OK. *(He does a funny chicken dance. She walks away. Calling after her.)* Hey, where are you going? Tiffany, I know you can't keep up with my best moves, but that's OK! I'll teach you! *(Beat.)* You don't know a good thing when you see it! Chicken.

Cool Counsel

TJ teaches his older brother, Darryl, how to be cool like him so Darryl can get Tanya to go to homecoming with him.

Darryl, look, if you want Tanya to go to homecoming with you, you need some serious advice from Lil Bro. Cause I'm it with the girls. This is whatcha gotta do. First off, get rid of that tacky outfit. You look like President Nerd! You should wear this fierce black tee with some krunk jeans and those fly shoes to go with it, so you're fresh, like me. And what's up with that jacked-up hair?! It looks like a hurricane just passed through! Get that thing under control. Now, when you see Tanya, ya gotta have confidence. Period. Like me. You've seen me working my magic. Look her in the eye, give her that sexy smile, and leeeaan. Nobody can do it like me, but you can try. Let's see what you're working with. *(Beat.)* Bro, that's just sad. You sure you weren't adopted?

Grade-A Flirt

Sean tries to get Kelly to let him cheat off her.

Hey Kelly, how ya doing? Are those new jeans? They look great! Did you by any chance do your math homework for today? *(Beat.)* Well, it's a long story . . . I had a really rough night . . . I didn't get much sleep or homework done. Sooo, I was wondering if there was any way you might let me copy yours—just so Mr. Reynolds doesn't fail me or something. *(Beat.)* Thanks. You're the coolest! By the way, your hair looks really good today. I mean it. You didn't happen to study for our history exam, did you? Cause since I sit right next to you, I was thinking maybe you could help me out a bit. I promise not to get you in trouble. How could I possibly do that to the prettiest girl in school? Don't blush—it's true. Hey, ya know the quiz we have in French class? *(Beat.)* What?! It's not my fault you were born a genius, and I was born a mooch!

The Innocent Troublemaker

Calvin tries to get out of trouble with the assistant principal.

Mr. Davis, it wasn't me! I wasn't even around you today, so how could I put a "Punch me—I'm only the Assistant Principal" sign on your back?! You're just picking on me because I'm always causing trouble. But this time, I swear I'm innocent. I can't even touch masking tape. It leaves a sticky residue on my fingers that makes me break out in hives all over! I almost died from it once! Mr. Davis, I'm serious! Don't you think if I was the one who put that sign on your back I'd be bragging? Cause you've got to admit that it was pretty funny. Anyway, I know it was Victor—not that I would rat on one of my friends—but he's not my friend! He got a date with Serena Lewis today, and just between us, he's one ugly dude. *(Beat.)* Detention?! That's not fair! I didn't do anything but stick it on your back! It was fear pressure! Victor threatened to kick my umm-hmm if I didn't! Fine. Next time it should be a "shoot me" sign!

Fouling Up the Field Trip

Zack and his classmates are on a field trip today. A few min-utes after getting off the bus, his friend Stephen loudly tells him in front of everyone that he is wearing girls' pants.

What Stephen? I can't hear you—everyone is so wired over this dumb field trip. Speak up! *(Beat. Looks horrified.)* Would you be quiet! *(Harsh whisper.)* What do you mean girls' pants? These aren't girls! Girls wear Capri's. These are in—they're gangsta! Check out the pockets. They— *(Tries to look at pockets in back. Is mortified. Pulls shirt down.)* Oh my gosh they are! What am I gonna do?! We're stuck here—it's not exactly like I can change now! Give me your pants! Well, this is your fault! You convinced me to sign up for this stupid field trip! You waited till we got off the bus to point it out! You probably planned this! You're jealous because I'm so stylish—normally—and you're not! You don't even know fashion when you see it! *(Beat. Gets idea.)* Ac-tually, I'm just joking. I handpicked these pants because I know they'll be the next big thing. They're avant-garde! Duh!

Sabotaged

Evan just lost a speech competition because he was distracted by a pretty girl. Here, he tries to get his speech partner, Steve, to forgive him.

Steve, hold up! C'mon, dude! I'm sorry, OK? I know how much our speech competition meant to you, but it wasn't my fault I ruined it! Marisa Ford winked at me— right when I was about to start, and whoosh—everything in my mind just left. Except her. When you elbowed me, I tried really hard to remember my lines, but then Marisa kinda leaned in on her desk, and she had this low-cut top on, and, and—what was I supposed to do? I was defenseless! But now that I think about it, it was probably sabotage. Like she purposely distracted me so we'd, ya know, lose. And we did! Because right when you slapped me on the back, she licked her lips, and that's why I sort of coughed out the word "hot." I think we should tell the judges and have some sort of do-over. To prove that she purposely threw me off. And they should make Marisa do those things to me again . . . and again, and again!

The Balancing Act

Ian tries to act cool to get Kristin to go out with him.

Yo, Kristin, 'sup? You're lookin' mighty fine today. Not like that's a surprise—you've always been a hottie. So, check it— Ashton's having a party at his crib Friday night, and I want you to go with me. So I thought I'd get your digits and call you later. Are you down with that or what? *(Beat.)* Conceited player?! Hey, listen, you've got me all wrong. I was just trying to like impress you with how cool I could be—I'm really a decent, somewhat geeky, nice guy! Maurice told me to ask you like that. He said chicks like cocky guys. But I am so not cocky. And I'm the furthest thing from a conceited player—I'm still a boy scout! I was planning on buying you flowers and I already wrote you a poem. *(Beat.)* "Eww, too mushy?" Um . . . OK . . . I'll rap you a rhyme instead, cuz you are the most beautiful girl that I, uh, really dig, yo. How does that combination grab ya?

The Baffling Blast

Gunnar's science teacher, Miss Lynch, has just accused him of causing the explosion in the science lab, which destroyed a row of lab tables. Gunnar defends himself.

Miss Lynch, I can't believe you think I would do that! You always blame me for everything. Think about it, how could I blow up a whole row of lab tables during third period when I'm in geography? Besides, I never pay attention to anything you teach us, so how would I know which chemicals would blow anything up? Blowing up a whole row of tables—how do you do that? I bet it was Brent Williams! He's acing your class—he'd know how! And he has extra credit lab time, by himself! *(Beat.)* A match? That's all? Well, seriously where would I get a match? They're hard to come by. I mean, my parents don't smoke or anything. I do, but I use a lighter. *(Beat.)* What do you mean I'm suspended?! This is so unfair! I should have blown up your ugly Volkswagen instead!

Love Signs

Isaac has a big crush on Jessica. Jessica has been playing all kinds of pranks on Isaac, which Isaac interprets as signs that she likes him. Today, after her biggest prank so far, Isaac decides to ask her out.

Hey Jessica, what's up? I've been wanting to talk to you cause I noticed all the little clues you've been leaving for me the past few weeks. Like last Wednesday when you accidentally tripped me in the hall. Accidentally, right. *(Smiles.)* And then in lunch when you knocked into my tray and spilled chili all over my sweater. Don't think I didn't notice. And the pictures of naked women stuck all over my locker that I got two detentions for? I knew it was you. That was really bold and sexy. But when I walked out to the parking lot and saw my toilet-papered car— the TP flapping in the wind, begging for my attention like a true sign, I just knew you wanted me to ask you out today! So Jessica, will you go out with me? *(Beat.)* "No way, freak"? You gave me a nickname already?! That's so cute!

Defeating Dudley

Luke tries to get out of trouble with the sheriff for basically ruining Officer Dudley's police car.

Sheriff, I don't mean any offense, but Officer Dudley is wrong. I didn't do any of those disrespectful things he said I did. First of all, I don't even like Krispy Kremes, so where would I get the Krispy Kreme sign to stick over his license plate? And why he would think I was the one who chained his car to a telephone pole is beyond me, because no offense, but there are a lot of folks who hate Officer Dudley. And the dead skunk . . . that wasn't me. I love animals! Sheriff, just between us, Officer Dudley's lazy eye makes him see things just a little bit different than how they really were. All I was doing was riding my dirt bike to the ice cream parlor, and the next thing I know a bumperless, blue-light, Krispy Kreme–tagged, foul-smelling cop car comes flying at me and nearly ran me over! He's lucky I'm not p ressing charges! If I may say so, Sheriff, Officer Dudley shouldn't even have a license the way he drives!

Mr. Smooth

Jarred teaches his younger brother, CJ, how to get girls.

You gotta be yourself. Give 'em that smile, that look. *(He demonstrates.)* Don't overdo it. CJ, you're my little brother— you can't be me. But you can try—you can come really, really close. Cause girls, they're falling out all over me. Here's what you gotta do. This girl you like? Go up to her and introduce yourself. Ya gotta lick your lips—make sure they're nice and moist. And when you're talking to her—now this is really important, CJ—make sure you're listening, not just checking her out. Cause you might actually have to answer a question. So do not look at her from the neck down cause it will throw you off! Wait till she walks away to do that. Look her in the eye and say, "Is your daddy a thief? Cause you're stealing my heart." *(Beat.)* What? That's good stuff! You think you got something better? Let's hear it. *(Beat.)* Wait, I gotta write that down.

Wipeout

Beau, a surfer dude, is on a first date in a local restaurant.

This is a rad place for a first date. Today I was surfing and the waves were so awesome! *(Looking at menu.)* They have cheese sticks here. I woke up this morning and there was a huge pool of drool all over my pillow. Hey, I rhymed. *(He laughs.)* Are you gonna eat that roll? Oh, dudette, I forgot my wallet. You've got money, right? Why'd you do that to your hair? Oh, dude, I was on my jet ski today. We were going off the waves on the beach, and we started racing. I totally won. I cheated, but hey, you do what ya gotta do. Like Nike says, "Just do it." You don't talk too much, do you? That's probably why you don't have a boyfriend. Speaking of me, doesn't my hair look awesome? *(Looking at menu.)* Whoa, chocolate! That's fattening—you can't get that. I'm gonna get the double-fudge supreme sundae with nuts. Hey look, they have multicolored sprinkles. I wonder if each color has a different flavor. I bet they do. Ya think they— *(Looks up and she is gone.)* Hey, where'd you go?

Boy Gone Wild

Anton took his little brother, Travis, to the fair today to have fun, but Travis is out of control.

Travis, I'm not taking you on the Ferris wheel again! Look what happened the first time—you threw up on that poor woman below us. I warned you not to eat ice cream and pickles. And I told you to stay off the skeeball ramp. You're lucky that policeman unwedged your arm from the fifty-point hole. You could have been stuck like that forever! I know you want a prize, and I'm sorry I didn't win that Sponge Bob you wanted, but who poked me when I started to throw the ball? You did! And it smacked that sad-looking game guy in the head! You're acting like a maniac. I think you should apologize. *(Beat. Anton sees a pretty woman.)* Whoa. You know what? Forget apologizing— I got a better idea. See that fine lady over there? Go tell her you're lost and come find me!

Students' Success Stories

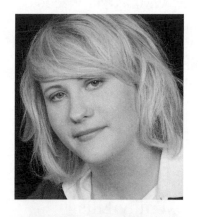

(Britni) Chole' Arrington

~ Top Ten, Monologue Competition (Div. A3) iPOP! NY 2006

~ Third Runner Up, Actress of the Year (Div. A3) iPOP! NY 2006

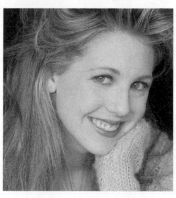

Karli Barnett

~ Winner, Monologue Competition (Div. A3) iPOP! NY 2006

~ Winner, Actress of the Year (Div. A3) iPOP! NY 2006

~ Signed with Abrams Artist, Los Angeles

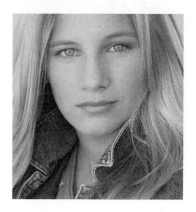

Keely Bilthouse

~ Third Runner Up, Monologue Competition (Div. A3) iPOP! NY 2006

~ Second Runner Up, Actress of the Year (Div. A3) iPOP! NY 2006

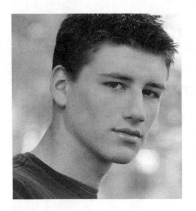

Mark Couch

~ Winner, Monologue Competi-
tion (Div. A2M) iPOP! NY 2006
~ Winner, Actor of the Year
(Div. A2M) iPOP! NY 2006
~ Signed with Wilhelmina Dan,
Nashville

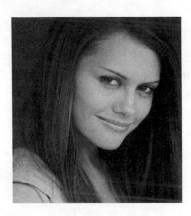

Emily Ellis

~ Second Runner Up, Monologue
Competition (Div. A2) iPOP!
LA 2007
~ Second Runner Up, Actress of
the Year (Div. A2) iPOP! LA 2007
~ Signed with Innovative Artists,
Los Angeles

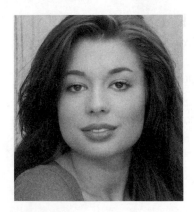

Amanda Freeman

~ Top Ten, Monologue Competi-
tion (Div. A3) iPOP! NY 2006
~ Top Ten, Actress of the Year
(Div. A3) iPOP! NY 2006

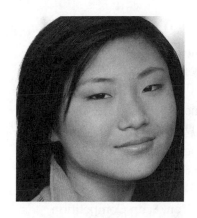

Anna Hou

~ Honorable Mention, Monologue Competition (Div. A3) iPOP! NY 2006

~ Honorable Mention, Actress of the Year (Div. A3) iPOP! NY 2006

~ Signed with Wilhelmina Dan, Nashville

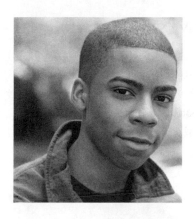

Marlon Hulett

~ Winner, Monologue Competition (Div. A3M) iPOP! NY 2006

~ Winner, Actor of the Year (Div. A3M) iPOP! NY 2006

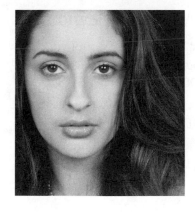

Celeste Iglesias

~ Honorable Mention, Monologue Competition (Div. A3) iPOP! NY 2006

~ Honorable Mention, Actress of the Year (Div. A3) iPOP! NY 2006

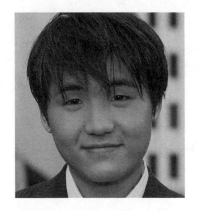

Young Kim

~ Honorable Mention, Monologue Competition (Div. A2M) iPOP! LA 2007

~ Honorable Mention, Actor of the Year (Div. A2M) iPOP! LA 2007

~ Honorable Mention, TV Commercial Competition (Div. A2M) iPOP! LA 2007

~ Top Ten, Soap Competition (Div. A2M) iPOP! LA 2007

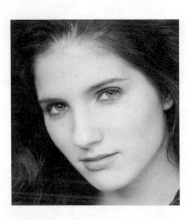

Megan Megahee

~ Honorable Mention, Actress of the Year (Div. A2) iPOP! LA 2007

~ Honorable Mention, Soap Competition (Div. A2) iPOP! LA 2007

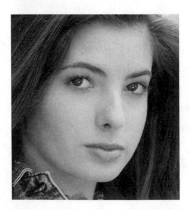

Amanda Olewicz

~ First Runner Up, Monologue Competition (Div. A3) iPOP! NY 2006

~ First Runner Up, Actress of the Year (Div. A3) iPOP! NY 2006

~ Signed with Carter Entertainment, Los Angeles

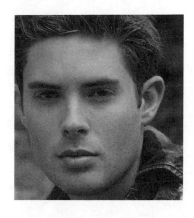

Andrew Olewicz

~ Top Ten, Monologue Competition
(Div. A2M) iPOP! NY 2006

~ Top Ten, Actor of the Year
(Div. A2M) iPOP! NY 2006

~ Signed with Carter Entertainment, Los Angeles

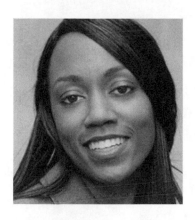

Jessica Palmer

~ Third Runner Up, Monologue
Competition (Div. A1) iPOP!
LA 2007

~ Top Ten, Actress of the Year
(Div. A1) iPOP! LA 2007

~ Top Ten, TV Commercial Competition (Div. A1) iPOP! LA 2007

~ Honorable Mention, Soap Competition (Div A1) iPOP! LA 2007

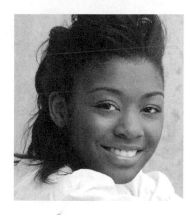

Shenell Watts

~ Top Ten Monologue Competition
(Div. A3) iPOP! NY 2006

~ Top Ten, Actress of the Year
(Div. A3) iPOP! NY 2006

~ Signed with Elite, Atlanta

Words from the Students

Karli Barnett

I think it was great to work with Janet Milstein one-on-one at the workshop. I liked having a monologue I inspired so that it was easier to relate to. Performing the monologue was fun because I also dressed in a costume or clothes that reflected my character. The judges thought it was hilarious! I received a wonderful response from the agents (judges). In fact, I won first place at iPOP! for my monologue in the teen division as well as Actor of the Year. What an experience! It has opened some doors for me, and I have signed with agents and managers in Los Angeles and New York City. Winning has inspired me to train more and to shoot for my goal of performing in a Disney production.

Keely Bilthouse

During my weeks of practice and preparing for iPOP!, Janet had me fill out a questionnaire giving some information about myself, my likes and dislikes. From that, Janet wrote an amazing monologue about cheese—a food that I thoroughly detest! It was really funny and perfect for me. So off to New York iPOP! I went. My experience at iPOP! was incredible. I had the amazing opportunity to perform in front of many agents from around the world.

At the end of the week, our group attended a gala where I received Third Runner Up for Best Monologue and Second Runner Up for Actress of the Year awards! It was so exciting for me to win these awards, and I was so amazed to have been chosen to receive them out of the hundreds of people who were

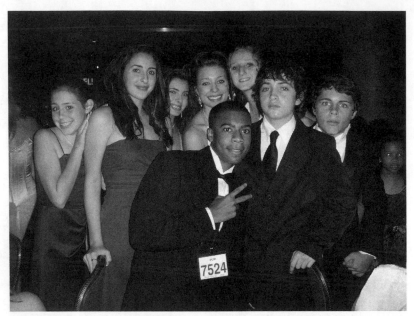

It's time to celebrate! Students at the awards banquet.

there! iPOP! was tons of fun, and everyone there was really nice. It was lots of hard work too, and I don't think I could have done it without all my amazing teachers. They were a huge help for me in getting prepared for iPOP!, and they always gave great tips and advice. And I can't thank Janet enough for giving me the "cheesy" monologue!

Mark Couch

Hello, my name is Mark Couch. I was just a country boy who loved to act, look good, work hard, go fourwheelin', and race dirt bikes. I heard about JRP, and I thought I might give it a try, so I did. I ended up going to JRP and taking classes for iPOP! I had to quit school to work so I could pay bills and rent out my house because my father was in a bad wreck and died twice, but is still living—the hospital brought him back to life. I am glad to have him.

Now my monologue was based on things that I did in my hometown in Ellijay, Georgia. My mind was blank at first, but then the wonderful Janet gave me a kick in the butt to get started. I have to say I could not have done it without her. We even stayed after class and worked on the floor outside JRP. When I did my monologue in New York, I was not scared because I had rehearsed so much, and it was so funny that everyone in the room laughed hard when I did it. I won first place for the Best Monologue, and I owe it all to Ms. Janet! *Thank you very much!*

iPOP! was awesome. I am moving to LA. I got over fifteen callbacks and—the biggie—I won Actor of the Year. I also won an Honorable Mention award for Commercial Print. That's not all: I also won four Top Ten Finalist in Top Ten Model! I also made showcase runway. I did not sleep much. I had a blast though. Can't wait till LA. Thanks for all your help!

Amanda Freeman

In March 2006, I was chosen to attend the International Presentation of Performers in New York. A one-minute monologue had to be pre p a red for the competition at the convention. Janet was brought in to write the monologue for each student selected. She met with us for several weeks and got to know each and everyone and wrote a monologue based on the personal experiences of each student.

We attended the convention in July 2006 where I competed and was chosen for Top Ten Best Monologue and Top Ten Young Actor of the Year 2006. It was an honor to be chosen for these awards as well as being able to work with Janet. Having a monologue written specifically for me gave me extra confidence to get up and perform my best. There were several students from our school who were awarded Top Ten Best Monologue honors, and our school won first place for Best School. This was an amazing experience from start to finish. Thanks, Janet, for your awesome work.

Marlon Hulett

My experience at iPOP! New York was one to remember for many reasons. I got to see many different styles of performers and learn my strong points and my weaker points. I also got a pretty good taste of what the business is like—the good and bad and how a lot of the people are straight-up blunt.

Originality helps and is something to have a lot of, which is one reason why I won Best Monologue in my age category. Janet Milstein came during iPOP! training and allowed us to have a say on our material, so it was more us, and it came out good. Because of her help, only three of the Top Ten girls' monologues *weren't* from Atlanta.

I also met nice and mean agents, but hey—that's how it is. Though there were many kids and little time, Janet worked hard to write the monologues and teach how us to say them. For a long time, I was very worried about my monologue. I couldn't get the flow of it just right. I attended extra practice and even cut some of it out to make it shorter. All the hard work paid off.

For those who are thinking about competing in iPOP! in the future, I say just have fun and be yourself. It will show and help in the long run. I got on camera a lot of times, so it can bring something out of you that you probably wouldn't have expected. I had fun and thank everybody for the learning experience.

Young Kim

Hi, my name's Young Kim, and I'm eighteen years old. I currently live in Forsyth County, Georgia, in a little town called Cumming. I've wanted to be an actor ever since I was six years old. Growing up, I lived in lots of small towns and couldn't find much opportunity. I did what I could growing up, but nothing's really taken me anywhere until I joined John Robert Powers Atlanta. Everything is slowly starting to happen ever since

I've been with this company. iPOP! LA was the *best* time I've ever had in my life. If you have any kind of passion or love for acting, singing, modeling, or dancing, you would probably feel the same.

I met so many different people from all over the country and even out of this country, and meeting all these people who all have the same kind of passion as I do made me feel really good. I tried comparing this iPOP! experience to all the other experiences that were fun for me, and I really couldn't compare it. Spring break vacations with friends and stuff like that is cool and all, but having an experience for something I really have a passion for and love doing meant sooo much to me that I can't even put it into words. Never in my wildest dreams did I think I would win any kind of award there.

I was expecting to just leave with a great experience but winning an award for something I love doing was overwhelming to me. Janet wrote my monologue, and it was very different, but Janet and I decided to take a chance, and it turned out to be great. It was so different that it was challenging in a way, but I think Janet did a *great* job writing it, and I can't thank her enough. The people thought it was funny, and I really think the agents liked it also. My scene and my commercial were a little less challenging, but I enjoyed them as well. Above being competitive and trying to get signed and get awards, I've met the most wonderful people in my life, and it really hurt me when we all went home in different directions.

Dale (owner of JRP Atlanta) made a really touching speech about what this experience is all about and things he's seen in the past (the Atlanta group knows). It really touched my heart, and I'm sure it touched other people there also. This experience was great, and it wouldn't have been the same without Dale, Charlene, Chad, Rachel Sale, Cassie Cope, Bethany Rountree, the London Group!, my roommate Dillon, Emily Ellis, my parents (especially), other parents who were really cool and supportive, the little ones from JRP Atlanta, and everyone else who put a smile on my face. Thank you!

Amanda Olewicz

My name is Amanda Olewicz; I attend John Robert Powers (JRP) School of Modeling and Acting in Atlanta, Georgia. After taking several lessons in acting and commercial print, I was one of the students selected to represent the JRP School at the iPOP! competition in New York City.

As I found out early on, one of the most important events for me at the iPOP! was going to be the Monologue Competition. During my preparation for the iPOP!, I met Ms. Janet Milstein. Management at JRP Atlanta invited Ms. Milstein to head up the monologue-writing workshop in an effort to help the iPOP! students in writing their own personalized and unique monologues. Ms. Milstein wrote a very humorous monologue for me, which was based on some of my own childhood memories and experiences. That monologue was unique and enjoyable for me to perform. The experience of working with Ms. Janet Milstein was amazing. She gave each of the iPOP! students the attention they needed in writing and performing a monologue that suited their own personal styles. I am also very thankful to all JRP teachers, our iPOP! director Amber and her assistant Chad, and the rest of the JRP Atlanta staff, who worked tirelessly to prepare us for the competition.

iPOP! was definitely an experience that I will never forget. From the meet-and-greet to the actual perfo rmances and award ceremonies, iPOP! was incredible. For me, just getting up on-stage and showing everyone what I have learned was so much fun. Having my family and everyone from my JRP group there to support me was very helpful. It was a great feeling at the end of iPOP! to find out that our JRP School received the first place award for the School of the Year. Everyone from the Atlanta school received either an award or a callback.

Thanks to the efforts of Ms. Janet Milstein and our acting teachers, eight Atlanta students placed in the Top Ten in the Monologue Competition. Out of the top four places, three were f rom Atlanta. All judges agreed that the Atlanta school's mono-

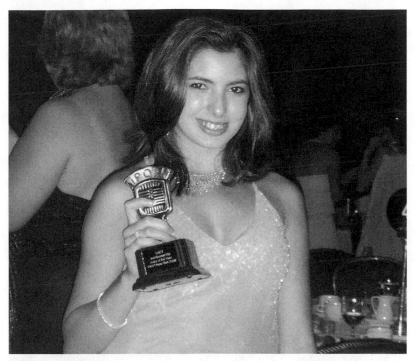

Amanda Olewicz with her trophy for First Runner Up, Actor of the Year.

logues were the best in the competition. I feel that the mono logues tipped the scale and got our school first place.

Personally, I have received three awards: First Runner Up for the Monologue, First Runner Up for Actress of the Year, and an Honorable Mention for placing in the top twelve in Scenes. Throughout this entire experience, I have learned that hard work and dedication pay out at the end.

The same day of my monologue competition, I received a callback from Ms. Bernadette Carter from the Carter Entertainment Management Company. I have signed a three-year contract with Ms. Carter and will be moving to the Los Angeles area in couple of weeks to train with her and continue to advance my acting skills. The entire iPOP! experience has definitely exceeded my expectations. I am thrilled about my new acting prospects and look forward to my acting career.

Andy Olewicz

Working with Janet was an awesome experience. It played such a huge role in the presentation of my monologue and added to a great iPOP! experience. Not only did we have an original monologue written for us, but we also received one-on-one training on how to perfect our monologue. She trained us on how to deliver our monologue, how to present ourselves, and how to become our character. After working with Janet, I was prepared and confident in how I was going to perform in front of any audience. Our monologues were witty and funny. They challenged us to take on a character role that was different from us but at the same time incorporated characteristics that highlighted our own personalities. At iPOP!, I won Third

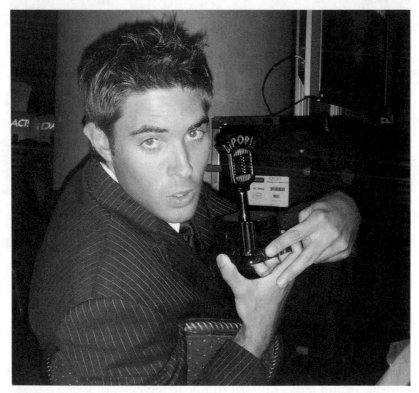

Andy Olewicz shows off his trophy.

Runner Up for my monologue. It was such an honor. I can't thank Janet enough for helping me. Janet did an amazing job developing my monologue, helping me become my character, and giving me the confidence I needed to succeed at iPOP!

Jessica Palmer

This was a wonderful experience for me. It amazed me how Janet could capture so much personality within my monologue. I received first prize in my division during iPOP! for my monologue and was also featured in the showcase at the end of the convention, which was a group of approximately twenty students chosen out of thousands to put on a performance at the closing banquet. The difficult part was keeping my composure when I saw a few giggles from the judges. Thanks, Janet, for aiding in a wonderful life experience!

Shenell Watts

Ms. Janet Milstein's monologue workshop during the preparation for iPOP! has definitely impacted and improved my acting skills. She taught that acting is more than trying to convey emotions, that it is also about who you are trying to convey the emotions to. This is one of many tips that can escalate your acting believability.

The monologue she created for me was the hardest to portray because I had to use nothing but my imagination. It was about how I dyed my friend's hair blue and burned off most of her long locks! However, pulling off the monologue wasn't impossible. Thanks to Ms. Milstein and her coaching, I did very well at iPOP! I was in the Top Ten for Best Monologue, was an Honorable Mention for Actress of the Year, and even got a personal callback from an exclusive agency in Los Angeles. She helped me strengthen and build confidence in a talent that I was unsure of. Thanks again!

Brandon White

My iPOP! experience was truly an amazing one! I had the time of my life because it gave me a chance to see what it was like to be famous. After we landed in LA, the first thing we did was get settled in. We took a tour of the convention center where we would be auditioning. My friends and I were not nervous because we had each other for support. We had so much fun in the hotel. Sometimes we just talked or hung out around the pool. We also went out to eat together. We all had a good time.

My first callback was for Actor I to appear in "True-Life, I'm an iPOP! showcase." Unfortunately, I did not make it. After I finished it, I had to perform in front of Paul and Jerry Morente for dance who were also working in the showcase. In the showcase, the best performers in dance, modeling, acting, and singing perform at the banquet in front of everyone. Well, I made it into the showcase for dance. The first audition was a scene. I was not nervous about that audition, but my partner was. I said, "Just calm down. It's going to be OK. I will be there. Just don't look at them, and you will do just fine." I was not able to perform with my group for the rest of the auditions because I had to practice with the showcase kids. It kind of ran overtime, so I had to make it up. It felt great to have a monologue written just for me that no one else had. No one's monologue came close to mine! *Thanks a lot, Janet Milstein!* It gave me a chance to put my own personal flavor to it, and everyone loved it. It was a real winner with the judges.

Well, the big day was finally here. The moment we all had been waiting for: Awards Night. It was also time for the showcase performers to show off, and I was ready. So everyone took their places. It was time for the show to start. Next, my friend Adam and I opened the showcase with a free-style dance routine.

Afterward, I went to change my clothes and joined all my friends at the banquet. Everyone I knew and didn't even know came up to say, "Good job, you were great. I did not know you could dance like that." All I could do was smile and say thank you. All awards had been given out except dance, which was the final category. Pictures of the Top Ten were shown on-screen. Can you believe it—I was one of them! Not only was I chosen, I won iPOP! Dancer of the Year. I received hugs, kisses, and praises. Finally, I knew what it was like to be famous. Everything about iPOP! was truly awesome. I hope I can go again.

In conclusion, my iPOP! experience was great. I felt like a VIP being in the showcase. It allowed us to move to the front of the line. When it was time to meet with all the agents, we were treated like royalty. It was outstanding!

P.S. I think that the entire iPOP! experience was phenomenal for both the children and parents. It especially gave my child the opportunity to see first-hand where hard work, dedication, and perseverance can take you in life. Life doesn't show favoritism. The iPOP! experience gave an ordinary child an opportunity to become an extraordinary young person. I know that he will always know what success feels like and choose not to settle for mediocrity—a memory that will last a lifetime. It was astronomical!
 —CHERYL WHITE-BRIGGS, MOTHER OF BRANDON WHITE

About the Author

JANET B. MILSTEIN is an actor, award-winning acting instructor, private acting coach, best-selling monologue author, and series editor. She received her MFA in Acting from SUNY Binghamton in New York and her BA in Theatre with Distinction from the University of Delaware. Janet has an extensive background in theater, having performed at numerous theaters with a variety of companies, including The Milwaukee Repertory Theater, The Organic Theater, Collaboraction, Bailiwick, The Artistic Home, ImprovOlympic, Tinfish Productions, Stage Left Theatre, Mary-Arrchie Theatre, Speaking Ring Theatre, Stockyards, Women's Theatre Alliance at Chicago Dramatists, Writers' Block at the Theatre Building, Symposium at National Pastime Theater, and Theatre Q. She has appeared in a number of independent films. She also works in industrials and voice-overs.

Janet has worked as a private acting coach in Chicago for the past twelve years. She trains beginning and professional actors in monologues, cold reading, career counseling, and high school/college theater audition preparation. She is listed in *The Book: An Actor's Guide to Chicago* under "Acting Coaches." She can also be found under "Coaches, Acting" at www.Chicago Actors.com, under "Best-Selling Authors" at www.smithand-kraus.com , and on her website at www.janetmilstein.com. Janet also offers specialized acting workshops nationally and oversees a number of projects for Smith and Kraus.

Other Books by Janet B. Milstein

Author

Cool Characters for Kids: 71 One-Minute Monologues, Ages 4–12.

The Ultimate Audition Book for Teens: 111 One-Minute Monologues.

Winners' Competition Series Volume I: Award-winning, 60-Second Comic Monologues, Ages 4 to 12.

Coauthor

Forensics Series, Volume 1: Duo Practice and Competition: Thirty-five 8–10 Minute Original Comedic Plays by Barbara Lhota and Janet B. Milstein.

Forensics Series, Volume 2: Duo Practice and Performance: Thirty-five 8–10 Minute Original Dramatic Scenes by Barbara Lhota and Janet B. Milstein.

Series Editor

Audition Arsenal for Women in Their 20s: 101 Monologues by Type, 2 Minutes and Under.

Audition Arsenal for Men in Their 20s: 101 Monologues by Type, 2 Minutes and Under.

Audition Arsenal for Women in Their 30s: 101 Monologues by Type, 2 Minutes and Under.

Audition Arsenal for Men in Their 30s: 101 Monologues by Type, 2 Minutes and Under.

Forensics Series, Volume 3: Duo Practice and Competition: Thirty-five 8–10 Minute Original Plays for 2 Females by Ira Brodsky and Barbara Lhota.

Forensics Series, Volume 4: Duo Practice and Competition: Thirty-five 8–10 Minute Original Dramatic Plays for 2 Females by Ira Brodsky and Barbara Lhota.

Want a Workshop?

JANET B. MILSTEIN offers various acting workshops locally and nationally. For information on workshops, please visit Janet's website at www.janetmilstein.com or e-mail Janet at Act4You@msn.com.